T0176471

Strengthening Young Bodies, Building the Nation

CEU Press Studies in the History of Medicine
Volume XII

Series Editor: Marius Turda

———— ⟶≈⟵ ————

Strengthening Young Bodies, Building the Nation

A Social History of Child Health and Welfare in Greece
(1890–1940)

Vassiliki Theodorou
and
Despina Karakatsani

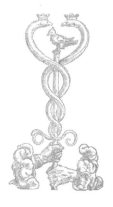

 C E U PRESS

Central European University Press
Budapest—New York

Published in 2019 by
Central European University Press
Nádor utca 9, H-1051 Budapest, Hungary
Tel: +36-1-327-3138 or 327-3000
E-mail: ceupress@press.ceu.edu
Website: www.ceupress.com

224 West 57th Street, New York NY 10019, USA

ISBN 978-963-386-278-0
ISSN 2079-1119

Library of Congress Cataloging-in-Publication Data

Names: Theodorou, Vasilike, author. | Karakatsani, Despina, 1967- author.
Title: Strengthening young bodies, building the nation : a social history of
child health and welfare in Greece (1890-1940) / Vassiliki Theodorou and
Despina Karakatsani.
Description: Budapest ; New York, NY : Central European University Press,
2018. | Series: CEU Press studies in the history of medicine ; Volume 12 |
Includes bibliographical references and index.
Identifiers: LCCN 2018025233 (print) | LCCN 2018037285 (ebook) | ISBN
9789633862797 | ISBN 9789633862780
Subjects: LCSH: Children--Health and hygiene--Greece--History. | Child health
services--Greece--History. | Maternal health services--Greece--History. |
Social medicine--Greece--History.
Classification: LCC RJ103.G74 (ebook) | LCC RJ103.G74 T44 2018 (print) | DDC
362.198920009495--dc23
LC record available at https://lccn.loc.gov/2018025233

Printed in Hungary

TABLE OF CONTENTS

INTRODUCTION

The political, cultural and social dimensions of the history of children's health and welfare have lately attracted much scholarly interest stimulated by the development of both childhood studies and the social history of medicine. The proliferation of studies on the history of public health and contagious diseases in the nineteenth century brought to light the special care taken for the protection of children. The history of tuberculosis reflects the great importance attached to children as a special and vulnerable age group which was not only "in danger" but also "dangerous" itself for the spread of the virus. The history of social hygiene institutions, which were established thanks to the initiatives of municipalities, voluntary organizations and state services across Europe, also points to the importance given to children's health at the beginning of the twentieth century. In addition, the history of education highlights the role that the enactment of mandatory education had in the regulation of student health. The study of the discourse on the degeneration of youth in the late nineteenth century shows a connection between the eugenic concerns voiced during this period by state officials and medical authorities and social policies concerning motherhood and childhood. Besides, historians who have studied child labor, street children, voluntary associations for the salvation of children and the demographic developments of various age groups have already highlighted the role that eighteenth and nineteenth century medical studies played in the perception of childhood. Therefore, it is not accidental that the first studies on the medical care of children come from the fields of historical demography and the history of social control.

In the 1990s, the gap between the history of medicine and the social and cultural history of childhood became evident. Although historians of health and social welfare had made some progress, especially with regard to the medicalization of child birth and infancy, the history of the institutions for the protection of the health of school-age children was still rather underresearched. Studies published in the 1980s and the 1990s on the history of motherhood delineated the mutually constitutive social and medical contexts in which the idea of motherhood was generated and politically deployed. These studies tended to examine social policy concerning mothers and children from the perspective of gender and women's emancipation.[1] Yet, they did not explore the medical supervision of children. Therefore, since knowledge on the historization of children's health was derived mainly from studies on education, psychology, social welfare, child labor, and legislation for the protection of children, as well as occasionally from the history of medicine, a series of issues still remained unexplored: the contribution of late nineteenth-century medical thought to the emerging understanding of children's health and its normalization through the application of psycho-medical terminology, the ways in which the newly emergent children's institutions marked a change in the medical and social perception of childhood, and the ideological and social conditions under which the institutions of child health and welfare took form.

It was this very connection between the history of medicine and the social and cultural history of childhood that some studies attempted to make, trying to move away from interpreting medicine within an evolutionary pattern in order to highlight the ways in which the change in adults' attitude towards the body of the child were part of wider socio-economic and cultural changes. Harry Hendrick's monograph *Child Welfare: England 1872–1989* and the volume *In the Name of the Child: Health and Welfare, 1880–1940* edited by Roger Cooter, among other studies, moved in this direction.[2] These seminal works discuss the changing aspects of intellectual, social, medical, political and professional interests in children's health and children's welfare, which transformed the idea of childhood at the end of the nineteenth

---

1 Jane Lewis, *The Politics of Motherhood: Child and Maternal Welfare in England, 1900–1939* (London: Croom Helm, 1980); Gisela Bock and Pat Thane, eds., *Maternity and Gender Policies. Women and the Rise of the European Welfare State 1880s–1950s* (London and New York: Routledge, 1994); Valerie Fildes, Lara Marks and Hilary Marland, eds., *Women and Children First. International Maternal and Infant Welfare, 1870–1945* (London and New York: Routledge, 1992).

2 Harry Hendrick, *Child Welfare: England 1872–1989* (London: Routledge, 1994); Roger Cooter, ed., *In the Name of the Child: Health and Welfare, 1880–1940* (London and New York: Routledge, 1992).

century. They mainly attempted to point out how medical discourse and practices helped assign a special nature to children and to the professionalization of children's health and welfare.

The notion of the medicalization of childhood that was adopted in these studies refers to the process that took place over forty years, roughly from 1880 until about 1920, during which the state regulation of child health and family issues was enhanced. Medicine informed all aspects of physical and mental classification, means of treatment, and the institutionalization of health, and medical discourse reinvented the child as both a subject/object and a problem. As the state intervened in the private sphere to improve health practices, factors like housing conditions, diet, hygiene and wages came to serve as analytical tools by which households, hygiene habits and lifestyle were scrutinized and moved out of the private sphere and towards the public. Therefore, the process of medicalization can translate into terms of improvement in the health of the population as well as into terms of vigilance.

These studies put great emphasis on the history of school hygiene in correlation with anthropometrics, physical education, social diseases and the construct of normality vs. abnormality. Historians have taken an interest in the period after World War I and doctors' efforts to correct the damage it had wrought. Doctors attempted this through the creation of social and racial hygiene institutions and the control of child birth. They examined the relationship between eugenics and puericulture in order to build optimism for the preparation of the youth from a biological perspective.[3] The history of the medicalization of children's health and especially the study of social hygiene and eugenics exemplifies the way doctors, politicians and civil servants in the early twentieth century imagined it was possible to create a robust, future generation that would contribute to "national regeneration." Because social policies on children's health intertwined with national anxieties in the early twentieth century, a thorough understanding of both is needed.

Most studies that came out in the 1990s made an attempt to understand the process of medicalization of childhood as a form of social control imposed by medical professionals. The history of the institutionalization of

3   Marius Turda, *Modernism and Eugenics* (New York: Palgrave Macmillan, 2010), 1–8.

medical care for children in western societies lends itself to the study of the microphysics of authority and the role that discipline plays in the transformation of subjects into obedient beings. A Foucauldian perspective is evident in these studies, which approach medicalization as a complex procedure, including not only the expansion and the improvement of medical services and hygiene institutions, but also the spread of a physical culture developed and controlled by medical professionals that gradually grew more and more powerful. In the context of this political anatomy, the enactment of the care taken for the body of the child leads to the obedient body, a machine-body that can be perfected and manipulated. The use of Foucauldian interpretative tools has shown how medical vision and practices construct subjectivity in medical terms and how they contribute to the imposition of a norm of physical being by introducing measurements. In the context of this norm, the individual turns into a medical case that is analyzable, describable, classifiable and comparable. In the case of the medical supervision of children on a mass scale, i.e., in the case of school, monitoring individual cases contributed to the development of a bureaucracy related to health. On the one hand, the latter allowed the supervision of health indices of the population as a total; on the other hand, it provided for the focus on the individual case seen against the general norm. In other words, bureaucracy allowed the transition from the general to the individual and vice versa.

Recent developments in the history of children's healthcare in the Balkans points to different aspects of the issue. Relevant studies focus mainly on two issues: firstly, on the importance that the transference of the western paradigm of children's healthcare by foreign-trained doctors had on the implementation of social welfare institutions at a local level; and secondly, the importance of the reception of child welfare institutions in strengthening the nation. The international movement for the protection of children was based on the existence of networks of doctors, jurists and social thinkers who took the initiative to establish local associations for the protection of children.[4] These associations promoted an international culture for the protection of children which had been cultivated in the context of the Geneva declaration while the institutional efforts for the welfare of children,

---

4   Kristina Popova, "From 'Save the Children' to 'Save the Tribe.' Child Care in Yugoslavia and Bulgaria 1919–1939," (Sofia: CAS Working Paper Series, Center for Advanced Studies Sofia, 2007), accessed July 5, 2015, https://tinyurl.com/ycmdnc9o.

developed in the aftermath of World War I, have been examined from the perspective of the state nationalism. The care taken for the health of children was aligned in these cases with the construction of the notion of the nation. As studies have already shown, the notions of national community and nationalism have been characteristic of the medical thought and the organization of public health systems in South-Eastern Europe since the end of the nineteenth century.[5] Health and hygiene were the main constituents of a wider bio-political agenda which led to the creation of a racially healthy nation conceptualized through eugenic terms.[6]

The present study takes up as its subject the understanding of the historical context of the medicalization of childhood attempted in Greece in the early twentieth century. More specifically, we seek to study the intellectual atmosphere within which the discourse on the need to set up special institutions for the protection of child health took place and the social and political conditions that contributed to the establishment of similar institutions. We are interested in exploring the ways in which children's health was turned into a scientific issue, how it was entwined with the social and national questions, and how it became part of government social policy in the first half of the nineteenth century.

We attempt to follow the development of these policies at both the level of state institutions and voluntary organizations, such as the Patriotic Foundation for the Protection of the Child. Since the institutions for the medical inspection of children were linked with a series of issues such as state welfare, nationalism, and eugenics, we examine them in correlation with both the social question and the discourse on the nation and the race. By looking into this issue over the span of fifty years, we are able to gain profound insights into how the political and scientific discourses on child health and motherhood were connected with wider social and political changes and how the professionalization of children's health and welfare were gradually attempted.

Our study covers the period from the 1890s until 1940. The 1890s witnessed mounting concerns over the health of children, while by the end of this period many of the efforts and pursuits for the medical supervision of

---

5   Marius Turda, "Ancients and Moderns: the Rise of Social History of Medicine in Greece and the Balkans," *Deltos: Journal of the History of Hellenic Medicine*, special issue: "Private and Public Medical Traditions in Greece and the Balkans" (Winter 2012): 13–7.

6   Christian Promitzer, Sevasti Trubeta and Marius Turda, eds., *Health, Hygiene and Eugenics in Southeastern Europe to 1945* (Budapest: Central European University Press, 2011), 14.

children had ended. Our working hypothesis is that during this period children's health gradually transitioned to being under the control of state services. Although the advancements in children's health largely disappointed the expectations of the doctors who led them and although these efforts were discontinued due to political upheavals, the progress they achieved contributed to the institutionalized medicalization of child health on a mass scale, mainly through school.

Our study looks into several issues: the procedures through which the changes in social policy regarding health were bought about; the way in which political upheavals affected the history of these attempts; the role played by doctors, social thinkers, state officials and educators in formulating this policy; the role voluntary organizations played in shaping schemes for children's health and welfare and the way these organizations acted in collaboration with state services; the process through which the cultural categories of children's physical health, mental health, and disease were constructed; and how the eugenic concerns of the early twentieth century were linked with policy concerning motherhood and childhood.

Since the attempt of the medicalization of childhood was inscribed in the context of the modernization of health and welfare services, we make extensive reference to the European paradigms from which the Greek case was derived throughout this study. This book consists of three parts, each of which examines various temporal dimensions of the issue. Part I of this study covers the period 1890–1920 and analyzes the development of medical thinking and social policy regarding the health of children in Europe at the end of the nineteenth century. It also looks into the public health problems that Greek society faced at the end of the nineteenth century and contextualizes the discourse surrounding the introduction of state institutions into the hygienic care of Greek pupils. In addition, we explore in this section the political conjuncture which made possible the introduction of school hygiene institutions to Greece in the 1920s, laying the foundations for the recording, monitoring and strengthening of students' health.

Since health problems revealed the dire living conditions of the working class, it was necessary to expand our research to include the first attempts for the social protection of children's health undertaken by a women's voluntary organization, the Patriotic League of Greek Women. The members of the league cooperated with state officials at the Ministry of Education in order to deal with the serious health problems pupils from Athens faced, and especially those who happened to suffer from trachoma, malaria and tuberculosis. We examine the problems in children's health revealed by morbidity statistics in correlation with the modernizing reforms introduced by the first liberal governments in the 1910s. These reforms concerned education and the improvement of the working class living conditions.

In Part II we attempt to contextualize the institutions for children's health between 1922 and 1935 i.e., from the arrival of refugees from Asia Minor until Metaxas's dictatorship. We attempt to investigate the changes that took place in child healthcare both at the European and national level. During the interwar period, the state dealt with children's healthcare more decidedly than it had previously, as the damage World War I had inflicted upon the population of European countries made state officials realize the future value of having healthy soldiers for national defense. The formulation of new institutions for the protection of motherhood and childhood in many European countries points not only to efforts made to repair the damage wrought by the war but also to mounting concerns about the degeneration of the race, a fear that allowed the state to gradually assume a central role in the private life of citizens. During this same period there was an attempt to internationalize child health and welfare issues. This internationalization occurred after the declaration of the Rights of Children in Geneva in 1924 and led to the emergence of international networks for the protection of children.

At a national level we follow the way the institutions for the health and welfare of children were run at a time when the state was obliged to come to terms with acute public health issues in the aftermath of the Asia Minor Disaster. We place great emphasis on the policy that the last Venizelos's government (1928–1932) implemented both in school hygiene and welfare since during this period children's health was given priority. An ambitious programme for the construction of new school buildings, the enactment of summer camps, an open-air school, and school meals as well as the introduction of hygiene as a school subject, all bear witness to the modernization attempt the Liberal Party undertook in the interwar period. The funding of the Patriotic Foundation for the Protection of the Child and its establishment as the main agent of social policy on motherhood and childhood can be inscribed in the same context. During this period two movements can be observed: first, the cooperation of local associations for the protection of children was initiated, many times by state functionaries who participated in these associations; and second, the emergence of a body of professionals who specialized in child welfare. During this fifteen-year period concerns about the racial degeneration of children were voiced more intensely.

Part III examines the policies of the 4th of August regime concerning the health and welfare of children in an attempt to understand how these policies were affected by the imposition of an authoritarian regime that tried to build up a special relationship with children and what similarities these policies present with the policies implemented by other contemporary fascist regimes. We assess both the projects undertaken in this period as well as their importance in strengthening the new regime. The dictator Ioannis Metaxas placed great importance on the social policy concerning children's health as evidence not only of the national regeneration but also of the cultural continuity of the Greek nation. His dictatorship sought to differentiate itself from previous governments, legitimizing itself in the eyes of the working class by increasing welfare projects for mothers and children. Great emphasis is placed upon the continuities, discontinuities and the renewed use of institutions that had been initiated by the previous governments. At the same time, we examine the demographic policy of the regime and the emphasis it laid on the welfare of rural childhood in the context of discourses and exchanges that took place during the two Balkan congresses on the protection of childhood.

Sources and Methodological Issues

Our study is an attempt to approach the emergence and the development of social hygiene institutions in Greece as this subject has been underresearched up until very recently. *Under the Threat of the Disease. Supervision and Control of the Population in Greece in the Nineteenth century* by Maria Korasidou, published in 2002, is the most important study in the history of medical supervision in general. Apart from the secondary sources of the period under discussion, our study draws on primary sources, especially in private and state archives. The archives of Emmanouil Lambadarios, director of the School Hygiene Service from 1911 until 1936 and of Apostolos Doxiadis, president of the Patriotic Foundation for the Protection of the Child in the interwar proved very useful for the purposes of our study. As far as politicians' archives are concerned, we mainly used Venizelos's and Metaxas's archives while the archives of the Ministry of Social Welfare and the Ministry of Education presented bigger deficiencies. Much useful information was derived from the special editions of agencies for the health of children and of relevant associations, from legal texts, constitutions and the minutes of associations as well as from journals such as *To Paidi* (The Child) and *Skholiki Ygieini* (School Hygiene). In many cases primary sources were inaccessible to us at the time of our research. Another problem the primary sources presented was the fact that they came from public services and therefore they reproduced governmental rhetoric.

Many thanks to the staff of the historical archives and the libraries we consulted in Athens, London and Paris for securing the ideal conditions for our research and for making available rare material. Special thanks to the staff of the Hellenic Literary and Historical Archive and of the General State Archives in Athens as well as to the staff of the National Academy of Medicine in Paris who kindly responded to our requests and questions. Discussions with colleagues in the field of the social history of medicine allowed us to widen our perspective in a period when the academic interest in similar issues was just beginning. We shared common concerns and exchanged information about the history of health with Katerina Gardikas, Despo Kritsotaki and Vassia Lekka while the critical eye of Sevasti Trubeta and the questions raised by Efi Avdela inspired and motivated further contemplations. We are indebted to Marius Turda not only for some challenging questions on the dissemination of eugenics in the Balkans, but also for his invaluable support and for providing us an international forum for our research. The publication of this study in English has been made possible thanks to the wholehearted support and the continuous effort of Vassiliki Vassiloudi who not only undertook the translation of our study but also solved various problems that arose during this long venture. Full responsibility for any weaknesses or unanswered questions lies with us. Lastly it is necessary to note that although this study has been the outcome of cooperation and joint research, the first and third parts were written by Vassiliki Theodorou while the second part was written by Despina Karakatsani.

PART I

Health and Children's Welfare in Greece
(1890–1920)

CHAPTER I

THE EMERGENCE OF INTEREST
IN CHILDREN'S HEALTH

In his 1863 treatise *Education: Intellectual, Moral and Physical,* Herbert Spencer, the English theoretician of social Darwinism, attempted to highlight the importance of the citizen's physical health not only for the individual but also for the nation, maintaining that "[t]he first term of well-being is for one to be a good animal while the first term of national prosperity is for the nation to be comprised of good animals."[1] This passage was commonly quoted in late nineteenth-century popular pedagogical leaflets in order to support the argument that the improvement of the citizen's health was not only the state's duty but also in the state's interest. The association of the physical health of future citizens with the nation's financial prosperity and combat readiness was characteristic of the emerging interest in the condition of children's health, conceived of as a vulnerable yet promising part of the country's population, in late nineteenth-century medical and pedagogical circles. At the turn of the century, the upsurge of militant nationalism rendered the robustness of the citizen a necessary prerequisite for the future viability of the nation. The state had to serve as the principal agent for the preservation and the improvement of this "physical capital" with the aim of

---

1   Herbert Spencer, *Education: Intellectual, Moral and Physical* (New York, 1863). Spencer quotes here a passage from the nineteenth-century American poet and philosopher Ralph Waldo Emerson to illustrate vividly the connection between physical, mental and intellectual health. Spencer was known in Greece through translations of his work that had been published in the journal *National Education* (*Ethniki Agogi*, 1896–1904) while in 1910 a Greek translation of his work came out. Herbert Spenser, *I Agogi, Pnevmatiki, Ithiki kai Somatiki* (Athens: Syllogos pros Diadosin Ofelimon Vivlion, 1910). The above extract comes from an anonymous article entitled "To Skholeion kai i Ygieini," which appeared in the journal *Ethniki Agogi,* no. 8 (April 15, 1901): 119–22.

national regeneration. As Marius Turda stressed in his *Modernism and Eugenics*, the interest of politicians, intellectuals and health scientists in the early twentieth century pointed to new conceptions not only of the body of the individual but also of the national community. Under the influence of growing racial concerns and new biopolitical discourses about the importance of the body to the national regeneration, the individual body was redefined while the collective body—the nation—came to be understood as a living organism that functioned according to biological laws.[2]

Concerning the quality of the race, the children's health in contemporary publications was associated with the biological ontology of the nation and the biological degeneration of the youth. In these contemporary interpretations the military defeats of European countries were attributed to the indifference of governments that had not taken proper care to invest in the physical health of youth.[3] The "national efficiency," a recurring term in many publications, took on not only a military but also a biological connotation at the end of the nineteenth century. As the state's intervention in the management of citizen's health gradually increased, voluntary organizations could only act within certain limits.

Exploring the historical circumstances that gave rise to the maintenance and improvement of children's health reveals the multifarious factors that contributed to the formulation of social policies on children's and mothers' health in many European countries during this period. Many contemporary studies on the history of childhood and the social history of health have attempted to shed light on the origin of this interest in the body of the child. The main questions such studies tackled can be summarized as: What social, economical and ideological circumstances gave rise to the interest in children's health? How did social policies on the health of lower classes which developed in various countries during the same period contribute to this interest? How is the institutionalization of compulsory education linked with the growing realization that children of school age encounter serious health problems? To what extent did medical studies on working children contribute to the rise of the medical interest in children? How did medical progress at the end of the nineteenth century, and especially the discoveries in

---

2   Marius Turda, *Modernism and Eugenics* (New York: Palgrave Macmillan, 2010), 5.
3   Virginia Berridge, "Health and Medicine," in *The Cambridge Social History of Britain 1750–1950*, vol. 3, ed. E.M.L. Thompson (Cambridge: Cambridge University Press, 1996), 218–19.

the fields of microbiology as well as the separation of pediatrics from general medicine, boost research that sought to fight child diseases and to the popularization of knowledge about the body and disease? How were policies on population and motherhood interconnected with eugenic concerns? What role did the discourse on the degeneration of the new generation play in the increasing state interest in the child? Finally, how did nationalism, liberalism and social democracy affect the implementation of policies on children?

THE EMERGENCE OF THE EMOTION OF CHILDHOOD

Most studies stress the role that wide cultural changes played in modifying the attitude of adults towards the body of the child. The development of family emotion among the middle class, traced back to the nineteenth century by historians of childhood, contributed to an increasing sensitization of parents to the health of their offspring.[4] At the same time, the spread of the romantic image of the child resulted in new parental responsibilities. Parents ought to secure the conditions that would allow their children to achieve happiness. Therefore, the maintenance of their health became the essential precondition for happiness.

The romantic understanding of childhood also affected the movement for the salvation of children. Thanks to the efforts of philanthropists, intellectuals and politicians, institutions for the protection of childhood were initiated in some European states; yet, these institutions came into conflict with older assumptions about the contribution of children's work to the industrialization.[5] These measures, which most of the time were directed against exploitative intentions of employers and parents, helped consolidate the idea that childhood was and ought to be "dependant." The concept of dependence in this case was identified with the protection of adults. Medical treatises on the harmful effects of industrial work on the health and especially on the development of the child's body played a crucial role in the new perception of childhood, which by then was linked with the future of the nation.[6] Statistics that showed the measurements of weight and height of chil-

---

4 Philip Ariès, *L'Enfant et la vie familiale sous l'Ancien Régime* (Paris: Éditions du Seuil, 1973).

5 Hugh Cunningham, *The Children of the Poor: Representations of Childhood since the Seventeenth Century* (Oxford: Blackwell, 1991), 64–95.

6 Viviana Zelizer, *Pricing the Priceless Child: The Changing Social Value of Children* (New York: Princeton University Press, 1985).

dren working in textiles were the most convincing proof of the effects that work had on children's development.

By the end of the nineteenth century, the view that every child should have a childhood had gained ground. In practice, this meant the enactment of laws that imposed restrictions on child work and provided for all-inclusive schooling, leisure time and the separation of children from the adult world. Despite the active role voluntary and philanthropic societies played in fighting the social problems caused by rapid urbanization, their intervention could not go beyond certain limits. To the extent this realization gained ground, the role of the state became more decisive since only the state was able to implement a child-centered policy that could secure satisfying living conditions for every child. At the end of the nineteenth and the beginning of the twentieth centuries, all European states went through a phase of institutionalizing children's health and welfare services, gradually restricting traditional philanthropic intervention.[7] Compulsory education enacted in most European countries until 1880 and legislation that restricted child work during the same period[8] stand as the most characteristic examples of the increasing intervention of the state for the benefit of children.

Advances in medicine also played an important role in the hygienic care of children. At the turn of the century, due to social changes, doctors gained a new perception of the child body.[9] Clinical research based on observation replaced theory when dealing with disease and the obsolete treatment methods followed by practical doctors. Practical medicine lost popularity among the working class. Although at the beginning of the eighteenth century children's diseases were not considered a separate category and children were not treated by doctors in a way different from adults, starting in the mid-nineteenth century, doctors turned their attention to the observation of the sick child body and to the factors that were responsible for child diseases. The discovery of vaccinations, the establishment of the first hospitals exclusively for child patients and the recognition of pediatrics as a sep-

---

7   Hugh Cunningham, "Saving the Children c. 1830–1920," in *The Global History of Childhood Reader*, ed. Heidi Morrison (London and New York: Routledge, 2012), 356–74.

8   Clark Nardinelli, *Child Labour and the Industrial Revolution* (Bloomington and Indianapolis: Indiana University Press, 1990), 109; Harry Hendrick, *Child Welfare*, 20–5. See also Pamela Horn, *Children's Work and Welfare 1780–1890* (Cambridge: Cambridge University Press, 1995).

9   For the social, economic, political and cultural conditions under which the medicalization of childhood took place at the end of the nineteenth century, see Cooter, *In the Name of the Child*, especially the introduction, 1–18.

arate specialty contributed to this change in how children's diseases were perceived. Around 1850, the first scientific studies that dealt with childhood in a medical context were published in medical journals and in 1860 the term "paediatrics" was coined in English by the American doctor Abraham Jacobi.[10] In the last quarter of the nineteenth century seats of paediatrics were established in Paris (1879), Berlin (1894) and at Harvard (1870). Around 1884, the term paediatrics was accepted by the international medical community. The establishment of scientific associations of pediatrics serves as evidence of the reception of the term: in 1888 the American Paediatrics Society was established, followed by the French one in 1890 and the Italian Paediatrics Society in 1898. The increase in the number of pediatricians serves as further evidence of this reception.[11] Laboratory research on microbiology, which led to the discovery of vaccines and other protective measures for children's healthcare, helped fight children's diseases and led to a decline in child mortality.[12] The isolation of bacilli in the laboratory led to the development of smallpox and anti-diphtheria vaccines. Yet, legislation that forced the compulsory vaccination of citizens was not adopted at the same time across Europe nor was this an easy question. Parents mounted opposition to vaccination either because they did not realize its importance for their children's health or because considered mandatory vaccination a violation of their personal rights.

Advances in medical science with regard to the treatment and protection from children's diseases contributed to the changing understanding of the child's body. As had been the case with other medical specialties in the nineteenth century, the development of medical statistics and innovative diagnostic methods contributed to the separation of pediatrics from general medicine.[13] Statistics that took into account the age of the deceased pointed to the high child and youth mortality rates due to conta-

10 Russell Viner, "Abraham Jacobi and the Origins of Scientific Pediatrics in America," in *Formative Years: Children Health in the United States, 1880–2000,* eds. Alexandra Minna Stern and Howard Markel (Ann Arbor: University of Michigan Press, 2002), 23–46.

11 Paul Weindling, "From Isolation to Therapy: Children's Hospitalisation and Diphtheria in Fin de Siècle Paris, London and Berlin," in *In the Name of the Child,* ed. Cooter, 124–45.

12 See, for example, the effects of vaccination on child mortality in nineteenth century France, Catherine Rollet-Echalier, *La politique à l'égard de la petite enfance sous la IIIe République* (Paris: PUF/INED, 1990). See also by the same author, *Les enfants au XIXème siècle* (Paris: Hachette, 2001).

13 For the factors that contributed to the separation of paediatrics, see Matthew Ramsay, *Professional and Popular Medicine in France, 1770–1830: The Social World of Medical Practice* (Cambridge: Cambridge University Press 1988), 9.

gious diseases.[14] "Child mortality" had been perceived since 1877 not only
as a separate category in medical statistics but also as an index that pointed
to social welfare.[15] The child constitution, which remained obscure until
then, started to attract the interest of doctors. Environmental factors like
packed housing conditions and infected air were held accountable for the
spread of contagious diseases among children. Statistics on housing, hygiene, nutrition conditions and family financial status served as analytical
tools by which state services attempted to gain access to the private sphere
with the aim of raising public health standards, thus transforming the private into public. Apart from tuberculosis, doctors' attentions were interested in diseases which presented epidemic breakouts and were accountable for high child mortality rates: diphtheria, smallpox, whooping cough
and scarlet fever. At the same time, medical authorities gradually replaced
the practical doctor in the fight against diseases among children. Protection and treatment of the child body, from birth to maturity, fell within
the doctor's responsibility.[16]

Since the late nineteenth century, different concepts of the body were
created in order to illustrate the various levels of health in child bodies: "delicate," "anomalous," "sickly" and the like. Within preventive medicine, research turned not only to the treatment but also to the protection of health
and the strengthening of the body. New hygienic means, i.e., sports and summer camps to strengthen children's constitutions, illustrate the tendency of
the medical community to protect future generations from the possibility
of illness. The results of this were reflected in the spread of compulsory vaccination and gymnastics, the diffusion of hygienic propaganda and the improvement of hygienic conditions in school, all designed to deal with infectious diseases more efficiently. The belief that children's health should be in
the care of scientists became increasingly acceptable towards the end of the
nineteenth century.

---

14 For child mortality in France, see Alfred Perrenoud, "La mortalité des enfants après 5 ans aux XVIII
    et XIXème siècle," in *Lorsque l'enfant grandit. Entre dépendance et autonomie*, eds. Jean Pierre Bardet,
    Jean Nicolas Luc, Isabelle Robin-Romero and Catherine Rollet (Paris: Presse de l'Université Paris-
    Sorbonne, 2003), 107–31.

15 For the child body as a social construct at the dawn of the twentieth century, see David Armstrong,
    Political Anatomy of the Body: Medical Knowledge in Britain in the Twentieth Century (Cambridge,
    Cambridge University Press, 1983), 15.

16 David Armstrong, "The Invention of Infant Mortality," *Sociology of Health and Illness* 8, no. 3 (1986):
    211–32.

The relationship between the individual and their own body changed as broad hygienic reform entered both the private and public sphere. Sanitary interventions in the urban landscape regarding air circulation, the removal of viruses and the creation of recreational areas formed part of a new perception that it was in fact possible to improve the body's functions. This cultural perception of the body was developed at the turn of the century and at its very heart lied the notion of bio-responsibility. Man was now considered to be capable of improving his health and elongating his life expectancy. This ability had yet to be further improved: the art of good nutrition, the art of breathing, compliance with hygienic rules, bathing, gyms and countryside retreats were pronounced as the classical prophylactic measures for the increase in the "individual biological capital" contingent on the individual's free will.

Individuals had to be persuaded that their fight against viruses was their own responsibility and necessary to bring their "body weapons" to perfection. These new theories on strengthening the body's defense have to be seen in the context of wider changes that initiated a new art: the art of well-being. Linked with the firm belief that the countryside air had an invigorating quality that gained ground at the end of the century, these theories pointed to new ideas on the use of one's own leisure time.[17] The spread of popular leaflets containing simple instructions for the protection of the individual's health as well as the proliferation of associations and societies for physical exercise and recreation serve as further evidence for the impact that this medical discourse had.[18]

The decline in infant mortality presented a great challenge not only for doctors but also for the state. The index of infant mortality, still high at the end of the nineteenth century in many countries, justified the concerns of politicians and state functionaries for the demographic future of their nations. In addition, the development of pediatrics and gynecology as separate fields signified the transfer of responsibilities from graduate midwives and the practical midwives to doctors. The medicalization of birth led to the establishment of maternity wards. Even though mothers would play the leading role in combating infant mortality, doctors nonetheless attributed high infant mortality rates to the indifference and ignorance of mothers. They had to be trained in

---

17 Georges Vigarello, *Histoire des pratiques de santé: Le sain et le malsain dépuis le Moyen Âge* (Paris: Éditions du Seuil, 1999), 266.

18 Jacques Leonard, *La médecine entre les pouvoirs et les savoirs* (Paris: Aubier, 1981), 187.

their duties not only towards their offspring but also towards the nation; doctors passionately involved in the campaign of instructing women emphasized that "instinct was not enough."[19] The eradication of unhygienic habits and superstitions was considered to be a necessary prerequisite for the spread of new knowledge and practices. In order to sensitize and instruct mothers in children's hygiene, modern methods of propaganda were adopted through agencies which funded campaigns for the improvement of public health, for instance the Rockefeller Foundation in the early twentieth century.[20] These campaigns used new methods like the establishment of special days and weeks, awards to the "most healthy babies" and National "Baby Day," films, information leaflets and stamps to raise the public's awareness of health.[21] Schools for mothers and for visiting nurses spread during this period, as well as consultation centers for mothers. Lessons on how to raise infants were introduced into girls' schools. It was their duty to make sure that working class families would follow the doctor's instructions at home. Social welfare institutions for mothers and infants were set up in the turn of the century in many states in the USA, as well as in some countries of Central, Northern and Western Europe. During the same period a dynamic international movement for children's welfare contributed to lowering infant mortality in various countries.[22] International scientific societies as well as the export of doctors educated in Western Europe helped circulate new medical approaches in even the most remote countries. Thus, despite vastly different cultural perceptions of hygiene in various settings, solutions ended up being more or less similar.

SCHOOL POPULATION UNDER THE MICROSCOPE: NEW THEORIES AND PRACTICES IN SCHOOL HYGIENE

Children attracted the interest of the state and medical community for two reasons. One, because they were a group considered likely of carrying contagious diseases. The second reason was related to the compulsory character

---

19 Alisa Klaus, *Every Child a Lion. The Origins of the Maternal and Infant Health Policies in the United States and France, 1890–1920* (Ithaca, New York and London: Cornell University Press, 1993), 142–3.

20 For the spread of the new practices and objects used for infant raising and the public reaction to them, see Patrice Bourdelais and Olivier Faure, eds., *Les nouvelles pratiques de santé: Acteurs, objets, logiques sociales (XVIIIe- XXe siècle)* (Paris: Belin, 2004), especially the introduction, 7–23.

21 Lewis, *The Politics of Motherhood*, 98–113.

22 The milk distribution centers ("Gouttes de Lait"), for instance, were spread after the international congresses in Paris in 1905 and in Brussels in 1907.

of education. Since the time of the establishment of compulsory education, many supported the idea that the state should ensure that school promoted children's health and imbued them with new hygiene habits. As the rates of school attendance had been on the rise since 1870, the medical inspection of school children was considered a necessary precondition for compulsory education in order to protect children's health from the effects of long school hours.[23] In fact, most late nineteenth-century medical treatises made references to unsuitable school buildings, poorly aired classrooms, and disproportionate desks that forced children to bend their bodies into uncomfortable angles.[24] Therefore, most European countries adopted medical inspection of school children in the last quarter of the nineteenth century, expecting that this would lower the danger of infection among the general populace that schools posed. Medical inspectors in schools devised new tools for monitoring the development of their bodies, and imposed new conditions for children's healthcare.

In this context it is not difficult to understand why late nineteenth-century medical literature and popular leaflets made such frequent references to the unhygienic conditions of school buildings and the harmful effects school attendance had on the physical and the mental health of children. The more schools were understood as an organic part of public health, the more the need to separate school hygiene from public hygiene was stressed. By the turn of the century, doctors had started to shape school hygiene theory and practice so as to control and improve not only children's bodies but also the school premises themselves. University textbooks for this new field were published gradually while research on school children, exploring the impact of school attendance on the physical development of students, was carried out.

"School hygiene," as this field was initially named, aimed to "decrease the harmful effect of school, showing the way towards the harmonious and healthy development of the intellectual and physical powers of the child attending school."[25] Since its inception, school hygiene, no less important

23 The number of children that attended elementary school rose from 24% in 1800 to 48% in 1880 and to 70% in 1900 in England and Wales; yet, numbers are not reliable since we do not know if they refer to registrations or to regular attendance. See Cunningham, *Children and Childhood in Western Society*, 159.
24 Cunningham, *Children and Childhood*, 157.
25 Emmanouil Lambadarios, "I Ygieini tou Skholeiou kai to Ergon ton Skholikon Iatron," *Ygeionomikon Deltion Iatrosynedriou*, Ypourgeion Esoterikon 6 (April 1, 1918) and also by the same author, *Skholiki Ygieini meta Stoikheion Paidologias* (Athens: 1934), 3–5.

than general hygiene, was perceived in a national dimension "since the vitality and welfare of the nation depend on the proper development during school attendance."[26] Johann Peter Frank, a German physician (1745–1821) considered the founder of the scientific school hygiene, in his nine-volume work *System einer Vollstaendigen medizinischen Polizei*, published between 1779 and 1827, described the harmful effects of school on children and suggested the problem be dealt with through scientific medical supervision. Frank's work was no longer remembered by 1836 when the German physician Carl Lorinser (1796–1853) managed, with the help of the studies and research of other doctors, to generate interest in school hygiene.[27] Academic positions for the study of school hygiene were gradually established in medical schools in the last decade of the nineteenth century. The congresses of hygiene in Geneva (1883) and Vienna (1887) stressed the need for systematic medical supervision in schools, but it took ten more years for the first systematic standard of school hygiene to begin in Germany (Wiesbaden, 1897).

Hygienist circles of the late nineteenth century were rife with speculation regarding the location, soil content, and size of the site where school buildings were to be constructed, as well as the direction buildings faced, the ratio of students to the seating capacity of classrooms, ventilation, light, furniture, and cleanliness. The first instructions given for school construction were based on hospital construction.[28] The school building had to be sunny, airy, in a central location that was easily accessible, and at the same time far from the hustle and bustle of markets, hospitals, military barracks, "deafening factories," and unhygienic or dangerous shops. Schools had to be built at least a hundred meters from the cemetery and, if possible, located in the fringes of the city to have access to the clean air of the countryside, but at the same time be reachable in a short time. The soil had to be uncultivated and dry, without any harmful substances. The school building had

---

26 See the inauguration speech of Jean Nicolas, professor at the seat of hygiene at the University of Lyon, entitled "School and Hygiene." In its translated version it featured in the journal *Ethniki Agogi*, no. 8 (April 15, 1901): 97.

27 For the contribution of the work of Frank and Lorinser to the development of the field, see Bernard Harris, *The Health of the Schoolchild: A History of the School Medical Service in England and Wales* (Buckingham: Open University Press, 1995), 24–5.

28 For the elements school architecture borrowed from hospital architecture and specifications, see Pierre Guillaume, "L'hygiène à l'école et par l'école," in *Les nouvelles Pratiques de santé. Acteurs, objets, logiques sociales (XVIII-XXe siècles)*, eds. Patrice Bourdelais and Olivier Faure (Paris: Belin, 2004), 215.

to be supplied with drinkable water of good quality, have modern lavatories connected with the water and sewage system, and a yard for students to rest and exercise.

It was the hygienists' responsibility to suggest which school furniture was most suitable for children's bodies. They attached great importance to the school desk which had to meet certain hygienic and pedagogic standards. They held desks accountable for high rates of myopia and scoliosis, conditions known as "school diseases," as many studies had shown the effect various postures had on the respiratory system.[29] A number of studies on anatomy concluded that it was student height that had to be considered when designing school desks, rather than age. Politicians adopted doctors' proposals on the basis of anthropometric measurements. Local committees were formed in towns and villages to decide on the size of school desks in proportion to the students' height.[30] Light was also essential. The distance between the student's desk and the source of light, as well as the light's angle had to be measured precisely. The school doctor even had to be capable of assessing the hygienic value of various heating equipments and the material used for heating. Similarly, the amount of viruses per cubic meter of air in the classroom had to be calculated. With the use of new tools, school doctors attempted to measure the carbon dioxide contained in the atmosphere of closed premises crammed with many people. The number of students, the type of food they had consumed at home, and the seating capacity of each classroom were linked with the level of noxious fumes in the atmosphere.[31] Most studies concluded that the air in the classroom had a harmful effect on student health. It was suggested that air in schools be renewed either through natural or mechanical means. The duration of recess was also determined in accordance with the time required to renew the air in the classrooms.

The panic over viruses instigated debate on the way viruses spread through dust in school buildings. The way the classroom was cleaned dispelled the fear of infection through the air. State intervention was required

---

29 Josette Peyrenne, *Le mobilier scolaire du XIXe siècle à nos jours* (Septenrion: Presses Universitaires de Septenrion, 2001).

30 For the adoption of similar measures by Jules Ferry in 1880 in France, see Peyrenne, *Le mobilier scolaire*, 167.

31 According to research carried out by American architects, fifty cubic metres of air per hour were required for each student under fifteen years while in classrooms lit up with gas an extra twenty cubic metres was required. See Georgios Vlamos, *I Ygieini tou Skholeiou* (Athens: P.D. Sakellariou, 1904), 213.

to issue regulations defining the way classrooms ought to be cleaned. They dictated prophylactic measures to avoid the spread of tuberculosis including dry sweeping, sprinkle school furniture with plenty of water, use antiseptic solutions for cleaning floors, and paint the walls regularly.

MEDICAL INSPECTION AND CLASSIFICATION OF THE BODIES

Defending the student against diseases required strict medical supervision. The school doctor was responsible for giving general physical examinations to the students and in charge of adopting disease prevention measures. En masse vaccinations in schools, starting in the end of the nineteenth century, aimed at the prevention of diseases among children that were responsible for high mortality rates, particularly scarlet fever and diphtheria. In the last decade of the century, medical journals specialized in school hygiene featured detailed instructions for vaccination. A few decades later vaccinations became more systematic and concerned the entire school population. Since parents were not always willing to comply with state-issued instructions, school vaccinations became necessary for disease prevention and necessitated school doctors. The development of medical examinations and measurements of students' bodies followed a similar course. In early years, medical checks were carried out for protective reasons and later on for monitoring student health.

It was in the 1880s that the first systematic medical examinations were conducted at schools. They aimed at spotting children who showed signs of infectious disease in order to detect the foci of infection, monitoring the students' sight and hearing to reduce the rates of short-sightedness and hearing impairment.[32] A few years later when student personal health cards—a very efficient tool for monitoring the health of the population—were introduced, medical inspection at school became more systematic. The personal health card was an objective data bank, a type of health identity card which made it possible to deal with each case individually. It also allowed schools to track down children who were not able to attend classes for health reasons.[33]

---

32 For the first medical studies carried out in schools in various European countries, see Harris, *The Health of the Schoolchild*, 27–33.

33 The personal health card for students was introduced in Germany by the school medical service in Wiesbaden and later in the early twentieth century it was adopted in France and England.

Tracking down children who were believed to cause the greatest problems in class instigated debate about a different pedagogical approach to address this problem. At the end of the nineteenth century, debate over the isolation and supervision of "mentally weak" or "retarded" students and the establishment of special schools for them had only just started.[34] Anthropometric indexes allowed classification into different categories, the estimation of average as well as the detection of deviant cases and isolation of problematic ones. The compilation of the personal health cards and their translation into statistics made it possible to record general trends in student health and define the average.

The medical examination of students gradually came to include all the body parts related to the function of the human body as a whole: the spine, heart, lungs, skin, glands, teeth and pharynx. Eugenic theories, which began to influence school doctors at the beginning of the twentieth century, contributed to the student development indices that were entered into their personal health card.[35] On the basis of these indices, it was possible to check whether the development of the child body fell within the category of normal. The rhythm each child body followed during its development was the subject of scientific pursuits. Student auxology grew into a special scientific field and auxological studies became more frequent towards the end of the nineteenth century. Diagnostic tests for the cognitive ability of students, which had first appeared in the mid-nineteenth century, were improved in the early twentieth century through experimental psychology studies on education. The IQ test devised by Binet and Simon in 1905 rapidly gained international recognition as a tool which could predict the potential of the child for cognitive development.[36]

Apart from the means of protection of youth from infectious diseases, it was the systematization of physical defense against diseases that brought

---

34 For the reception of mentally retarded children by the medical and pedagogical circles in England in the beginning of the twentieth century, see Mark Jackson, "'Grown-up children': Understanding of Health and Mental Deficiency in Edwardian England," in *Cultures of Child Health in Britain in the Nineteenth and Twentieth Century*, eds. Marijke Gijswijt-Hofstra and Hilary Marland (Amsterdam and New York: Rodopi, 2003), 149–68.

35 For the contribution of eugenics to the organisation of the school medical service in England, see Roy Lowe, "Eugenicists, Doctors and the Quest for National Efficiency: An Educational Crusade, 1900–1939," *History of Education* 8, no. 4 (December 1979): 293–306.

36 Serge Nicolas and Bernard Andrieu, eds., *La mesure de l'intelligence (1904–2004)* (Paris: L'Harmattan, 2005); Theta H. Wolf, *Alfred Binet* (Chicago: The University of Chicago Press, 1973).

doctors to schools. Academic books on school hygiene published between 1880 and 1900 reflect this trend for accurate calculations and "numerical-ization" of care. Nothing could elude the doctors' examination. They had to pay attention to a wide range of issues from the composition of the soil where the school building was to be erected, the site where the lavatories would be built, the type of desks, the detection and suspension from school of the students suspect of ailment, the type of gymnastics required for the "national" type of physical development. One can detect in school hygiene treatises the invention of discipline regulations and the links between po-litical power and scientific knowledge. A political technology of the body was devised in order to place the student under the microscope and mea-sure the effects of a series of parameters on his health. Some of these param-eters concerned the school environment—composition of the surround-ing soil, angles of light, the content of oxygen and number of viruses in the air—, while others concerned the student himself—diet, manner and num-ber of breaths, as well as hygienic habits and private life. A total control of the student's physical behavior was attempted in individual examinations, the observation of their bodies, the completion of health card with informa-tion about measurements, the emergence of indices, the detection of devi-ant cases, the crosschecking of information and, last but not least, the com-pilation of statistics.[37]

Why then did schools draw the attention of doctors in this period? School offered the opportunity for observation and experimentation "since [school] is the space were the gathered bodies of children can more eas-ily be observed, examined, described and be put under the microscope of attention."[38] The school doctor was concerned with the classification of bod-ies according to indices, distinguishing among different cases, the dictation of suitable corrective means and the effectiveness of the suggested hygienic measures. With the optimism that follows the newly-enlightened, school doctors attempted to compile statistics of child development, define nor-mality, impose the norm, prevent the spread of infection and in general con-trol children's health. Doctors were responsible for exercising discipline on student bodies according to what was considered the health norm in schools

---

37 Michel Foucault, *Surveiller et punir: Naissance de la prison* (Paris: Gallimard, 1975), 192–3.
38 Foucault, *Surveiller et punir*, 143.

for the benefit of society. Thus, school took on a higher importance at the end of the nineteenth century.

THE STUDENT AS HYGIENE APOSTLE:
HYGIENE PROPAGANDA IN SCHOOL

The student population lent itself to the spread of innovative practices regarding the body, hygienic way of living and protection against disease. Students were instructed to wash their hands and brush their teeth, among other hygienic habits. This campaign, which was launched in school, was targeted not only at the student but also at his family. Attempts to eradicate the old regime of "dry" hygiene at the turn of the century targeted children with the publication of informative materials about the value of cleanliness and the danger of infections.[39] Thus, the child was perceived as the "apostle" of new hygienic principles. In addition, the introduction of innovative institutions such as the visiting nurses "for the systematic control of private and domestic life of children," as well as the introduction of hygiene as a school subject, which became more systematic in the early twentieth century, would further reinforce this trend.

Doctors attempted to penetrate into hygienic practices in people's private lives, a sensitive area considered to be an uncontrollable factor for the spread of contagious diseases, especially of tuberculosis. The lack of hygienic habits or the agricultural model of cleaning practiced by many student families aroused doctors' concern. Hygienists attempted to regulate these attitudes through instructions, yet with no spectacular results. Clean clothes, the washing of hands, mouth rinsing, and hair care were crucial for the removal of suspect contagion carriers and offered a shield of protection against the spread of viruses. Daily hygienic checks of students conducted by teachers to make sure they complied with the new instructions testified to the popularization of hygiene rules and the authoritarian manner in which it was attempted. In many English and German cities, school baths were built with municipality funds not only to insure cleanliness, but also to reduce bad odors in classrooms. Teachers supervised student group baths according to grade.

---

39 Vigarello, *Histoire des pratiques de santé*, 273.

The development of medical views on tuberculosis affected the way schools were equipped with new objects and furniture, designed according to hygienic standards. The introduction of novelties such as lavatories with running water, fountains with drinkable water and "spittoons" reflected concern over mouth contact with the school objects. The spread of popular leaflets about tuberculosis and the signs "Do not spit on the ground" put up in classrooms were a response to similar concerns. In addition, experience led doctors to bring public attention to new dangers, meaning more checks had to be conducted on children's bodies. The individual use of certain objects by students such as glasses, pencils and even books was highly advisable. Touching these objects with the mouth was prohibited to prevent the transference of viruses with saliva as there had been recorded cases of infection from books and pencils that were in common use.

Strengthening the Body and Open-Air Teaching

The school not only had to spread the new habits of private hygiene, but also to teach new attitudes towards health and healthy living. The familiarization of students with new means of recreation, i.e., countryside walks, exercise in the open air, games and sports, beneficial to both the body and the mind, aimed at the spread of the new hygienic way of living. New terms such as open air teaching, sun-bathing and air-bathing were introduced into the educational system, signifying a new attitude towards aspects of nature like sun, air, and water, but also towards the body itself. New institutions such as school meals, summer camps, student clinics and school baths would also be devised during this period to strengthen children's constitution against viruses.

Doctors placed great emphasis on transporting weak children from industrial cities to the countryside, as these children were considered to be susceptible to tuberculosis, a finding supported by student morbidity. General weakness, anemia, bronchitis, malaria, respiratory problems, scrofula and other health problems were symptoms thought to make one predisposed to disease. The first answer to this problem was the establishment of summer "countryside colonies" where a growing number of children suspected of infection were transported. Yet, these three or four-week stays in the countryside colonies did not prove to have long-term effects on children who were thought to be carriers of tuberculosis. The establishment of "alternative" schools located in the countryside by the sea or in the woods, but still close to the big cities where children could spend the day and return home at night, included the hygienic sojourn without having to remove children from their family environment. The main aim of these schools was to strengthen students' bodies through appropriate exercise in the countryside, a healthy diet, rest and the acquisition of hygienic habits.

Open-air schools (*école de plein air*, or "forest schools"—*Waldschulen* and *escuela del bosque*) were rapidly expanding in number until the mid-twentieth century. The medical origins of this educational institution can be traced to attempts made within the sanatoria. Such was the case of the school which operated in the Davos sanatorium in 1878. Similar "sun schools" were set up where children who suffered from surgical tuberculosis were taught outside in the sun while naked in accordance to open-air teaching principles. Air convalescent homes or *prevantoria* were also set up. In the same period innovative educators stressed the beneficial effect of the countryside on the intellectual development of healthy children, operating experimental, open-air schools like Hermann Lietz who set up such a school in Germany in 1898, Cecil Reddie in England and Edmond Demolins in France.[40] These educational experiments paved the way for the New Education which aimed at balancing students' physical and mental development, and placed emphasis on the free communication of teachers and students. Guided learning experiences, community life, isolation in the countryside, agricultural and manufacturing activities were common to all of these attempts.

The first open-air school was the "forest school" (Waldschule) in the area of Charlottenburg, near Berlin. The school was the result of the cooperation of the doctor Bernhard Bendix and educator Hermann Neufert, who suggested a hygienic educational programme specially adjusted to the needs of sickly children. Although the German model of the "forest school" spread widely and provided the international standard, the contribution of the French doctor Joseph Grancher to the promotion of open-air schools for pretubercular children was also crucial. In 1903, Grancher attempted to place children of tubercular families from Lyon with peasant families in the

---

40 For the experience drawn from the reform in the countryside schools of Lietz, see Peter Littig, *Reformpädagogische Erfahrungen der Landerziehungsheime von Hermann Lietz und ihre Bedeutung für aktuelle Schulentwicklungsprozesse* (Frankfurt: Peter Lang, 2004).

countryside. Since then the notion of "the salvation of the young generation" coincided with their removal from the unhygienic urban atmosphere
and their placement in the healthy environment of the countryside.[41] Open-
air schools proliferated in Europe and America in the 1910s thanks to municipal funds and allotments from school funds, parents' associations, charities, and local and regional councils. The venture of the open-air school
spread from Germany to Austria (with the establishment of the open-air
school in Freiwaldau), Switzerland (with schools in Glarisegg and Grünau
near Zurich), Italy and France, while in England forest lands were given to
settle garden cities. In the USA the view that some classrooms should be
transformed in semi-open air spaces also gained ground. Finland made considerable advances in the medical supervision of special schools with the establishment of open-air schools for blind and mentally retarded children.

The open-air schools were simple constructions with only sheds and pavilions or houses in the woods, in a garden or in seaside areas. The organization
of teachers' associations and congresses for open-air education contributed
further to the exchange of ideas and experience. Not only doctors and educators participated in these congresses, even mayors attended. These congresses
in the early twentieth century commonly found that open-air schools were
important not only for individuals, but for the very nation and race as well.
The third School Hygiene Congress in Paris in 1910 lauded Germany's success in the field for its establishment of forest schools and the Society of School
Trips to the countryside. The strong influence the German forest school had is
evidenced by the English, Danish, Swedish, French and Spanish officials who
traveled to Charlottenburg to study the way the school operated.

Open-air schools rested on the adoption of a new pedagogy which was
adjusted to the intellectual abilities of the weak and sickly children, whose
brains could not be overexhausted. This model dictated measures for dealing with students' mental exhaustion, school work load and the systematic measurement by school doctors of students' physical development. The
measurements of students' weight, height, and blood cells before and after
attending the open-air school was an attempt to translate into numbers the
beneficial effects the countryside had on weak children. Physical exercise

41 Jean Houssaye, "Le centre de vacances et de loisirs prisonnier de la forme scolaire," *Revue française de
pédagogie*, no. 125 (October–November 1998): 95–107.

(gymnastics, walking, games, gardening, and manual work) in nature and naps had shortened the duration of lessons. Teaching was only a small part of the curriculum and was orientated towards hygienic education, as well as teaching principles of autonomy, self-action and discipline, evidencing the influence the New Education movement had on open-air schools, although a number of scholars have pointed out the military and disciplinary character of these schools as well.[42]

Physical education at school served the same objective, namely strengthening the defense of the body through air-bathing. The discourse about the effects of physical education on children's health points to the large say doctors had in daily school routine. Since the beginning of the nineteenth century, exercise was considered the doctors' responsibility. Doctors had to decide on the type of exercises, their duration and their suitability according to the age of the students. Exercise was expected to contribute not only to physical development but also to the correction of the bad body posture, the training of the nervous system and the strengthening of children's morality. Under the influence of this hygienic discourse, gymnastics began to lose its military character and complexity which had been prevalent since the 1870s, in order to widen the circumference of the thorax.[43] Doctors tended to value either the entertaining character of physical education, which compensated for mental exhaustion, or its ability to prevent tuberculosis. The medical community regarded respiratory exercise as a suitable type of physical exercise since it involved the expansion of the chest, thus better supplying the body with oxygen.

Pedagogical Exaggerations and Medical Interventions in the School Curriculum

The effects of teaching on the health of children in general gradually became a subject of medical practice. Issues such as mental exhaustion, the duration of school lessons and recess, the age of admission to elementary education and the synthesis of the everyday school schedule played important roles in

---

42 For an alternative reading of the aims British open-air schools served, see Linda Bryder, "'Wonderlands of Buttercup, Clover and Daisies': Tuberculosis and the Open-air School Movement in Britain, 1907–39," In *In the Name of the Child*, ed. Cooter, 72–92.

43 Georgios Koromilas, "Peri tis mi en Khrono kai Rythmo Physikis Ekpaidefseos os Aitiou Prodiathetontos eis Nosous kai di eis Fthysin," *Dimotiki Ekpaidefsis*, no. 16 (February 15, 1903): 246–53.

the normal development of the child's brain. Mental exhaustion, the second important issue after contagious diseases, brought doctors to schools. To define mental exhaustion, new methods, new tools of measurement and new terms would be used. The term "intellectual fatigue" (fatigue intellectuelle, over-pressure, cachexia scolastica) denoted the condition of "chronic fatigue caused by study load" which manifested in sickness due to the disproportionate ratio between the physical and intellectual powers of the child.[44] Extreme mental fatigue disrupted the normal development of the child. Doctors were not hesitant to point out the harmful effects of school on children's development. To the extent that mental work impeded the normal development of the child, medicine should intervene to restore balance. The priority given to school hygiene regarding issues of bodily functions led to a rift between doctors and educators, especially when the latter attempted to have a say on issues of brain physiology or mental health.

Applying the first experimental methods in the field of experimental psychology, doctors attempted to determine with numerical accuracy the stages of exhaustion caused by the requirements of school curriculum in order to define the standard and predict the damage done to the body. Measurements taken during lessons or during completion of school homework attempted to estimate the symptoms of fatigue in the students in correlation with various parameters, i.e., sex, age, social origin, duration of lessons, difficulty of the subject, teaching method, and the cognitive ability of students, etc.[45] Doctors examined the pace at which mental strength of students deteriorated over time, how their concentration fell in relation to the difficulty of learning, the incidence of mistakes, the impact of various durations of recess, the impact the order of subjects in the school schedule had on the performance of students, etc.[46] The first studies on students for the measurement of mental fatigue were carried out by the Russian neurologist Sikorsky in 1879. In the 1880s measurements in the school population of European countries raised the percentage of students who displayed symptoms of fatigue—headaches, anaemia, scrofula, myopia—between 29 and 46%. Even those who took issue with the manner of measurement agreed that a high

---

44 Dr. A. Jacquet, "I Somatiki Agogi ton Paidon," *Ethniki Agogi*, 9, no. 2 (February 29, 1904): 49.

45 Classic studies on this issue include Alfred Binet and Victor Henri, *La fatigue intellectuelle* (Paris, 1898) and Angelo Mosso, *La fatigue intellectuelle et physique* (Paris: F. Alcan, 1905).

46 P. Malapert, "Les récherches expérimentales sur la mésure de la fatigue intellectuelle et sur les conclusions pédagogiques qu' on peut en tirer," *L'Hygiène scolaire*, no. 14 (April 1906): 83–95.

percentage of students—almost one third—were not healthy and the most aggravating factor for them was school fatigue.[47] From all the bodily functions disturbed by the grueling work of the child's brain, respiration was the one that physiologists were most interested in. According to the medical thought of the times, the body was becoming more vulnerable to infectious diseases due to poor circulation of blood and pressure applied to the lungs. The papers of the French Medical Academy in the 1880s lashed out against the tendency of the teachers to overload children's brain with abstract and useless knowledge, which apart from straining the children's mental powers, exhausted them, thus putting them on the path to tuberculosis and other fatal diseases.[48] The medical measurements of the students' stamina led to speculation about the aims and the quality of teaching. The long-run damage worried some doctors who began asking: "Is teaching possibly harmful?"[49]

Among the therapeutic measures that had to be taken to inflict less damage on students, experts recommended: the decrease in the material taught; the time allotted for teaching, study and exams; the time students should arrive at school. In general, the overall school schedule was likewise influenced by medical views.

FROM THE MILITARY DEFEAT TO
THE "DEGENERATION" OF THE YOUNG

Medical discourse held stronger appeal when it stressed the national dimensions of unhygienic education. The high rate of soldiers who were rejected on the grounds of being physically unable appeared to continue the trend of students who had been characterized as "weak," "anemic" and "fragile" in morbidity statistics. Mental fatigue, pedagogical exaggeration and the absence of medical supervision were held accountable by some intellectuals for the military defeat. The Boer War for the English[50] and the defeat of the

---

47 For these measurements in various European countries, see Harris, *The Health of the Schoolchild*, 29.

48 The issue of mental fatigue recurs in many medical congresses and articles in the end of the nineteenth century. See among others, Jacques Léonard, *La médecine*, 320–21.

49 Georgiou Konti, "Mipos Vlaptei I Didaskalia?" *Dimotiki Ekpaidefsis*, no. 1 (September 1, 1901): 3–5.

50 In 1904 in England an Inter-departmental Committee on Physical Deterioration was set up so as to investigate the reasons of the physical weakness of the English soldiers in the Boer War. See Virginia Berridge, "Health and Medicine," in *The Cambridge Social History of Britain, 1750–1950*, vol. 3, ed. Francis M. L. Thompson, 171–242.

French in the French-Prussian War in 1870 were presented in the press as symptoms of the "gradual degeneration" of weak, nervous-natured people whose health suffered irreparable damage during their school years.[51] The concern for the health of future citizens and soldiers and consequently for the "national efficacy" brought forward the issue of children with mental deficiency, mental problems and other mental and physical disabilities. Although the distinction between various types of mental deficiency had not been drawn yet and the means of detection had yet to be defined, the attempt to distinguish this group from the general student population can be seen in the legislation passed in various countries in the late nineteenth century. Special classes began to be established for children with learning difficulties, the "less gifted,"[52] or the "abnormal children" (enfants anormaux) as well as for the deaf and the blind.[53]

Although the main national eugenics societies had not been set up until the 1910s, the request for "national efficiency" meant that the state had to assume new duties concerning children's health. Under the threat of degeneration, state control of youth health was very desirable and to a certain extent expected. In the context of these concerns, medical supervision at school was legitimized for contemporaries in that medical supervision was considered to contribute to the preparation of a robust future generation. The healthy well-trained bodies of students was a guarantee of preparedness for war, important for every nation interested in building a powerful army. It was generally believed that the "vitality and welfare of the nation"[54] was contingent on the healthy development of children while at school.

SPREADING THE NEW INSTITUTION: THE SCHOOL DOCTOR

The first attempts to organize school hygiene were made in the 1880s and became more frequent in the course of time. Thus, by the turn of the century school doctors were already an institution in most European counties.

---

51 For the military defeat of France in 1870, see Guillaume, "L'Hygiène à l'école er par l'école," 221.
52 For the social welfare services for children with special needs in England, see Hendrich, *Child Welfare*, 95–101.
53 For children with special needs in the nineteenth century, see Monique Vial, "Enfants handicapés du XIX au XXe siècle," in *Histoire de l'enfance en Occident*, eds. Egle Becchi and Dominique Julia (Paris: Éditions du Seuil, 1998), vol. 2, 331–60.
54 For this issue, see many references in the journal *Ethniki Agogi* for the years 1898–1904.

At the same time, doctors and educators participated in international congresses on supervising child development and the protection of children's health, laying the foundations for school hygiene. The way school medical supervision was organized in each country reflects the sort of speculations raised among local medical circles, the level of public health, the status of doctors and the relationship between doctors and the state.

Although Belgium was the first country to introduce school doctors in 1874, Germany stood as the model for this despite infrastructural differences from town to town.[55] The German doctors Baginsky and Gruber were considered in the early twentieth century the founders of school hygiene since they were the first to systematize the institution of the school doctor while the School Hygiene Service in Wiesbaden provided the model for most European cities. Studies on the school population by Kräpelin, Griesbach and Meumann established Germany as the leader in the field of experimental psychology. The Institutes of Applied Psychology set up by teacher associations in collaboration with important paedologists in Leipzig, Berlin and Munich testify to the spread of the experimental methods among teachers. In addition, studies on various health problems were conducted on samples of student population in Germany at the end of the nineteenth century. Cohn's studies on myopia in 1886 after the examination of 10,000 students in Breslau pointed to the harmful effects bad lighting and unsuitable desks had on the health of the students. The supervision of 1,000–1,200 students assigned to each school doctor, the personal health card and the fortnight inspection of schools were considered the ideal quota for securing the health of the student population. At the end of the nineteenth century, the influence of German social policy on schools was visible in other European countries.

In general, between 1874 and 1906 school hygiene services had been set up in at least twenty countries. In Scandinavia and in Austria the establishment of the School Hygiene Service dates back to 1900 with the exception of Sweden where the service was set up earlier (1878). The School Hygiene Service began in 1897 in the USA, 1898 in Denmark, 1902 in Portugal, 1890 in Japan, 1904 in Argentina, which is considered to be a pioneer among the

---

55 In Belgium a special preventive treatment for sickly children in summer camps and the separation of children with physical and mental problems in special classes were implemented. Also a great boost was given to the experimental pedagogy in the paedology institutes and psycho-physiological laboratories of Antwerp and Brussels. See Emmanouil Lambadarios, *Paidologia kai Skholiki Ygieini* (Athens: Ypourgeion ton Ekklisiastikon kai tis Dimosias Ekpaidefseos, 1916), 12–3.

countries of Latin America, while in the Balkans the School Hygiene Service began in the early twentieth century with Bulgaria in the lead following the German model. In England in the 1880s, despite the appealing discussion on fatigue and degeneration, only independent schools had introduced school doctors. In the 1890s the school boards of certain boroughs in London, Edinburgh and Manchester appointed doctors who provided advice to school principals. Yet, it was only in 1907, when a law was passed, that school doctors were appointed by almost all local education councils. School and dental clinics assisted the school doctor in an attempt to improve the health of working-class children. The role of English school nurses in checking the personal hygiene of both students and their families set the model for other countries. In France, although interest in the supervision of students' health dates back to the French Revolution, schools were only gradually staffed with doctors. In 1879 the local council in Paris organized for the first time the school medical service of the city, and in 1883 the Minister of Education Jules Ferry addressed prefects requesting that doctors in their areas be assigned to public schools.

What were the duties of school doctors in the early stages of the school medical service? Despite the differences noticed from country to country, school doctors had to perform quite similar duties. The school doctor was in charge of the examination of the students' health and of the school premises. It was his duty to examine all schoolchildren soon after their admission, to conduct regular measurements of their weight, height and thorax circumference, to examine certain organs—the mouth, the nose, the ears, the eyes, the heart, the glands—to take down the medical history of each student, to complete the student's personal health card, to gather statistics on the hygiene of the students in his assigned area, to conduct vaccinations, to check the sanitary facilities of the school, to visit the school during epidemics, to examine the children who did not attend school because of illness, to locate the foci of infection, to publicize the manifestation of contagious diseases in the area, to classify students according to the level of their health and to assume responsibility for special schools and to teach the subject of hygiene.

The need to control contagious diseases and to detect the initial disease carrier required collaboration between school doctors and the families of the students and the teachers. This increasing power over the body of the students was not always favorably received by parents. As the role of the family was considered important for imparting information, it was necessary to improve the communication of parents with doctors and educate them. New ideas on the hygiene of the body were met with strong resistance. Popular publications, lectures, posters, brochures and films were circulated to inform parents. The introduction of hygiene as a school subject in schools since the end of the nineteenth century was meant to inculcate hygiene principles in students and to indirectly communicate this knowledge to their families.

The speed at which the network of school doctors spread in each country was contingent on a series of factors, most importantly the legislation passed by the state and the presence of eminent medical figures in the field of school hygiene were decisive to its growth. The French school doctors Riant, Mayet, Mosso and Dufestel, the English school doctors Kerr and Newman, the Belgian female doctor Jyoteco, the Swedish doctor Key, the German doctors Baginsky and Gruber became famous for their initiatives to improve students' health and for their publications that set the model for School Hygiene Services in other European countries. On their own initiative, international congresses on school hygiene and paedological institutes were organized to carry out research based on anthropometric measurements while indices of physical and mental development of students were named after these doctors. The spirit of international collaboration that characterized the field of hygiene can be detected in the establishment of international societies such as the Open-Air School Society and in the organization of international congresses on school hygiene (Nuremberg 1904, London 1907, Paris 1910). In addition, in the international hygiene reports, school doctors were able to observe and compare the advances each country had made and the possibilities offered for the supply of their services with technical and material equipment.[56]

At the beginning of the twentieth century, the scope of school hygiene expanded in the fields of psychology and pedagogy to cover the wider field of paedology, an otherwise undefined interdisciplinary field that included all the sciences that dealt with the development of the child. Under the influ-

---

56 M.E. Fustel, "L'Hygiène scolaire à l'Exposition internationale de Dresde," *L'Hygiène scolaire*, no. 38 (April 1912): 121–40 and no. 39 (May 1912): 213–28.

ence of the American Oscar Chrisman—student of the pedagogue and psychologist Granville Stanley Hall—paedology aspired to study the physical, mental and moral development of children's constitution.[57] This trend developed mostly in the first half of the twentieth century, aimed at their normal development as the designated "healthy" standards of normality dictated. The developmental trend that left its stamp on these attempts gave a new orientation to the experimental dimensions of education. The paedological institutes that operated in Belgium, Germany and America starting at the end of the nineteenth century were the first agencies to promote this trend as they carried out experimental psychological research mainly and designed the first tools for the measurement of the mental and intellectual development of children.

The Student as "Biological Capital" for the Nation

The end of the nineteenth century—as a growing portion of Western society realized that the state should fervently involve itself in protecting children's health—witnessed the gradual medicalization of childhood. As knowledge about children's health contributed to a better, overall understanding of national health, services that monitored children's health became all the more important. Thus, as long as the discourse on hygiene drew a growing audience, students were considered to represent a form of capital whose value increased provided that its physical and mental health was constantly improving. The school should take action to grow this capital to its maximum value so that, in turn, students would be able to come up to societal expectations. School became a privileged space for exerting control over the bodies of working class children, while allowing doctors greater access to the health of the general population.

At the beginning of the twentieth century school doctors were expected to inspect school buildings, deal efficiently with common diseases and physical weakness and control contagious diseases. In combination with the teaching of hygiene, the school doctors would spread new concepts and practices for strengthening the body and students' well-being. In a time when greater priority was given to developing means of protection against

---

57 Oscar Chrisman, *Paidologie* (Jena: 1896).

contagious diseases, schools were expected to play a key role in the spread of new hygienic practices. School could also contribute to the improvement of the health of the race and to the confirmation of the innovative character of hygiene as a practice by which man could improve his future.

The above analysis has shown that the introduction of doctors to schools correlated with wider changes in the attitude of European society towards childhood at the end of the nineteenth century. The emergence of family emotion among the middle class, the rising state concern for declining child mortality, and advances in pediatrics strengthened the conviction that children's health must be doctors' responsibility. Medical discourse offered cognitive schemata for children's health that shaped views on its "normality," protection, the patterns of the development of the child's body and the dangers threatening children's health. The establishment of the developmental patterns of the child's body contributed decisively to the definition of the physical and mental health of children and to the construction of pertaining notions of normal and abnormal. Medical science also provided political power with measurement tools and shaped the educational and social policies. Under the influence of medical discourse, the physiology of the child's body started to be understood in different terms compared to adult physiology, and this difference started to affect the planning of health social policy. Thus, the political, national and social meaning which childhood took on at the turn of the century was reflected in the development of social welfare systems for children.

The firm belief that the emerging twentieth century would be the "century of the child" pointed not only to the title of the well-known book *The Century of the Child* published in 1900 by the Swedish feminist educator Ellen Key, but also to the general perception across Western society at the end of the nineteenth century that children were its ultimate value and therefore the protection of children's health took on a great significance for the future.

CHAPTER II

CONCERNS ABOUT STUDENT HEALTH
AND THE FIRST HEALTHCARE STEPS
IN THE EARLY TWENTIETH CENTURY

1. Public Health and Student Morbidity

In the 1890s, voices of protest were increasing in Greece, calling for the introduction of healthcare provisions at schools. These provisions would aim at improving the health of schoolchildren and involve the construction of new school buildings in compliance with hygiene standards. Other European countries provided the model for the development of school hygiene and school architecture. The institutionalization of school hygiene in European universities at the turn of the century also indicated the academic recognition this field had begun to attain.

As the interest of the medical profession began to swing away from the individual and towards vulnerable population groups, children became the heart of the debate over public health. Although the concerns of Greek physicians about high infant mortality, which had been recorded since the first decades of the Greek state, had not diminished by the turn of the century, fresh data had begun to stoke a new round of concerns. These concerns were related as much to the question of racial degeneration and national efficiency as to the problems arising from the lack of a public health system. At the beginning of the twentieth century, public discussion focused on the spread of serious contagious diseases among students, the lack of protective health institutions and, more centrally, the so-called "weakening of the young generation." Discussants were particularly concerned about the risks threatening the health of children and young people, and consequently the future of the nation.

During the same period educators had also begun to associate school attendance with student health. Reports by emergency school inspectors, sent to the provinces in 1883 by the Ministry of Education to tell of the problems facing the Greek educational system, revealed for the first time the poor health of students.[1] Scant student attendance at school, the filthiness of children and the miserable conditions of many classrooms, were three facets of one, greater problem that would attract the interest of both doctors and educators throughout the following decades.

Medical studies on the student population brought to light the extent of these problems and stressed the importance of monitoring and improving this vulnerable group. As medical professionals blamed school buildings and school attendance for the morbidity of students, debates waged in Greece over the systematic monitoring school children's health at the end of the nineteenth century.

1.1 Concerns about Infant and Child Mortality

Since the beginning of the nineteenth century, statistics have been a powerful tool for medical positivism and often been used by healthcare policymakers. During the 1890s, high levels of child mortality and morbidity recorded in the Greek medical press led to skepticism about the physical health of students, their future and that of the nation. Although doctors were not unanimous in accepting official morbidity statistics, since the Ministry of Health did not set up a special service until 1923, the high proportion of child deaths among the overall population was again and again recognized during the nineteenth century. Although Greek physicians were interested in informing the public about prevention and cure of contagious childhood diseases since the establishment of the Greek state—their interest was mainly expressed through publications and translation of medical treatises—yet treatment of fatal infections was still at an embryonic stage.[2]

As there is currently no study available on nineteenth century childhood illnesses, the papers given by doctors published in the meeting minutes of

---

1   *Ektheseis ton kata to 1833 pros Epitheorisin ton Dimotikon Skholeion Apestalmenon Ektakton Epitheoriton* (Athens: n.d.), 22.

2   Childhood diseases had been addressed in a number of publications by eminent Greek doctors during the eighteenth and the beginning of the twentieth centuries. See Giannis Karas ed., *Istoria kai Philosophia ton Epistimon ston Elliniko Khoro (17th-19th century)* (Athens: Metaikhmio, 2003), 629–36.

the Athens Medical Society between 1835 and 1900 constitute the prime source for the study of nineteenth century child mortality.[3] Studying these minutes enables the historian to grasp the seriousness of certain childhood diseases and the extent of infant mortality. Dysentery, diphtheria and scarlet fever appeared time and again in the minutes of the Society. As to precautionary measures against these illnesses, opinions were divided among university professors of pediatrics. A large number of medical competitions launched from 1833 were concerned with how to deal with epidemics that targeted the child population, mostly infants.

It was not accidental then that before the 1890s the attention of medical professionals focused on infant mortality: "the terrible hecatomb of early childhood."[4] Doctors maintained that an infant's first year was decisive for children's survival, since, as statistics had shown, infants accounted for a significant proportion of child mortality. For instance, between 1860 and 1870, children under 10 made up 10,000 out of 22,000 deaths across all ages, while between 1880–1890, out of a total of 28,589 deaths across all age groups throughout Greece, 48.13% were children under the age of 10. Among those, 66.19% were younger than one year old.[5] In 1892, infant mortality in Ermoupolis, on the island of Syros, accounted for 29% of deaths among the entire population, a proportion nearing the highest level recorded in any town during the same period.[6]

According to the Royal Medical Council[7] (*Vasilikon Iatrosynedrion*) which was the Supreme Hygiene Board within the Ministry of the Interior established under Otto's reign, the most common contagious diseases in Greece, such as scarlet fever, smallpox, diphtheria, meningococcal meningitis, typhoid fever and dysentery, caused high mortality rates among chil-

---

3 Konstantinos B. Khoremis, "I Paidiatriki en ti Iatriki Etaireia," *Elliniki Iatriki* no. 4 (1930): 400–90

4 Anastassios Zinnis, *Études sur les principales causes lethiferes chez les enfants au dessous de cinq ans et plus spécialement chez eux de 0–10 ans à Athènes* (Athens: 1880).

5 Alkiviadis Papapanagiotou, "I Thnitotis ton Paidon en Athinais," *Imerologion Efimeridos ton Kyrion tou 1891* (Athens: 1890), 36.

6 Lyntia Trykha, "Synthikes Ygeias kai Ygieinis kata ti Diarkeia tou 1880," in *O Kharilaos Trikoupis kai I Epokhi tou: Politikes Epidiokseis kai Koinonikes Synthikes*, eds. Kaiti Aroni-sikhli and Lyndia Trikha (Athens: Papazisis, 2000), 379–400.

7 The Royal Medical Council published monthly tables of mortality statistics based on data collated from perfects. However, the means of collection was far from uniform and as such the information provided was considered unreliable. Daily and weekly reports on deaths within the area of Athens were published in newspapers, medical journals and the special supplements of the Government Gazette (*Efimeris tis Kiverniseos*). Starting in 1900, the mortality of urban population is more detectable since the Ministry of the Interior published reports on deaths occurring in the twelve largest urban Greek centers.

dren up to 10 years old.[8] On more than one occasion, Greece witnessed outbreaks of scarlet fever, meningitis, dengue and typhoid fever epidemics in the 1880s. Smallpox epidemics were the most common, and accounted for the highest number of victims, although the smallpox vaccine had been in use in Greece since the beginning of the nineteenth century.[9] Between 1880 and 1888, epidemics continued to spread across several regions in Greece, from Corfu to Crete. In 1884, 40% of deaths in Heraklion were caused by smallpox. Between 1882 and 1883, the epidemic hit Athens and Piraeus and caused 1,400 deaths, 400 of which were children and young people under thirty.

The vaccination campaign had not been organized effectively. Closing the university and schools was the most common preventive means. Strict legislation passed in accordance with the Decree of 1835, which imposed fines on parents who did not have their children vaccinated during their first year, had not been successful in containing the disease. At the end of the nineteenth century, smallpox was still the main children's disease. Diphtheria, the second most serious childhood illness, claimed a high number of victims. Starting in 1895, doctors began to fight it with the use of anti-serum and even then this was only true of some Greek doctors.[10]

Gastroenterological disorders, acute respiratory diseases and diarrhea—the latter accounting for about one in three cases—were cited as the most common causes of death at an early age and had been the concern of Greek doctors since the establishment of the Greek state.[11] As early as 1840, the Athens Medical Society was issuing calls for a competition for writing a treatise on the symptoms, strains and causes of diarrhea among children up to the age of two.[12] Innovative practices proposed by some pediatricians

---

8   Konstantinos Savvas, "Ypomnima peri Idryseos Ypourgeiou Ygeias kai Koinonikis Pronoias Ypovlithen eis ton Kyrion Proedron tis Kyverniseos kata Mina Dekemvrion 1920," *Arkheia Iatrikis* no. 3 (March 1922): 65–72.

9   The vaccine was first applied on patients in Constantinople in 1800 and within the next years on patients in the Ionian Islands. See Karas (ed.), *Istoria kai Philosophia ton Epistimon ston Elliniko Khoro*, 632–33.

10 Serum therapy for diphtheria was first applied to patients in Greece in 1895, only two years after its discovery by Behring and Wernicke. Georgios Tsoukalas, Panagiota Mexi and Ioannis Tsoukalas, "I Paidiatriki mesa apo ti Drasi tis Iatrikis Etaireias Athinon 1835–1930," *Deltio A' Paidiatrikis Klinikis Panepisthmiou Athinon* 50, no. 2 (2003): 170–79.

11 Between 1880 and 1890, gastroenterological disorders accounted for 32.37% of child deaths up to the age of ten. Among them, the percentage of infants 0–12 months old reached 78%. Alkiviadis Papapanagiotou, "I Thnitotis ton Paidon en Athinais," 34; Anastasios Zinnis, *I en Athinais Thnitotis ton Vrefon* (Athens: 1877), 4.

12 "Peri tis Epikratousis eis tin Ellada kata to Theros Diarroias ton mi Dieton eiseti Nipion," *O Neos Asklipios* (March 1842): 93.

in the last quarter of the nineteenth century like the introduction of flour-based foodstuffs and "artificial" infant feeding were still received with sus-picion by mothers. The mortality rate was even higher among abandoned infants housed in the Athens Public Foundling Home since 1859. In certain years it reached 58%. For this reason, the first pediatric clinic of the Univer-sity of Athens began operation in 1879 within the premises of the Athens Public Foundling Home.[13]

Compared with other branches of medicine, pediatrics, which broke away from mainstream pathology relatively early, was important for the popularization of medical knowledge. Two doctors who carried out re-search and published many studies on child mortality during that pe-riod—Anastasios Zinnis, Professor in the Medical School and first Di-rector of the Foundling Home, and Alkiviadis Papapanayotou, Lecturer in the Pediatrics School—considered the ignorance of hygienic practices among mothers as the main cause of infant death. Premature weaning, an unhealthy diet, superstitions, and high temperatures during summer all contributed to the infant hecatomb. Educating mothers in their du-ties, fighting their superstitions, learning the rules of hygiene and, chiefly, propagating breast-feeding, were the focal points of doctors' fight to re-duce infant mortality since the 1870s. During the second half of the nine-teenth century, the popularization and dissemination of medical knowl-edge to the lower class was considered one of the most effective means of intervention by the medical community in order to address the morbid-ity of the population. Educating the public in the principles of hygiene and changing the attitude of the lower class towards medical authorities, were given a "moralizing" dimension that pervaded nineteenth century percep-tions of charity in Greece. This tendency—also common in other coun-tries—to attribute the high morbidity rate to lower class ignorance was the main characteristic of medical thought during this period. Linking morbidity causes with sociological factors related to the health of the pop-ulation rather than with ignorance would not become an integral part of medical rationale before the 1920s.

---

13   Eleftherios Skiadas, *Dimotikon Vrefokomeion Athinon: 1859–1899* (Athens: 1899), 70.

1.2 Infectious Diseases and Other Childhood Scourges

Infant mortality monopolized the interest of the medical profession in the middle of the nineteenth century, but towards the end of the century doctors' attention shifted to combating the acute infectious and contagious diseases proliferating within the school environment. Infectious diseases such trachoma, an eye disease that leads to blindness, malaria and TB were considered the scourges of the school population.

Malaria, a "national curse" that hit entire populations in certain lowland areas of Greece, although not leading directly to death, exhausted the constitution of young people through frequent bouts of fever rendering them vulnerable to other illnesses.[14] At the turn of the century, intermittent fevers were common among schoolchildren and attracted the attention of pediatricians.[15] According to Papapanayotou, between 1888 and 1897, deaths from malaria accounted for 49% of all deaths in the 0–10 age group and certain districts in Athens posed a particular threat to the child population.[16] Ioannis Kardamatis (1857–1942), consultant at the Pediatric Clinic of Athens University and a prominent medical figure in the fight against malaria since the end of the nineteenth century, was the first to deal with the problem of malaria systematically, collating data on the effects the disease had on children's constitution.[17] The outbreaks of malaria in Athens in 1901 and 1907 were the subject of his research. His efforts to limit malaria were reflected in the activities of the Anti-Malaria League, established in 1903 on his and Konstantinos Savvas's initiative. The pale face, swollen spleen and general sickliness observed among schoolchildren suffering from the disease resulted in their dropping out from school. The number of dropouts, especially in certain lowland areas, reached alarming rates.

---

14 According to Konstantinos Savvas, in 1907, the morbidity rate for malaria in a considerable number of towns reached 80, 90 and very often 100%. See Konstantios Savvas and Ioannis Kardamatis, *I Elonosia en Elladi kai ta Pepragmena tou Syllogou* (Athens: 1907), 13.

15 Tsoukalas, Mexi and Tsoukalas, "I Paidiatriki mesa apo ti Drasi tis Iatrikis Etaireias Athinon 1835–1930," 176.

16 Alkiviadis Papapanagiotou, *De la Morbidité et de la Mortalite des Enfants* (Athens: 1899), 76.

17 For the action of Ioannis Kardamatis, see Lazaros E. Vladimiros, *Ioannis Kardamatis: O Protergatis tou Anthelonosiakou Agona* (Athens: 2006). For a review of the history of malaria in Greece, see Grigorios A. Livadas and Ioannis K. Sfaggos, *I Elonosia en Elladi (1930–1940): Erevnai – Katapolemisis* (Athens: 1940); Katerina Gardikas, *Landscapes of Disease: Malaria in Modern Greece* (Budapest, New York: Central European University Press, 2018).

However, among the endemic illnesses of most concern to the medical community, TB was considered to be the most dangerous due to its high mortality rate across the general population. The disease attracted the attention of doctors for two main reasons: it was one of the prime causes of death among teachers, and almost all pupils were carriers of the bacillus by the age of 12. Prevention was highlighted as the best means of safeguarding public health and protecting children's health.

According to conclusions Vassilios Patrikios drew from mortality statistics, compiled by the Ministry of the Interior, TB was responsible for 16–18% of all deaths around 1900.[18] Although this percentage was average among European countries, the infectious nature of schools and, more worryingly, the probability of the disease spreading from schools to the wider population, made students the center of medical attention. Concerns regarding the infectivity of the school building were repeatedly raised at the first medical conferences organized in Greece (1901, 1903 and 1906). During the 1901 conference particularly, TB was referred as one of the top three scourges to strike Greek society. At the same conference, the Medical Council entrusted Patrikios with studying the causes of the disease, the possibility of establishing a sanatorium in Greece, and presenting his proposals to the medical community. In his study, Patrikios reached the conclusion that, even though wretchedness and poverty of the lower class in Greece had not reached the levels found in industrial centers in the West, the upward trend in the number of those affected by TB, together with the high percentage of young people who fell prey to the disease, justified the determination of doctors. Doctors demanded that the state launch a campaign against the disease. Since the establishment of sanatoriums was considered untenable for financial reasons, Patrikios proposed a number of direct, everyday precautionary measures be taken against TB.

The establishment of the Pan-Hellenic Association against TB in December 1901 enabled the doctors leading the movement pay more attention to the issues of unhealthy working and schooling conditions. The school building, with all its shortcomings emerged as a prime site of infection. For this reason, school students and professional groups, would be among those

---

18 Patrikios was an active doctor who led the Anti-TB campaign in Greece in the early twentieth century. Vasilios Patrikios, *I Phthisis en Elladi (meta Khartou)* (Athens: 1903). See also the newspaper *To Asty* (May 6, 1901), 1.

mostly studied.[19] Between 1908 and 1909, Georgios Trokhanis and Konstantinos Papayannis, lecturers in Pediatrics at the University of Athens, carried out significant research on schoolchildren in many regions throughout Greece in order to identify TB victims and carriers of the disease.[20] They presented their conclusions at the first conference against TB in 1909 which were useful in launching the fight against TB. According to this research, students demonstrated high levels of morbidity in the large urban centers of Athens, Piraeus and Ermoupolis. Although the proportion of schoolchildren suffering from TB was no greater than 20%, the number of suspected cases ranged from 9% to 25% approximately. "Scrofulous" schoolchildren who formed a multitudinous group, were not included in the category of suspected cases, although doctors admitted that even mild "scrofulous tendencies" could, under certain conditions, lead to TB.

During this research, the doctors were able to ascertain the unhygienic condition of most school buildings. Unsuitable classrooms, poor ventilation, crowding, lack of cleanliness and the poor condition or total lack of school furniture, made up the bleak picture of Greek school buildings at the end of the nineteenth century. In the following decades this picture which would be further implicated by the morbidity of the school population. Doctors noted that the spread of infectious diseases was more likely in Athens schools, "whose classrooms where many childhood years are crushed, are totally unsuitable, and certainly do not contribute to preserving the health and growth of the human body; instead, they damage it."[21]

The basic principles of school hygiene were completely absent from school life. Schoolchildren in Athens "were swarming into small, sunless and poorly aired rooms, full of dust, sitting at old and entirely unsuitable desks. In some classrooms, dampness reached 2 meters up the walls."[22] Almost no school was found to have a clean and spacious playground, while the "stinking lavatories" consisted of a row of 4–6 holes in the ground.

---

19   For the morbidity statistics published by the Association, see Vassiliki Theodorou, "Oi Giatroi apenanti sto Koinoniko Zitima: O Antiphymatikos Agonas stis Arkhes tou 20ou Aiona (1901–1926)," *Mnimon* 24 (2002): 145–78.

20   The sample of the research included 6,560 students from Athens, 2,090 from Pireaus, 3,358 from Patra, 1,137 from the island of Syros, 2,344 from Volos, 750 from Kalamata, 1,813 from Tripoli and 442 from the island of Zakynthos. See the paper presented by Georgios Trokhanis and Konstantinos Papayannis in *Praktika tou A'Synedriou kata tis Phymatioseos. 6–10 Maiou, 1909* (Athens: 1909), 82–107.

21   *Praktika tou A' Synedriou kata tis Phymatioseos*, 84.

22   *Praktika tou A' Synedriou kata tis Phymatioseos*, 84.

This unsalubrious picture was completed by parental indifference towards the health of their offspring and defiance of personal hygiene rules. Most children were found to be pale, anemic and scrawny. They came for their medical checks unwashed and wearing dirty clothes, "visible from afar by the dirt on the nape of their necks, with rheumyeyes, displaying extensive eczema and ulcerations on the neck and other parts of the body."[23] Such conditions left doctors with no doubt that schools were failing to contribute to the intellectual and physical development of schoolchildren.

1.3 The State of Public Health

In the early twentieth century, Greek medical professionals tended increasingly to criticize the state's indifference towards the supervision of schoolchildren's healthcare. These concerns are more understandable if one takes into account that the organization of the county public health system, institutionalized since 1833, was far from ensuring the effective medical inspection of schoolchildren. Health inspection of school buildings was essentially non-existent. County medical officers, burdened with various responsibilities ranging from checking county medical staff and monitoring welfare institutions, to supervising slaughter-houses, public baths and schools, so as to identify the initial carrier of the infection, were unable to monitor whether or not pupil absenteeism was due to childhood illnesses or infectious diseases. They were also unable to carry out vaccinations on a mass scale. Moreover, debarring children with infectious diseases from school, a measure enforced by the police, had questionable results.[24]

As far as hospitalization was concerned, some efforts were made at the end of the century. Thanks to funding from private donations, the special children's hospital *Saint Sofia Children's Hospital* (Nosokomeion Paidon Agia Sofia) began operating in 1900, and a small number of beds were made available for children in the pediatric ward of the Clinic of the Greek Women's Union, a charitable organization. In order to understand why children's hospital facilities were limited to these two institutions, it is essential to out-

---

23 *Praktika tou A' Synedriou kata tis Phymatioseos,* 85.
24 Vasiliko Diatagma (Royal Decree), "Peri Empodismou tis Metadoseos ton Molysmatikon (Kollitikon) Arrostion," Efimeris tis Kyverniseos A' no. 83 (December 31, 1836): 426–29. Also Theodoros Flogaitis, *Parartima ton Dikastikon Nomon,* part B' (Athens: 1887), 1184–96.

line the general condition of the public health system in Greece. Indicators such as cumulative morbidity of the population, the stage of development of the healthcare system and state provisions, healthcare legislation and the standard of public health infrastructure, are indispensable for contextualizing the issue of the children's health.

Both medical treatises and popular publications in the second half of the nineteenth century emphasized the appalling health conditions of the general population. According to Konstantinos Savvas (1861–1929), president of the Royal Medical Council, official doctor of King George and the first professor of Hygiene and Microbiology at the University of Athens since 1900, mortality was high in Greece compared with other European countries despite its healthy climate. Most studies on the morbidity of the population tended to associate poor public health with the lack of healthcare institutions and infrastructure, meagre funding and the state's general indifference towards health issues. Since current historians have not yet systematically addressed public health issues during the nineteenth century, we have to rely on available sources derived mainly from administrative and legal records to provide a more complete historical account of all these correlations. These sources, including appeals by voluntary associations, preambles to laws, regulations issued by county councils on how to deal with epidemics, and medical topographies, tended to foregrounded certain health issues and omit others.

Nevertheless, most sources concur that at the beginning of the twentieth century, and even earlier, Greece was ravaged by malaria and TB, smallpox was on the way to acquiring the status of a "Greek disease," typhoid fever was responsible for a steady number of deaths, and the spread of sexually-transmitted diseases had reached worrying proportions. Appropriate services had not been set up to combat these diseases. The urban working class who lived in poor health conditions suffered mainly from TB, while rural populations displayed symptoms of emaciation due to periodic malarial fevers. As these "intermittent fevers" broke out from April to October, i.e., during the harvest, their impact on the performance of farmers was more than evident: Exhausted by sickness, they had less stamina for work and often fell prey to TB or other epidemics.[25]

---

25 Antonis Liakos, *Ergasia kai Politiki stin Ellada tou Mesopolemou: To Diethnes Grafeio Ergasias kai I Anadysi ton Koinonikon Thesmon* (Athens: Idryma Erevnas kai Paideias tis Emporikis Trapezas tis Elladas, 1993), 319.

At the beginning of the twentieth century, people were beginning to connect issues of nutrition, living conditions and sanitation in towns to the health of the population. According to newspaper articles and reports by work inspectors, high rates of morbidity and mortality were related to a diet lacking in healthy nutrients.[26] In both urban and rural areas, the poor nutrition of laborers and farmers' families reflected their meagre incomes. In towns, laborers' low income led to malnutrition, while in villages the meagre incomes of farming families were insufficient to satisfy their nutritional needs. Those meagre earnings were supplemented by credit, remittances from abroad and undeclared sources. Housing problems—most acute in Athens and Piraeus—worsened due to the refugee influx as a consequence of war events in the 1910s, as well as due to the rise in rents. Many working-class families were crowded into one-room houses, most often basements, where sanitary conditions were appalling. The "War on the Slums" became the main slogan of the anti-TB campaign, while references to the cause and effect link between habitation and contagious diseases became commonplace in the contemporary press.

Improving public health was not among the state's priorities, at least until the early twentieth century. Economic difficulties and political unrest stood in the way of setting up institutions for the prevention and treatment of diseases. The very concept of public health as a political issue was not understood as such by the political leadership during the nineteenth century. The first attempts to draw the legislative framework for health issues were undertaken by the Bavarian jurists[27] who accompanied the young King Otto, son of King Ludwig I of Bavaria, following the foundation of an independent Greek state under the protection of the great powers. These attempts were followed by a period of stagnation from 1864 until the Balkan Wars (1912–13), when the shortcomings became more obvious. During these fifty years, governments were often forced to curtail public spending on health care in order to balance their budgets.[28] The reduction in public healthcare funding from 1859 to 1908 tells of the state indifference. Thus, the state limited itself

---

26 For the purchasing capacity and the living conditions of the working class as they were outlined in the work inspectors' reports, see Mikhalis Riginos, *Paragogikes Domes kai Ergatika Imeromisthia stin Ellada, 1909–1936* (Athens: Idryma Erevnas kai Paideias tis Emporikis Trapezas tis Elladas, 1987), 240–8.

27 This framework was drawn according to the model of the conservative Bavarian state.

28 For the history of the hygiene services in Greece, see Nikolaos Makridis, *Ai Ypiresiai Ygieinis en Elladi: Apo tis Idryseos tou Ellinikou Vasileiou mekhri ton Imeron mas* (Athens: 1933), 15–6.

to funding charity organizations and associations that fought endemic diseases, such as the Pan-Hellenic Association Against TB and the Anti-Malaria League. Despite efforts undertaken by the presidents of these associations, who were eminent physicians, the scope of these organizations was rather limited. According to Konstantinos Savvas, as far as healthcare was concerned, Greece was "on the bottom rung of the scale of civilized nations."[29]

The legislative measures to combat epidemics adopted by the Bavarians were still in effect in 1900. The Royal Medical Council convened when an epidemic broke out. Outbreaks of cholera, swine fever, typhus fever and smallpox, were commonplace in the nineteenth century, highlighting deficiencies in water supply and lack of sanitation in urban centers. The operation of slaughterhouses in city centers—until around 1890 in Athens and Piraeus—the use of open spaces as lavatories, the lack of a sewage system, the poor state of stone aqueducts which dated back to the Romans, and ineffective dust and rubbish collection, all contributed to the spread of epidemics and brought about insurmountable problems for the local councils.[30] Articles on health and hygiene appeared very often in the Athens and Piraeus press testifying to these deficiencies.[31] According to the Athens Hygiene Society, health conditions in Athens at the beginning of the twentieth century were far from favorable. Most unsanitary dwellings were located in the center of the town, where densely-populated narrow streets blocked air and sunlight to the houses. Emergency measures taken during wartime attempted to address these problems, which had been exacerbated by the overcrowding of refugees, but did not produce any spectacular results. During the Balkan Wars from 1912–13, 466 people died in the Public Hospital for Infectious Diseases in Thessaloniki in the span of a single year: 204 from smallpox, 55 from typhoid and 207 from Asian cholera. Most of the victims were soldiers and refugees.[32]

---

29 Savvas, "Ypomnima peri Idryseos Ypourgeiou Ygeias kai Koinonikis Pronoias," 70–2.
30 For the public health problems in Athens, see Ioannis Vamvas, *Peri tis Katastaseos en I Diatelei I Dimosia Ygieini en Athinais* (Athens: 1882). For the problem of water supply in Athens, see Ioannis Lambrou, *O Ydatinos Ploutos tis Attikis Gis* (Athens: Agricultural Bank of Greece, 1998). On the means the local council of Piraeus used to deal with epidemics at the end of the nineteenth century, see Giannis Giannitsiotis, *I Koinoniki Istoria tou Peiraia. I Syngrotisi tis Astikis Taxis 1860–1910* (Athens: Nefeli, 2006) 214–25.
31 See, for example, the hygiene measures taken in Piraeus in 1883 to deal with the cholera epidemic in the newspaper *Sphera*: "Kholera," *Sphera*, June 28, 1883, 1; "Kholera kai Perithalpsi," *Sphera*, July 12, 1883, 1–2 and "Igieina Metra," *Sphera*, July 22, 1883, 1–2.
32 For the hygiene problems in Thessaloniki at the beginning of the twentieth century, see Kyriakos N. Kyriakidis, *I Thessaloniki apo Ygieinis Apopseos* (Athens: 1917).

As far as sanitation works in cities were concerned, much remained to be done at the turn of the century, with information on health issues still in its infancy. Traditional perceptions of treating disease went hand in hand with lack of personal hygiene, thus expediting the spread of contagious diseases. The level of medical knowledge at the time must be analyzed alongside the lag in state welfare. Despite advances in hygiene and microbiology, combating many childhood illnesses or epidemic diseases was far from feasible. For some diseases vaccinations had not yet been discovered, while for others the use of vaccines was negatively received, as was the case with the smallpox vaccine. Nevertheless, there had been changes regarding children's health and hygiene: as the sick body of the child gradually took a distinct place in medical statistics, precautionary health was proclaimed a national issue.

2. The Health of Schoolchildren: a Matter of 'National Efficiency'

The Greco-Turkish War (1897) brought to the fore the issue of 'national efficiency' and the comparison of Greece with other countries, particularly in terms of health care of the young people. The war revealed the gap between the country's irredentist goals and its military preparedness. The high proportion of youth declared unfit for enlistment highlighted the deficient national vitality of Greece. Adopting the interpretations prevalent in France and England following their defeats during the Franco-Prussian War (1870) and the Boer Wars (1880–1881, 1899–1902), respectively, attempts were also made in Greece to connect national defeat with the educational system and the latter was held responsible for the 'unprepared' young body. Attempts to attribute the defeat to the deficiencies of the educational system, not only in terms of teaching, but also its material conditions, were evident in the press, and, in particular, in educational treatises, stamped with national concern, during the years following the Greco-Turkish War. The impact of the defeat of 1897 is evident on the educational reform attempted by the Theotokis government in 1899. As mentioned in the preambles of the educational bills, this reform would build up "a strong army capable of removing the stigma of 1897."[33]

---

33 *Ekpaifeftika Nomoskhedia. Aitiologiki Ekthesis kai Agorefseis peri Dimotikis Ekpaidefseos* (Athens: Ethniko Typographeio, 1899): 3.

Greek doctors and educators held the poor state of school buildings, the unsanitary conditions of schooling and the inadequacies of the infrastructure responsible for stunted physical development and national decline. Sentencing children's bodies to long-term deformity, sickliness or unfitness and 'anemic constitution' and the lack of personal hygiene rules did nothing to ensure the regeneration of the race and preparation of a well-trained army. Military preparations would be insufficient, were they not accompanied by the construction of new school buildings, that were true 'soldier-producing factories.'[34]

The debate on school health rendered educational reform and national regeneration inextricable elements of the contemporary national rhetoric. Thus, the regeneration of the Greek race was unimaginable without a school system that would guarantee the health of future soldiers and the development of hardy and robust bodies. The issues of constructing sanitary buildings, the inadequacy of desks, physical education and the mental fatigue of students would be linked to the educational reform that was expected to lead to national recovery. Comparison with neighboring Balkan countries, then regarded as national rivals, highlighted the backwardness that could have an impact on the outcome of national conflicts. Most references in the daily press cited Bulgaria, a neighboring newly established state that, in the early twentieth century, claimed not only the territory of Macedonia but also the sympathy of Europeans. Apart from its military preparation, Bulgaria could boast of a significant administrative organization. According to the articles hosted in the journal *National Education* (Ethniki Agogi), Bulgaria, having followed the German model, had a special infrastructure set up for school hygiene inspection, which had been conducted by school doctors since the beginning of the twentieth century. Progress in Bulgaria, Serbia, and Romania, three countries distinguished in international hygiene exhibitions for their efforts to reform primary education and establish medical inspection, contributed to a Greek public debate that tended to infuse the issue of medical inspection of schoolchildren with a nationalist tone. As Drosinis highlighted, "Of course our consciousness will be raised too, but I am afraid it may be raised too late. Unfortu-

---

34 Anonymos, "Ta Nea Ktiria ton Dimotikon Skholeion," *Ethniki Agogi* no. 2 (March 15, 1898): 17–9 and Georgios Drosinis, "Ta Skholeia tou Dimou Athinaion," *Ethniki Agogi* no. 19 (January 1, 1903): 223–24.

nately, our downfall in 1897 proved that the scalding metal of war did not burn our flesh sufficiently."[35]

During the 1890s, two educational journals, which often featured articles on the harmful effects schooling had on the physical and mental well-being of schoolchildren, began to inform the educational community about the value of school hygiene and the advances in this field in Western Europe. *National Education,* published by George Drosinis, a renowned poet, since 1898, and *Primary Education* (Dimotiki Ekpedefsis), published by Spiros Doukakis since 1901, hosted articles by doctors, educators and social 'thinkers,' such as Herbert Spencer, Aimé Riant, Phillippe Tissié, Luis Dufestel, Henry Guillaume, Jacques Tessier and others. These articles discussed issues such as the mental fatigue and other health risks the young generation would face due to the unhealthy conditions of schooling and they stressed the importance of physical exercise and personal hygiene to the health and well-being of the individual. The articles reflected the fact that Drosinis and Doukakis had come under the influence of the European experience in school hygiene while studying in Western Europe. *National Education* highlighted achievements in the field of student health, like the adoption of medical inspection programmes in Germany, Switzerland and France, while simultaneously emphasizing the obligation of the Greek state to the health of Greek schoolchildren. These journals informed the Greek public about experts' views on school hygiene expressed at international conferences, innovations in the healthcare and welfare of students and opinions held by renowned hygienists on preventative health care for schoolchildren. Student fatigue, ways in which diseases spread, the most appropriate types of physical exercise, the first 'school colonies,' school baths and school meals were recurrent issues in translated articles, which, despite their pedagogical slant, placed significant emphasis on preventive measures.

A quantitative analysis of the issues tackled in these journals demonstrates a focus on two key-themes: the health risks posed by the infectivity of the air in closed spaces and the overloaded school curricula which led students to mental exhaustion caused by overloaded school curricula. The

---

35 Drosinis, "Ta Skholeia tou Dimou Athinaion," 224. For the inferiority feelings towards the means of state organization in Bulgaria, see Elli Skopetea, "I Katastasi tou Ethnous sti Arches tou Eikostou Aiona," in *Istoria tis Elladas tou 20ou aiona: Oi Aparkhes 1900–1922,* ed. Christos Khatziiosif, vol. A2 (Athens: Vivliorama, 1999), 19–20.

crowding of young bodies into unhygienic classrooms for hours on end had been proved to be the main factor contributing to student morbidity, while references to school fatigue and the 'unnatural' character of education were common in contemporary publications in Greece. During this time, similar approaches in European medical thought were beginning to gain popularity in Greece and causing people to increasingly blame poor health on schools: "[No schooling is free of harmful effects on the physical development of the child,] because any such schooling keeps a child in the contaminated atmosphere of a classroom all day long, tied to a desk, instead of running out and about in the open air, as age and nature command."[36]

In addition to doctors, educators also contributed to these journals, suggesting practical ways to disinfect schools in an effort to minimize the incidence of TB. The dust in the classrooms, the children's unpleasant body odors and dirt carried in from city's streets on children's shoes, chalk dust and even childish spontaneity, were all suspected of spreading the disease. Teachers published articles proposing new ways of cleaning classrooms and lavatories, while doctors experimented with forms of physical exercises that would contribute to strengthening the respiratory system and the chest.

Similar concerns were raised in medical and pedagogical conferences in Greece at the beginning of the new century. The risks that the sluggishness of the Greek state on the issue of school hygiene posed to student health came up in many papers presented around 1900s. During the first Pan-Hellenic Medical Conference, held in Athens in 1901, doctor Konstantinos Papayannis presented the basic principles of school hygiene, examining a series of issues such as the suitability of the grounds where the school was to be built, the right schooling age, appropriate physical exercise and the avoidance of fatigue. It was the first time in Greece that the need for health reform in the field of school hygiene had been emphasized. The conference adopted Papayannis's suggestion for the establishment of the High Board of Hygiene in the Ministry of Education, with the participation of doctors who "possessed expert knowledge" and the appointment of a school doctor to the Prefectural Supervisory Board (Nomarkhiako Epoptiko Symvoulio).

---

36 Emmanouil Lambadarios, "I Ygieini tou Skholeiou kai to Ergon ton Skholikon Iatron," *Ygeionomikon Deltion Iatrosynedriou* no. 6 (April 1918), Ypourgeion Esoterikon (edited by B. Patrikios, K. Kyriazidis, E. Lambadarios).

A few years later, Konstantinos Savvas made a more systematic presentation of the principles of school hygiene to teachers. He had studied in Vienna and London and he later organized the state hygiene service. Having presented a paper, entitled "Some thoughts on the improvement of School Hygiene in Greece," he caused a stir at the first Greek educational conference in 1904.[37] His paper highlighted the necessity of introducing such a service in Greece and set out its goals. Savvas referenced a series of issues that had caused concern among other European school hygienists.

For the first time in Greece, he presented the benefits of open-air teaching. He argued that the country's mild climate meant that classes could be conducted in the open air almost all year round with the construction of a shed in the schoolyard. At the same time, he put forward the introduction of baths in schools. Making reference to the installation of the first school baths in 1884 in Göttingen, Germany, he set out the beneficial effects of bathing on students' bodies and the consequent improvement in the atmosphere of the schoolrooms. According to Savvas, the introduction of school baths in Greece was expected to be of wider social significance, as it would contribute to the dissemination of the principles of hygiene to all social classes. He also considered the introduction of sports as part of physical education to be necessary to improve the function of bodily organs as well as to contribute to the development of a brave and bold nation.

As far as school hygiene was concerned, Savvas placed greater emphasis on the consultative and essentially preventive role of school doctor, rather than on the role he could play in treatment. He held that the recruitment of school doctors would come up against insurmountable obstacles and therefore proposed that the duties of school doctors be temporarily assigned to future doctors of the municipalities and county councils. This would be the first step towards the appointment of "special independent doctors, as is the case in Western Europe."[38]

Finally, he recommended the training of educators to teach in health and hygiene so that they could understand and support the efforts of doctors, as well as disseminate knowledge of hygiene to the public. Teaching hygiene as an independent subject in the final year of primary school

---

37 Konstantinos Savvas, "Nyxeis Tines pros Veltiosin tis Skholikis Ygieinis en Elladi," *Dimotiki Ekpaidefsis* no. 22 (April 1904): 337–57.

38 Savvas, "Nyxeis," 356.

could be effectively enhanced by knowledge of hygiene being dovetailed into other school subjects. The link between hygiene and national discourse was reflected in the importance Savvas attached to the collaboration of doctors with educators so as to prepare a healthy future generation endowed with the necessary strength and stamina both for work and war. The same conference emphasized the need to reduce the workload in the curriculum of girls' schools. The argument, based on medical discourse, that school workload could pose a threat to the female reproductive system had already gained ground in some educational journals in the late nineteenth century. The concern that too much mental work could lead young women to become sterile was expressed in many articles. Headaches, scrofula and anemia were indications of this morbid condition that, according to measurements by certain school doctors, affected 40% of girls attending women's schools. In an article published in *National Education* in 1900 on the impact of education on girls' fertility and, by extension, the biological quality of the race, Herbert Spencer claimed that taxing the brain brought about greater imbalance in the female body, mainly in terms of reproductive function, since reproduction was of greater significance to the female body than the male.[39] Thus, the curriculum of female schools called for review. Limited course material in physics and math, reduced teaching hours, and selected non-taxing literary works, combined with artistic subjects and physical education, would safeguard the health of future mothers.[40]

The first books on school hygiene were published in the first decade of the twentieth century, with the exception of a book on combating student myopia published in 1898.[41] The Maraslis Library published G. Vlamos's *School Hygiene* in 1904.[42] Vlamos, a doctor from Smyrna who had studied in Germany, was familiar with the existing literature. In a massive 945-page volume he set out all known theories of school hygiene up to the early twentieth century and the policies implemented in many European countries. Although his contemporaries considered his work to be an adaptation of

---

39   Herbert Spencer, "I Fysiki Agogi," *Ethniki Agogi*, no. 41 (August 15, 1900): 253–55.
40   Eleni Fournaraki, *Ekpaidefsi kai Agogi ton Koritsion: Ellinikoi Provlimatismoi (1830–1910): Ena Anthologio* (Athens: IAEN, 1987), 52–3.
41   Giorgos Karapanagiotis, *Ygieini Proliptiki tis Mathitikis Myopias* (Athens: 1898).
42   Georgios Vlamos, *I Ygieinitou Skholeiou* (Athens: Sakellariou/Vivliothiki Marasli, 1904).

a similar work in German by Leo Burgerstein and August Netolitzki, Vlamos's book later became the standard reference for the manuals on school hygiene, written at the beginning of the twentieth century.

Greek doctors in the Ottoman Empire also wrote about the need of physical education and medical inspection in schools. Both papers given at conferences and relevant publications attest to this interest. *The Hellenic Literary Society of Constantinople* led efforts to spread knowledge of hygiene. At the beginning of the twentieth century, the Society launched a competition for a school textbook on hygiene.[43] The paper on school hygiene Thalia Flora presented at the Educational Conference of the *Hellenic Literary Society of Constantinople* in 1908 attracted the attention of experts to a series of measures that would become widespread over the next decades, such as the need to measure school fatigue and compile statistics on the physical development of students.[44] Physical education classes were introduced into primary schools in Constantinople in 1900, while medical inspection of students at the Great School of the Nation (Megali tou Genous Skholi) was institutionalized in 1902.[45] In 1903, on the initiative of the physician A.S. Matlis and Karaia, a school principal from Vitolia in Macedonia, *School Hygiene* was published. The *Illustrated Manual of School Hygiene* by N.A. Triantafilidis came out in Constantinople in 1911.[46] The author put particular emphasis on the preventative value of school hygiene to safeguard students against contagious diseases and the need for classrooms to be equipped with spittoons and ventilation systems.

The medical discourse built up in conferences, medical and educational journals, as well as school hygiene textbooks contributed towards raising public awareness of the ways the health of schoolchildren could be improved. The national defeat at the end of the nineteenth century made this discourse to seem all the more timely.

43 Kharis Exertzoglou, *Ethniki Taftotita stin Constantinoupoli ton 190 Aiona: O Ellinikos Filologikos Syllogos Constantinoupoleos 1861–1912* (Athens: Nefeli, 1996), 76.

44 *O en Constantinoupolei Ellinikos Filologikos Syllogos: Praktika ton Ekpaideftikon Synedrion 1907–1908*, vol. 31 (Constantinople: 1909), 3–28.

45 On the relationship between church intelligentsia and school hygiene supervision institutions in Constantinople, see Giorgos Kokkinos, "Ygeia, Alki, Kalokagathia: Orthodoxi Ekklisia kai Somatiki Agogi. Oi Anstistaseis kai i Vathmiaia Prosarmogi," in *Praktika tou Diethnous Symposiou Oi Khronoi tis Istorias: Gia mia Istoria tis Paidikis Ilikias kai tis Neotitas* (Athens: IAEN, 1988), 317–39.

46 Nikolaos A. Triantafyllidis, *Enkheiridion Skholikis Ygieinis met' Eikonon* (Constantinople: 1911).

3.1 Physical Education: Healthcare and Recreation

State interest in student healthcare began during the 1890s and manifested itself in two ways: firstly, a Royal Decree was issued in 1894 that laid down hygienic standards in the construction of school buildings;[47] and secondly, the introduction of physical education classes and sports competitions at all grade levels in 1899.[48] Both measures, innovative as they were, reflected the criticism that physicians and educators had levelled at the state regarding the effectiveness of the educational process.

Until the late nineteenth century, physical education in Greek schools was linked to the nation's preparation for war. Following the French example, Harilaos Trikoupis's government introduced physical education classes into secondary schools in 1884, emphasizing military drills. The School of Physical Education was founded in the same year.[49] However, attempts by subsequent governments to introduce physical education classes into primary schools failed. In the 1890s, progress in the field of physical education was most apparent in women's gymnastics and in the organization of school competitions by the Hellenic Athletics Club. The introduction of "educational gymnastics," as opposed to competitive sports in girls' schools, reflected perceptions that the degree and content of physical exercise should be differentiated according to gender. In the case of girls, gym was considered to support the weak female constitution, strengthen the nervous system of the fragile female, shield her from the passions of the soul and, in general, enable her to acquire the skills considered proper for her feminine nature—so that women would be able to live up to their natural calling.[50]

In 1899 the Minister of Education Athanasios Eftaxias introduced gym and sports competitions into primary and middle schools and teacher training colleges.[51] The innovative element of Eftaxias's bill was the abolition of mili-

---

47 Eleni Kalafati, *Ta Skholika Ktiria tis Protovathmias Ekpaidefsis, 1821–1929* (Athens: IAEN, 1988), 167–78.

48 On the institutionalization of physical education at all levels of education and its importance to the school curricula, see Khristina Koulouri, *Athlitismos kai Opseis tis Astikis Koinomikotitas: Gymnastika kai Athlitika Somateia, 1870–1922* (Athens: IAEN/KNE, 1997), 65–9.

49 In order to follow the changes taken place in the teaching of physical education, see Eleni Fournaraki, "Somatiki Agogi ton dyo Fylon stin Ellada tou 19ou Aiona," in *Praktika tou Diethnous Symposiou Oi Khronoi tis Istorias: Gia mia Istoria tis Paidikis Ilikias kai tis Neotitas* (Athens: IAEN, 1988), 293–317.

50 Fournaraki, "Somatiki Agogi," 303–17.

51 For the importance of the Eftaxias's bills, see David Antoniou, *Ta Programmata tis Mesis Ekpaidefsis (1833–1929)*, vol. 1 (Athens: IAEN, 1987), 396–410; Stratis Bournazos, "I Ekpaidefsi sto Elliniko Kratos," in *Istorias tis Elladas tou 20ou Aiona: Oi Aparkhes 1900–1922*, ed. Khristos Khatziiosif, vol. A2, 189–281.

tary exercises and the introduction of competitions and games. These changes were designed not only to strengthen the body and contribute to a balanced physical development, but also to boost a vigorous character and, finally, to reduce the harmful effects of school on the constitution of students. Thus, gym was expected to fulfil a multi-faceted mission with regard to "health, ethics and nation."[52] The preamble of the bill described the cultivation of discipline, the spirit of equality, and allegiance to the community, as the essential elements of preparing schoolchildren for socialization. Cultivation of character and healthy exercise were considered to be equally important.

Interest in the physical exercise of children and young people increased in the late 1890s, due in part to the aftermath of the Olympic Games which were held in Athens in 1896, as well as to the national defeat in the 1897 Greco-Turkish War. Health and national goals went hand-in-hand, and were considered to be the "perfect preparation for patriotism."[53] Thus, even though reference to the preparation of students for military life went unmentioned in the royal decree of 1899, a new attitude towards physical exercise is manifest as the emphasis was placed on national games and team sports. Organization of the first school gymnastics competitions in 1899 and the replacement of old school buildings with new ones, some of which had outdoor areas for physical education, were warmly welcomed by the medical community.

Sports competitions and games as a type of physical exercise in the open air, in contrast the inertia of sedentary life were considered beneficial not only for the harmonious development of the body but also offered pleasure and amusement, and further contributed to the cultivation of an active character.[54] In the same vein, school trips were introduced and we planned to take place out of town every Thursday afternoon when high schools were closed. The circular on "physical education trips," sent out by Ministry in 1898, emphasized that the health and well-being of the body was of prime importance to human happiness and that children's bodies should not be confined to the narrow environment of the school, "bent over their desks, in a stifling and

---

52 Vasiliko Diatagma "Peri tis Didaskalias tis Gymnastikis en tis Skholiois tis Dimotikis kai Mesis Ekpaidefseos kai en tois Didaskaliois Ekaterou Fylou," *Efimeris tis Kiverniseos* A′, 255 (November 20, 1899): 939–949. See also Antoniou, *Ta Programmata*, vol. 1, 398–408 and Koulouri, *Athlitismos*, 66.

53 Vasiliko Diatagma "Peri tis Didaskalias tis Gymnastikis" 942.

54 The change in the content of physical exercise at the turn of the century was connected with the gradual prevalence of British sports in most European countries and the emergence of new values. See Koulouri, *Athlitismos*, 68–9.

contaminated atmosphere, but instead they should be free to venture out-side, in the fresh air, as often as possible."[55] Both the circular on physical edu-cation trips and the preamble on teaching gym at schools indicated the influ-ence of medical discourse, as they stressed the imbalance in schoolchildren's development as a result of mental exhaustion.[56] Thus, physical education was expected to serve as "the necessary counter-balance to mental activity, [...] as well as the soundest basis for a healthy and manly upbringing."[57] It was not only the Ministry of Education but also charity organizations dedicated to the popularization of medical knowledge that pushed the same priorities as they promoted good health and attempted to protect society from infec-tious diseases. As new perceptions about the body, innovative physical activ-ities, and recreational education spread among the working class, they took on an ethical dimension. Medical campaigns to combat alcoholism and TB, undertaken by voluntary organizations at the turn of the century, juxtaposed physical exercise that strengthened the body's immune system with the un-healthy habits of the coffee-house and alcohol. Gym classes were linked to physical health and stamina both in medical discourse and health books, and were expected to provide an antidote to the degeneration of young people.

However, the medical press noted that the complexity of the physical ex-ercises and the monotonous way in which they were performed made school-children averse to exercise. Discipline and walking in file, along with lack of spontaneity, even during walks in the countryside, took away the pleasure, while good cheer and joy "escaped" children's faces. "How is it possible to re-main cheerful, in the face of such physical activity?" a columnist in an edu-cational journal wondered at the beginning of the twentieth century, "joy is missing even from those walks in the country, and seeing schoolchildren in the countryside is unwittingly reminiscent of a funeral."[58] This combination of pleasure and physical exercise when running in the open air, climbing trees, or playing traditional games such as leap-frog, wrestling, running races, curl-ing, and prisoner's base were "frivolous fun" expected to satisfy the schoolchil-dren's natural instincts for play and give them an appetite for physical exercise,

---

55 Circular 2361 - Ypourgeio ton Ekklisiastikon kai tis Dimosias Ekpaidefseos, February 1898 "Peri Gymnasiakon ekdromon," in David Antoniou, Ta Programmata tis Mesis Ekpaidefsis (1833–1929) (Athens: IAEN, 1987), 378–82.

56 Vasiliko Diatagma, "Peri tis Didaskalias tis Gymnastikis" 939–40.

57 Vasiliko Diatagma, "Peri tis Didaskalias tis Gymnastikis" 940.

58 Vassilios Kontis, "Peri Gymnastikis Palin," Dimotiki Ekpaidefsis, no. 4 (October 1, 1902), 53–6.

without causing mental exhaustion. Outdoor games tempered the harmful effects of sedentary school life because they fulfilled a dual purpose: exercising the muscles and providing more air to the lungs. At the end of the nineteenth century, educators and doctors were considered the best authorities on the appropriate games for each gender, though a special committee chaired by the Minister of Education in 1900 identified the most suitable games for high school students, among them cricket and football, and a second committee recommended the most suitable locations for games in Athens.[59]

Doctors argued that the transition from games to gymnastics should take place gradually, depending on the pupil's physical development. Because of this, gym teachers had to have some knowledge of physiology to determine the physical condition and temperament of each pupil and the appropriate exercises, according to age, for each of them individually. Doctors were quick to criticize abuses in physical education, when for instance: smaller schoolchildren were subject to "labors much greater than their bodily capacity and age" during their preparation for sports competitions; when gym teachers tended to put weak and robust children or children of different ages together; when there were no recess to break up exercise; or when the nature of the exercises was too complex, involving a series of successive movements, while "only 6 to 8 movements at most are necessary for healthy exercise."[60] Thus, despite positive medical opinion on the founding of the School of Physical Education and the introduction of games and school sports competitions, difficulties arose in their implementation. Doctors felt that gym teachers' lack of knowledge on health issues and the absence of paediatricians during competitions were largely to blame.

Replacement of the complex German-Swiss physical education system with its Swedish counterpart in 1909 meant that these efforts had come full circle. Introduction of the Swedish system would enhance the health benefits of physical exercise in schools, as emphasis was placed on respiratory exercises and strengthening of the chest. The German-Swiss gym system was replaced by simpler exercises that aimed to strengthen respiratory capacity. The Swedish gym system was a better fit according to the medical community in the fight against TB among the young. As the size of the chest cavity became

---

59 Georgios Vlamos, *I Ygieini tou Skholeiou* (Athens: Sakellariou, Vivliothiki Marasli, 1904), 596–97.

60 Konstantinos Papayannis, "Peri tis Ygieinis ton Skholeion en Elladi," *Praktika Panelliniou Iatrikou Synedriou, 6–11 Maiou 1901* (Athens: Sakellariou, 1903), 148.

the prime indicator of sound physical health, doctors investigated methods of expanding it. The way in which schoolchildren breathed was considered to play an important role in this. The combination of physical exercises and singing was considered to be an appropriate way for schoolchildren to achieve correct breathing. In 1903, a Greek physician, Georgios Koromilas, proposed a "respiratory workout with chants," to be performed at regular intervals during the course of the day in order to expand the chest cavity, strengthen the lungs and cultivate patriotic sentiment. This method could contribute to preparing young TB-free men who could serve their country well.[61]

At the same time, the fact that the goals of gymnastics were clearly divided into educational and athletic ones reflected new attitudes towards physical activity in school, as was concluded in the report filed by the school competitions committee, in 1907, that proposed the adoption of the Swedish system.[62] On the one hand, gymnastics served a pedagogical goal, namely to prepare boys so as to become healthy, orderly and law-abiding citizens and girls to be healthy mothers; on the other hand, competitive sports and athletics were expected to instil mental virtues, happiness, and pleasure. Leisure time, thus, acquired a health dimension. The founding of sports and gymnastics clubs in the early twentieth century also illustrated a new attitude towards games as a source of pleasure. Furthermore, the development of sports in this period contributed to the spread of new attitudes towards the body that linked the cultivation of moral qualities with physical exercise.

3.2 The Construction of Hygienic School Buildings: Standards and Conditions

Not only physical education but also the construction of hygienic buildings was directly linked to the material and moral development of the nation. The problem of unsanitary school buildings, known of since the first decades of the Greek state, concerned both the medical and educational community and led to the introduction of health inspection in schools in the 1890s. In both educational and medical texts, the condition of school buildings was referred to as a "national issue" since, more than any other educa-

---

61 Georgios Koromilas, "Peri tis mi en Khrono kai Rythmo Fysikis Ekpaidefseos os Aitiou Prodiathetontos eis Nosous kai di eis Phthisin," *Dimotiki Ekpaidefsis*, no. 16 (February 15, 1903), 246.
62 Koulouri, *Athlitismos*, 72.

tional matter, the impact the building had on the health of schoolchildren was associated with the national defeat in 1897 and the vitality of the race.

The *National Education* journal became the platform for fierce attacks on the "miserable and literally brutal state of the primary school building,"[63] where children of a "tender" age withered away. It was estimated that 160,000 children spent approximately eight thousand hours during the years of compulsory school attendance suffering in decrepit, stifling and unhealthy schoolrooms that resembled prisons more than places of learning. Data demonstrating the lack of compliance with hygiene regulations were related mainly to the soil, the proximity of the school to sites of unhealthy activities (i.e., factories, slaughterhouses), the cramped spaces as well as inadequate lighting and poor ventilation. Together these issues rendered school attendance a major health risk. Konstantinos Papayannis stressed at the First Pan-Hellenic Medical Conference in 1901 that schools had been constructed on moist and contaminated soil close to drains and did not comply with any hygiene regulations.[64] The decrepit interior of the buildings and their insufficient equipment also bore witness to the indifference of the state. The lack roofing or flooring, the presence of water tanks, and the dampness that eroded the walls of the school, all put the physical safety of schoolchildren at risk and were often denounced in the press.[65] The crowding was overwhelming. For example, at around the turn of the century in Athens the space available in schoolrooms could not accommodate even one third of the pupils.[66] The school inspectors emphasized in their reports that "these classrooms cannot provide sufficient air for even half or, in many cases, a quarter of the poor schoolchildren to breathe," implying that the atmosphere was contaminated.

According to an official report, this outrageous situation was due to the fact that most schools—55% in 1888—were housed in rented buildings totally unsuitable for the purpose.[67] George Drosinis, the editor of *National Education*, reported that out of 1,800 primary schools in operation in 1898 approximately 1,000 were housed in rented buildings, while several oth-

---

63   Anonymos, "Ta Nea Kritia ton Dimotikon Skholeion," *Ethniki Agogi*, no. 2 (March 15, 1898): 17–9.
64   Papayannis, "Peri tis Ygieinis ton Skhoeion en Elladi," 155.
65   Georgios Drosinis, "Ta Skholeia tou Dimou Athinaion," *Ethniki Agogi*, no. 19 (January 1, 1903): 224.
66   Papayannis, "Peri tis Ygieinis ton Skhoeion en Elladi," 136.
67   Georgios Theotokis, *Ekpaideftika Nomoskhedia Ypovlithenta eis tin Voulin ton Ellinon ypo tou epi ton Ekklisiastikon kai tis Dimosias Ekpaidefseos Ypourgou 4 December 1889* (Athens: 1899), 65.

ers were set up in pig farms, barns, monastery cells and cemetery chapels.[68] Drosinis led a campaign for the improvement of conditions in schools. He highlighted the political dimensions of the issue in the *National Education*. Even though many of the rented buildings were completely unfit to be used as schools, their owners had secured multi-annual leases thanks to their political power and connections with the local government. It seems that this kind of relationship was mainly true for school buildings in large towns, particularly Athens. The image of ruined, dirty and miserable primary schools, like the "the damp Karamanou stable," sharply contrasted the neo-classical mansions housing the National Library, the University and the Academy. Fears were expressed in the press that state indifference would expose those in political power who had created this unequal situation and provoke the ridicule of foreign visitors.[69] To grasp the situation, we must take into account the fact that until the 1894 law was passed, authorities did not pay any attention to hygiene regulations in the construction of school buildings. Most nineteenth century schools were built through minimal means because the teaching methods in use, the Lancasterian system (1834–1880), placed no particular emphasis on building sanitation. The lack of sufficient resources and the contracting of construction and maintenance of school buildings to local municipalities resulted in the simple, small school premises, similar to village houses, without any particular regard to hygiene standards.[70] Indifference to the location, soil, natural light and ventilation of the schools can partly be attributed to the fact that the choice of the construction plot or rented building was in the hands of the County Prefect, the local police or magistrate— i.e., people ignorant of hygiene regulations.

In the 1880s, Trikoupis's reforms reflected a change in intentions. In 1880, the institutionalization of the co-teaching method brought about changes in the spatial organization of schools.[71] Each class now only comprised schoolchildren of similar age. As such, the issue of securing adequate material conditions for children's bodies was more than critical. *Moraitis's Guide*, which laid the foundations of the co-teaching method in Greece, was

---

68 Theotokis, *Ekpaideftika Nomoschedia*, 19.
69 Drosinis, "Ta Skholeia tou Dimou Athinaion," 223.
70 Kalafati, *Ta Skholika Ktiria tis Protovathmias Ekpaidefsis*, 141.
71 Spyridon Moraitis, *Didaskaliki i Syntomoi Odigiai peri tis Khriseos tis Neas Methodou* (Athens: 1880), 9.

the first to include clear regulations on the hygiene of school premises in 1889. The influence of Prussian regulations on school construction was evident in *Moraitis's guide* regarding the choice of the school's location to ensure ample sunlight and ventilation, emphasis on the classroom's capacity, and the dimensions of the windows; all in order to ensure the necessary amount of air and light per child.[72] The dimensions of the desks were estimated according to the age of the pupils, even though these were based on anthropometric measurements in other countries.

In the same decade, the issue of schoolrooms began to attract criticism from educators, politicians, and doctors. Building up hygienic school premises will be a recurrent issue that educational reforms will attempt to address at the end of the nineteenth century but to no avail. The preamble to a law, submitted to the Parliament in 1889 under minister of Education George Theotokis, stated that school buildings operated in annexed cow sheds, sheep folds and stables.[73] The first references to school buildings date back to hygiene manuals published in 1880.[74] During the same period, Greek educators and doctors visited international hygiene exhibitions that demonstrated the progress achieved in the field of school hygiene.

The new law on construction of school buildings marked a breakthrough in school hygiene policy. The decree passed on May 17, 1894, "concerning the way schools are constructed," laid down for the first time in a coherent way the technical details and guidelines on sanitation standards. These details had been recommended by Dimitrios Kallias, an engineer who had studied at the University of Ghent in Belgium. According to Lambadarios, Ghent had had a model system of medical inspection of schools since 1874. Kallias proposed the French model of constructing and equipping school buildings. The bill was a translation of the corresponding French regulation of 1880. It followed the same structure, while the accompanying plans were copies of the corresponding French ones.[75] The new law strengthened centralized control over the planning of buildings, whereby the plans and bud-

---

72 Moraitis, *Didaskaliki*, 3–5 and Kalafati, *Ta Skholika Ktiria tis Protovathmias Ekpaidefsis*, 154–7.

73 *Ekpaideftika Nomoskhedia ypovlithenta eis tin Voulin ton Ellinon ypo tou epi ton Ekklisiastikon kai tis Dimosias Ekpaidefseos Ypourgou 4 Dekemvriou 1899* (Athens: Typografeio, 1899).

74 Georgios Vafas, *Ai Athinai apo Iatrikin Apopsin: I Polis*, vol. 1 (Athens, 1878), 149 and Nikolaos Saliveros, *Ygieini ton Oikodomon, itoi Anegersis, Exygiansis kai Syntirisis ton te Idiotikon kai Dimosion Ktirion* (Athens: 1893).

75 Kalafati, *Ta Skholika Ktiria tis Protovathmias Ekpaidefsis*, 167.

get for every future school building were submitted to the Ministry of the Interior and approved by the Board of Public Works.

The provisions of the 1894 decree took into account the desiderata of school architecture, as they had been developed under the influence of hygienic discourse at the end of the nineteenth century. Following the French model, the principle of central location was adopted in order to ensure good ventilation, adequate natural sunlight and a suitable distance from unhealthy, dangerous or noisy activities.[76] As far as surface area was concerned, a minimum of 10 square meters was allotted to each pupil, while the capacity of each classroom was estimated on the basis of 0.90–1.25 square meters per pupil. This was the first time the volume of air allocated to each child in the classroom had been calculated; five cubic meters of air per schoolchild was comparable with international capacity standards as such measures apparently ensured the volume of air necessary to meet individual respiratory needs.[77] The dimensions of the schoolyard were also defined according to the number of pupils while construction of a covered pavilion reflected the importance attached to physical activity. Particular reference was made to lighting and ventilation of the schoolrooms: the location of the school, the height of the rooms and dimensions of the windows served to provide lighting from the left or lighting from both sides and create the necessary draught of air.

This regulatory model established a common typology for schools in both urban and rural areas. However, it reflected more the intentions of the legislator rather than the realities of the school buildings at the end of the nineteenth century. Very few municipalities conformed to the decree or proceeded to construct healthful school buildings over the next few years. The implementation of the decree was met with difficulties such as fundraising and the lack of an administrative structure, thus revealing the need for supervision of the construction process by a specialized architectural service in the Ministry of Education. Knowledge of technical construction in the design of school building, along with the medical inspection of school-age children made the expertise of both architectural engineers and school doctors a necessary component of a modern educational system. Two laws

---

76 Phocion Barbatis, *De l'inspection médicale des écoles* (Paris: Vigot Frères, 1916), 26–27 and Guillaume, "L'Hygiène à l'école," 225.

77 This regulation was derived from the corresponding French law as of 1880. See Kalafati, *Ta Skholika Ktiria tis Protovathmias Ekpaidefsis,* 169.

passed in 1895 ("on primary education" and "on school fees") laid down the details related to the expropriation of land and the construction of school buildings. Construction would be funded by a specific account of the Ministry of Education.[78] A new committee for the examination and the approval of the design of school buildings was struck in the Ministry of Education to take responsibility for compiling plans of schoolrooms in compliance with the provisions of the 1894 decree by promoting the legal provisions on hygiene and sanitation of school buildings.

For the first time in Greece, educators, architects and doctors collaborated to develop a uniform type of school building, providing for four types of classrooms—single, double, four and six class respectively—according to local educational needs. The first Pan-Hellenic Medical Conference in 1901 approved the classroom types elaborated by the committee in 1898 as these were found to fulfil hygienic standards. In 1898 the decree on equipping classrooms with double desks was also passed. This decree defined the dimensions and construction of desks, suitable for Greek schoolchildren in accordance with measurements made by school inspectors.[79] The appointment of Konstantinos Savvas, who offered his services free of charge as school doctor in Attika, indicated significant advances in health supervision in schools.

The legislation of 1894 and complementary laws related to the means of securing school fees marked the dawn of a new era in education policy. Between 1898 and 1911, 407 new school buildings were constructed along neoclassical lines in compliance with health and hygiene standards, mostly in the provinces. However, new buildings accounted for just 11.5% of all schools in Greece, while the majority of pupils continued to be housed in unhealthy buildings. For instance, in the municipality of Athens, in 1912, only 5 out of a total of 33 school buildings were hygienic.[80] According to the reports of school doctors, most of the primary schools in the capital were still housed in rented buildings in the decades to come, with small rooms lacking in light and ventilation, damp, with unhygienic lavatories, small and dirty yards without sufficient space for the schoolchildren to do gymnastics or breathe fresh air.

---

78 In 1888 the Fund of Primary Education was established, financially supported by municipalities and the state while in 1892 expenditure on primary education was entered in the state budget.

79 Emmanouil Lambadarios, *Skholiki Ygieini meta Stoikheion Paidologias* (Athens: 1934), 19.

80 Anonymos, "Entyposeis apo ta Skholeia tou Dimou Athinaion," *Deltio tou Ekpaideftikou Omilou*, vol. 2 (Athens: 1912), 176–201.

CHAPTER III

THE SCHOOL HYGIENE SERVICE
AND THE SPREAD OF HYGIENE

1. The Establishment of the School Hygiene Service

The School Hygiene Service and the Architectural Department at the Ministry of Education, founded by the royal decree September of 1908 under Minister Spyridon Stais, were institutional breakthroughs in the health inspection of school buildings and students.[1] The decree was issued two months before the tabling of education bills which would introduce changes on a series of issues, such as female education, the organization of the central service of the Ministry of Education, and the implementation of the Kallias Decree.[2] The 1908 decree complemented the earlier legislation of 1894 concerning the construction of healthy schoolrooms since, as the medical community had declared, the lack of a School Hygiene Service posed an obstacle to the implementation of legislation regarding the choice of site, the renting of healthy schoolrooms as well as compliance with health and hygienic rules in the construction and maintenance of school buildings. In addition, key issues related to the health of schoolchildren remained unresolved, due to the lack of specialized personnel: Teachers, for example, were unable to apply anti-epidemic measures, i.e., to identify the initial carriers of the infection or to decontaminate the school building. The only thing that could be done following an outbreak was to close the schools. Overuse of this mea-

---

1 Vasiliko Diatagma "Peri Systaseos en to Ypourgeio ton Ekklisiastikon kai tis Dimotikis Ekpaidefseos, Grafeiou tis Skholikis Ygieinis," *Efimeris tis Kiverniseos* A', no.239 (September 17, 1908): 1053.

2 "Ta Ekpaideftika Nomoskhedia," *Empros*, November 25, 1908, 1–4 and David Antoniou, *Diadromes kai Staseis sti Neoelliniki Ekpaidefsi 190s-200s Aionas* (Athens: Metaikhmio, 2008), especially the chapter entitled "To ekpaideftiko ergo tou Spyridonos Emm. Stai," 689–711.

sure led to prolonged interruption of schooling in some areas. The institutionalization of medical inspection in schools in many European countries in the 1910s and, in particular, the progress made by neighboring Balkan states regarded as national competitors to Greece at the time, such as Bulgaria and Serbia, contributed to public debate that tended to imbue the issue with a nationalist tone.[3]

The goals of the School Hygiene Service encompassed the key issues targeted in the criticism put forth by doctors and educators during the last decade. According to 1908 decree, the new service was to undertake the inspection of the premises, equipment and utensils of both private and public schools. It was also charged with the protection of schoolchildren from contagious and infectious diseases, the monitoring of their mental and physical development and the dissemination of basic health and hygiene knowledge. In brief, these were the essential lines along which school health services would develop in Greece, from 1910 until around 1940. However, the systematic organization of the Architectural Department and School Hygiene Service came about only two years later, when the qualifications required for their personnel were laid down in detail.

The School Hygiene Service was subject to the General Inspector for Primary Education. The post was held by Georgios Drosinis, a renowned poet who likely exercised some influence over the ministerial decision to found the Service in the first place. Drosinis, in a series of articles published in the *National Education* journal,[4] often criticized the deficiencies of the school health and hygiene system, attributing the defeat of Greece in 1897 to the indifference of the state towards addressing these deficiencies. He further supported that national priority should be given to the physical development of the young generation. He himself had also inspired the operation and equipping of the Sevastopoulio Labor School in Athens that did comply with the health and hygiene standards of European school buildings.

---

3   Comparison with other Balkan countries continued even when school doctors were appointed in Greece. The comparison was both quantitative and qualitative. According to the school doctor of the first educational district, Ioannis Fassanelis, while in Bulgaria there were 400 school doctors and in Serbia 200, in Greece there were only 12. Ioannis Fassanelis, *Ta Pepragmena kata to Skholikon Etos 1914–1915* (Athens: 1915), 4.

4   For the collaboration of Drosinis and Stais in the Ministry of Education during this period, see Georgios Drosinis, *Skorpia Fylla tis Zois mou*, vol. 2 (Athens: Syllogos pros Diadosin ton Ofelimon Vivlion, 1982).

Drosinis sought to equip the newly-established School Hygiene Service with instruments that were "pioneering in the service of the Ministry," as he himself noted, to measure, weigh and monitor the health of schoolchildren. But, despite this optimistic start, no progress was made in improving schoolchildren's health for a two-year period. Perhaps this was due to the political unrest during 1909, which signified a political crisis. Thus, the decree on the organization of the School Hygiene Service and the Architectural Office remained a dead letter until 1911. In March 1910, under Minister Andreas Panayotopoulos, the government passed legislation on a series of pending educational measures: Law no. 3721, "on organization of the central headquarters of the Ministry of Education," stipulated the establishment of the School Hygiene Service.[5] The law provided for the post of a school doctor to be appointed through open competition,[6] "preferably a Doctor of Medicine specializing in School Hygiene and Paedology."[7]

However, once again the relevant provisions remained inactive and it was not until the first government under Venizelos had come to power that the service began operation. In the parliamentary discussion of 1911, when the first Liberal government submitted bills to reform school building policies, known as the Alexandris Bills[8] the Minister of Education, Apostolos Alexandris, outlined once again the bleak state of the health of schoolchildren and the deficiencies in school buildings and furnishings. He cited the need for the construction of 2,300 buildings and 3,000 desks, as 3,000 pupils "are obliged to remain standing or sit on the floor."[9] The details of the Service's launch were ultimately laid down by the Royal Decree of October 5th, 1911. This legislation complemented the school hygiene goals set in 1908. A paedology laboratory was established, equipped with the instruments required to carry out the observation and research of schoolchildren at all

5   Law no. 3721 "Peri Organoseos tis Kentrikis Ypiresias tou Ypourgeiou ton Ekklisiastikon kai tis Dimosias Ekpaidefseos," *Efimeris tis Kiverniseos*, A', no. 178 (May 24, 1910): 1029–32.

6   Emmanouil Lambadarios, *Kodix Skholikis Ygieinis* (Athens: 1922), 25.

7   Law no. 3721, "Peri Organoseos tis Kentrikis Ypiresias tou Ypourgeiou ton Ekklisiastikon kai tis Dimosias Ekpaidefseos," 1030.

8   Law no. 3827 "Peri Didaktirion en Genei kai tis Organoseos tis Skhetikis Ypiresias" *Efimeris tis Kiverniseos*, A', no.191 (July 18, 1911): 893–96. The new law "on school buildings and the organization of the relevant service" provided for the adoption of different types of school buildings according to location. For the work of Alexandris, see Antoniou, *Diadromes kai Staseis*, 714–34.

9   *Efimeris ton Syzitiseon tis Voulis*, B' Anatheoritiki Vouli, vol. 2 (1911), 1051–52.

levels of education.[10] Its aim was to provide therapeutic advice to teachers, monitor the vaccination of pupils and inspect the health and hygienic conditions of school camps, an innovation introduced for the first time in Greece.

At the beginning of the twentieth century, only a few countries had established paedological institutes and these countries had taken the lead in setting up Schools of Hygiene and already had a history in the field of experimental pedagogy, such as the United States, Belgium and Germany. 42 large paedological laboratories were in operation in the United States at the beginning of the century. In Germany, well-known paedologists such as H. Griesbach, E. Kräpelin, August Mayer, and others, headed up psycho-pedagogical institutes in Leipzig, Berlin and Munich, while in Belgium the paedological institutes in Brussels, Antwerp and Ghent were directed by well-known pedagogues and psychologists, such as Jean-Ovide Decroly, J. Joteyko and J. Van Biervliet. Belgian paedologists played an important role in the international reception of this new interdisciplinary field.[11] It is worth noting that the International Society of Paedology was established in 1909 in Brussels by Alfred Binet and Jules-Jean Biervliet, and the first International Paedology Conference also took place in Brussels in 1911. The founding of a paedological institute alongside the organization of the School Hygiene Service may reflect the intention of the newly-elected liberal government to introduce innovative institutions in the field of school hygiene.

2. EMMANOUIL LAMBADARIOS: A PIONEER IN SCHOOL HYGIENE

The most important provision of the new law was related with the appointment of a school doctor as head of the School Hygiene Service. This post was taken up by Emmanouil Lambadarios (1885–1943) in November 1911, following a competition conducted by the Medical Council. Lambadarios was a young hygienist who would become the uncontestable founder and guiding spirit in the science of school hygiene in Greece. Emmanouil, son of the assistant professor of Medicine Nikolas Lambadarios, had studied medicine

---

10 See the third article of the Vasiliko Diatagma "Peri tis ypo tou Grafeiou tis Skholikis Ygieinis Askoumenis Epopteias dia tou par'afto Skhokikou Iatrou epi tis Skholikis Ygieinis tou Kratous,"*Efimeris tis Kiverniseos*, A', no. 279 (October 5, 1911) : 1449–50.

11 Marc Depaepe, *Zum Wohl des Kindes?: Pädologie, pädagogische Psychologie und experimentelle Pädagogik in Europa und den USA, 1890–1940* (Weinheim: Deutscher Studien Verlag; Leuven: University Press, 1993).

in Athens and Bern. He specialized in pediatrics and apparently was the first to introduce the term "paedology" into Greek. During his return to Greece from 1909 until 1911, he worked as assistant to K. Savvas, the main rapporteur on school hygiene in Greece, President of the Royal Medical Council and the first Professor at the Seat of Hygiene.[12] This apprenticeship with Savvas must have helped prepare him for his tenure in the field of hygiene.

Having laid the foundations for the operation of the School Hygiene Service, Lambadarios can justly be considered the father of the science of school hygiene in Greece. He strove to raise funds and worked for the passing of bills that contributed to improving the health of students. He remained head of the Service and later director of the School Hygiene Service until 1936, when he became Professor of School Hygiene and Paedology at the University of Athens. Nevertheless, he continued to take part in and direct all relevant projects, at least until 1940, shortly before his death. His prolific scientific work also contributed to the establishment of paedology in Greece. He taught paedology and school hygiene at the Secondary Teacher Training College and to undergraduates at the University of Athens trained to become school doctors. He was director of the Social Hygiene Center in the interwar, organized by the American Red Cross, which operated in Athens during the 1920s. It was in this center that the BCG vaccine against tuberculosis was applied to patients. Lambadarios worked for the dissemination of hygiene principles throughout Greece as a member of the Supreme Healthcare Council of the Ministry of Health, vice-president of the Greek Junior Red Cross, and advisor to the Greek Red Cross.

In his capacity as the government's delegate and as a member of many international scientific associations, he participated in many congresses and exhibitions held in Europe. He presented the work of School Hygiene Service in some of them to show the progress Greece had achieved. The Association Internationale pour la Protection de l'Enfance had organized the most important congresses in Liège in 1930, in Brussels in 1935 and in Paris in 1937. He was interested in the open-air school movement and therefore took part in the Conférence internationale des colonies de vacances et œuvres de plein air in Geneva in 1931.

---

12 For Lambadarios's bio, see Emmanouil Lambadarios, *Megali Elliniki Egkyklopaideia*, vol. 15 (Athens, 1926), 747.

Since the mid-1930s, he must have been in contact with American scientific associations such as the American Child Health Association and the Health Section of the World Federation of Education Associations (WFEA); he was Greece's representative in the latter. The WFEA aimed at the promotion of the health of students, adolescents, and teachers across the world; the collection of comparative data; the introduction of common school hygiene regulations; and the forging of strong bonds with state delegates from various countries to promote progress in school hygiene. Drawing on his correspondence, we infer that his papers must have been presented in congresses that took place in Tokyo in 1937 and in Rio de Janeiro in 1939. Lambadarios was familiar with popular hygiene leaflets that had been widely circulated in America probably through the work of the WEFA.

In the 1920s and 1930s, he published papers in international scientific journals such as *Médécine Scolaire, Pensée médicale, Bulletin de l'A.I.P.E, Revue Internationale de l'Enfant, Annales de l'Institut Pasteur, Revue Internationale de l'enfant, Journal of the International Committee on Open Air Education, Vers la Santé, Revue de l'Institut Internationale pour le Cinema educative* (Istituto Internationale per la Cinematografia Educativa). Most of his papers looked at the organization of school hygiene in Greece, open-air institutions and child TB.

As a member of various international networks Lambadarios was in contact with important medical authorities who played a significant role in the development of theories and international schemata of hygiene, i.e., Albert Calmette, whose method was applied by Lambadarios,[13] René Sand, general secretary of the Ligue des Sociétés de Croix Rouge, Dr. L.de Feo of the Istituto Internationale per la Cinematografia Educativa and G. Barnu, editor of the journal *Revista de Igiena Sociala* in Bucharest.

Through Lambadarios's voluntary work, speeches and special publications, he contributed a great deal educating the public on hygienic practices. His prolific writing ranged from studies on scoliosis, infectious diseases, school camps, and open-air schools, to general approaches of social hygiene. His books, *School Hygiene* and *Paedology and School Hygiene*, reprinted several times between 1916 and 1934, were the standard reference

---

13 He was the first doctor to give the BCG vaccine to new-borns in Greece at a time when this practice was received with suspicion by the international medical community.

on issues of school hygiene for educators and school doctors in Greece during the interwar. His participation in international conferences and scientific associations, as well as his collaboration with major journals of hygiene and paedology, reveal the breadth of his intellectual concerns and his devotion to keeping up-to-date on scientific issues.

Convinced of the importance of school hygiene to the health of the population overall, Lambadarios secured the collaboration of charitable associations and international organizations in order to overcome the hurdles posed by the meager finances of the Ministry of Education. In collaboration with voluntary societies, such as the Patriotic League of Greek Women, the Society for the prevention of TB, the Greek Junior Red Cross, and the Social Hygiene Center in Athens, he endeavored to create the necessary infrastructure to combat major childhood diseases, in particular TB and trachoma. His numerous publications and his wider activities illustrate his interest in combating these diseases. Bills for the establishment of school camps, open-air schools and student soup kitchens, the introduction of hygiene as a school subject to schools, and the bill establishing the Ministry of Health and Welfare in 1921, all bear his signature. Although most of his plans for the inspection of children's hygiene materialized when the liberals were in office, Lambadarios collaborated with governments from across the political spectrum during his long service as an expert on hygiene.

Apart from organizing the health inspection of schools and students, Lambadarios took initiatives to establish institutions for wider social intervention, aimed at enhancing the health of homeless and sickly schoolchildren: Children's polyclinics, student soup kitchens, school bathrooms, school camps, special popular publications, together constituted a huge contribution to the mobilization of public awareness. The institutionalization of school camps and school meals testified to his ongoing dedication to helping sick children.

3. School Medical Inspection before 1920

The appointment of Lambadarios as head of the School Hygiene Service at the Ministry of Education in November 1911, marked the beginning of state enforcement of school hygiene in Greece. The head of the School Hygiene Service exercised overall supervision of school hygiene. This was an ambitious project that included a wide range of services: inspecting school buildings, monitoring the physical and mental development of schoolchildren, informing teachers of hygiene issues and vaccinations, and the hygienic inspection of summer camps. In time, the publication of hygiene guides and the establishment of a paedological laboratory were added to the responsibilities of the Service.[14]

Nevertheless, in the first years of its operation, the work of the Service was limited, as it totally relied on its head. The law providing for the appointment of school doctors had not been passed until 1914. It was only in 1918 that the School Hygiene Service was established as an independent department. Thus, due to the lack of staff between 1911 and 1914 the Service gave priority to the inspection and improvement of hygiene regulations concerning the construction of school buildings, and to combatting the spread of contagious and infectious diseases among school children.

3.1 Hygienic Buildings and Furnishings: a Matter of Urgency

In 1911, the School Hygiene Service and the newly-established Architectural Service of the Ministry of Education designed two series of model buildings for four types of schools and made proposals for the improvement of the sanitary conditions in older buildings. Thereafter, doctors and architects would determine the details of school construction, the alterations and leasing of school buildings and would choose school furnishings. However, most of the plans elaborated at that time did not differ significantly from those of 1898. In addition, despite the freedom conferred by Law no. 3827/1911 on the adoption of different types of school buildings according to location, the two sets of plans that had been elaborated would in fact constitute, with certain variations, the standard models for the construction of school buildings until 1920, as they reflected the generally accepted rules of hygiene and pedagogy. In the new plans, the influence of the hygiene perceptions formulated by the School Hygiene Service was most evident on issues of lighting and space.

The layout of the schoolrooms along the façade, to ensure even distribution of natural light from the south or southeast, was one of the elements

---

14 Vasiliko Diatagma, "Peri ekteleseos ton Nomon 3721, 412" and no. 238 "Peri Organoseos tis Kentrikis Ypiresias tou Ypourgeiou ton Ekklisiastikon etc.," *Efimeris tis Kiverniseos*, A', no. 398 (October 27, 1915): 3197.

that Lambadarios insisted on. Countries such as Greece, without artificial heating in schools, favor south-facing spaces because of the solar heating benefits. The same care was taken in determining the position of the corridor as well as the size and position of the windows.[15]

Law no. 2442/1920 on "the establishment of educational welfare funds for the construction of school buildings across the state and supply of school furniture and teaching instruments," transferred the financial burden of constructing schools from the state to local authorities and the educational welfare funds.[16] The poor state of the school buildings in territory annexed to Greece after 1913 due to the Balkan wars seems to have led to this financial decentralization. According to the new law, an Educational Welfare Fund (EWF) was to be established in every municipality and village, administered by a five or seven member committee. The funding would be raised through local taxes, state grants, funds from church committees, municipalities and village councils, bequests and donations. Although the commitment of funds by municipalities and local councils accelerated the pace of construction, the financial difficulties faced by the village councils, the educational welfare funds and the Ministry of Education did not permit the ambitious project to be completed. According to data from the School Hygiene Service, in the eight years since its inception, 54 new school buildings approved before 1911 were constructed and 52 were completed. Another 976 were completed from 1920 to 1928.[17] Although progress was evident, Greece's need for school buildings was not sufficiently met.

Despite the repeated protests of the School Hygiene Service, before 1928 less than half of all pupils were accommodated in school buildings considered to be sanitary. In a series of reports submitted in 1919 by school doctors in the 12 educational districts, the majority of school buildings were deemed unhealthy. The school doctor in the first educational district, Ioannis Fassanelis, reported 48 primary school buildings to be healthy, 67 moderately healthy and 77 unhealthy.[18] The extremely crowded classrooms fea-

---

15 Lambadarios, *Skholiki Ygieini meta Stoicheion Paidologiaς*, 34–5.
16 *Deltion Ypourgeiou Ekklisiastikon kai Dimosias* no. 23 (January-February 1921): 141–55 and Lambadarios, *Kodix Skholikis Ygieinis*, 184–93.
17 Lambadarios, *Skholiki Ygieini meta Stoicheion Paidologiaς*, 107.
18 Anonymos, "Pinax tis Ygieinis Katastaseos ton Didaktirion tou Kratous kata tas ypo ton Skholikon Iatron Ypovlithisas Ekthesis Mekhri Telos Iouniou 1916," *Deltion tou Ypourgeiou Ekklisastikon kai tis Dimosias Ekpaidefseos*, no. 3 (March 1919): 12–3.

tured in the reports submitted to the School Hygiene Service from 1915 onwards, testified to the lack of schoolrooms. This lack was attributed by Lambadarios to the financial difficulties that begun in the Balkan Wars.

Political and national upheavals also had an impact on the condition of the school buildings. In 1919, following the occupation of eastern Macedonia by the Bulgarians, major problems were noted in the schools. The problems were bound to continue and hinder the normal operation of schools, as the state prioritized housing and feeding the repatriated students from Bulgaria. In order to meet basic needs, government officials suggested the requisition of premises and temporary housing of students in churches. The destruction of the educational services' records and furniture at this time paints a dire picture of the difficulties faced in reorganizing schools.[19]

Part of the problem was the fact that many schools were housed in rented premises. In 1911, 45% of primary schools were in rented locations. In directives to the county prefects and school heads, the School Hygiene Service defined the hygiene standards to be fulfilled by rented premises, as well as the obligations of the owners as far as cleanliness and building materials were concerned. The directives also placed emphasis on the supply of clean, healthy water, the provision of taps—3 per 100 students—and the means of tap construction, so that "the child's lips would not come into contact" with the tap.[20] Following the American model, construction of jet-fountain water taps were considered the most suitable means for protecting children from infection. Detailed instructions for cleaning lavatories and floors were also included in the directives. The floors had to be made of wood, concrete, or be covered with linoleum but with a smooth surface "without cracks or holes" to prevent penetration by dust or urine.

In 1911, new double-desks were manufactured in eight sizes depending on the stature of students in accordance with guidelines provided by the School Hygiene Service. For the first time, the placement of students at the desks depended on the measurement of their height by teachers. "Healthy" desks were first introduced in Greece at the end of the nineteenth century by the primary school inspector, Theodoros Mikhalopoulos, who, with the

---

19 "Apospasma Ektheseos tou Genikou Epitheoritou Georgiou Khatzikyriakou peri Katastaseos ton Skholeion tis Anatolikis Makedonias," *Deltion tou Ypourgeiou ton Ekklisiastikon kai tis Dimosias Ekpaidefseos*, no. 1 (January 1919): 17.

20 For the connection between taps and the spread of contagious diseases, especially of TB, see Lambadarios, *Skholiki Ygieini meta Stoicheion Paidologias*, 29.

assistance of an engineer from the local municipality, manufactured an improvised double-desk. However, the results of this initiative are not widely known. The "Greek" desk, proposed by the School Hygiene Service in 1911, used the "internationally reputed 'Retting-Müller' desk as a model.[21] No part of this type of German double-desk, which was widely used in Europe, particularly in Belgium, was movable, so that students were not "tempted" to play about. It differed from other types of desks in that it had a special faucet at the bottom, to facilitate cleaning the schoolroom floor. The School Hygiene Service gave instructions on the arrangement of desks in the classroom, so that the distance between desks necessary for proper ventilation was observed, to ensure the minimum of 0.90 square meters per child and to provide natural lighting on the left of the students. In 1920, the Architecture Department of the Ministry of Education designed three types of desk, depending on the individual student's height, and issued a manual demonstrating the appropriate type of desk according to the size of the room. The particular timber to be used and the means of manufacturing were specified in a form sent to schools. The color of the desks had to be "the deep green of the olive leaf."

Although, according to reports of the School Hygiene Service, 10,000 desks were manufactured between 1911 and 1920, it is doubtful whether the needs of schools in equipment were indeed satisfactorily met. During the 1920s, multi-seat desks were still in use and quite a few students must have needed to stand. The first reports compiled by school doctors in 1914–15, emphasized these deficiencies, especially the lack of double desks for younger students. One school doctor, Ioannis Fassanelis, reported in 1915 that in the First Educational District (Athens, Piraeus and the nearby islands, and Cyclades) he had found a large number of pupils still seated on the floor.[22] It seems that the situation did not improve over time. On the contrary, the population movement due to war aggravated the problem. According to a report by the same school health inspector for the first three months of 1921–1922, in the same area, out of a total of 22,000 students approximately 5,000 were on their feet in the classroom. In some schools students sat on chairs, stools or on the floor without any desks at all. "For example, in

---

21 Lambadarios, *Skholiki Ygieini meta Stoicheion Paidologias*, 100–3.
22 Fassanelis, *Ta Pepragmena kata to Skholikon Etos 1914–1915*, 8.

Kallithea boys' school, many were seated on a few seats of an adjoining theatre, most of them on the floor, etc."[23]

3.2 Health and Hygiene Education in School:
Combatting Contagious Diseases

The protection of students against major infectious diseases was the second group of health care measures in schools at that time. During the first
phase, over the four-year period 1911–1915, protection from the most threatening diseases was implemented with directives by the head of the School
Hygiene Service to the teaching staff. Information circulars are an interesting source on the way the service operated, while they simultaneously
provide a picture of the main health problems the school population faced.
During the first period of the operation of the School Hygiene Service, staff
shortage resulted in assigning the medical inspection of pupils to the teachers. Thus, these directives opened new lines of communication between the
school doctor and teachers.

3.2.1 The First Directives (1911–1915):
Decontamination and Precautions

A few months after Lambadarios's appointment, the Minister of Education
issued a general circular on January 12, 1912 addressed to teachers. It laid
down regulations for health checks conducted on schoolchildren. Teachers
were informed of current advances in medicine concerning the prevention
of infectious diseases and the precautions necessary to protect the health of
both schoolchildren and their families. Apart from compliance of schools
with hygiene regulations—ensuring ventilation of schoolrooms and cleanliness in all areas—the teachers also became responsible for checking
whether student absenteeism was due to an infectious or contagious disease. Identification of the primary carrier of infection was considered crucial in the fight against childhood diseases. Students thought to be suffering
from infectious diseases were expelled by the teacher in order to protect the

---

23   "Pinax Synoptikos Ektheseos a´ Triminias ypo tou Ygeionomikou Epitheoritou ton Skholeion tis A´ Ek-
     paideftikis Periphereias I. Fassaneli," Januuary 22, 1922, unclassified archive of Emmanouil Lambadar-
     ios, Hellenic Literary and Historical Archive (ELIA).

rest of the class. Moreover, pupils absent for more than four days were not permitted to return to class unless they provided a certificate of good health issued by a doctor.

Special measures were taken in cases of diphtheria, scarlet fever, small-pox, typhoid and meningitis, which were considered to be the most severe infectious diseases claiming many victims among the school population. In the case of contagious diseases, a specific time period had to be met before a pupil was readmitted to school, and a specific decontamination process had to be carried out. Thus, students could return to school after a period of forty days, "but only following systematic decontamination of their home, clothing, and books, etc. and thorough bodily cleansing with soap. Infected books and objects of minor value, such as toys, notebooks and other items, should preferably be burnt."[24] During sickness students as well as teachers and caretakers who either lived or communicated with the patient were suspended from school. Teachers also had to decontaminate the school building. Should there be repeated outbreaks of the afore-mentioned illnesses, the school had to remain closed for a short period of time, in order to be properly decontaminated. Detailed instructions were also given for other less severe childhood diseases. In such cases, it was the task of the teacher to check the personal hygiene of the student upon his/her return to school. Teachers were also obliged to check if the students had been "recently vacci-nated" and remove those who had not.

In an attempt to modernize the fight against contagious diseases in schools, efforts were made to replace the practice of suspending classes with the identification of the prime carrier. In case there was an outbreak of an infectious disease, teachers were obliged to notify the School Hygiene Service, which stands as an example of the close cooperation between teach-ers and the responsible doctor. Furthermore, the instructions given in the circular illustrated how to plan the service and set the standards to be ap-plied. At the beginning of the twentieth century, the international medical community was concerned with the planning of such services, including for instance the presentation by the student of a medical certificate following

---

24 Circular no. 2101 Ypourgeion ton Ekklisiastikon kai tis Dimosias Ekpaidefseos, Grafeion Skholikis Ygieinis, "Peri Profylaxeos ton eis ta Skholeia Foitonton apo ton Oxeon Loimodon Noson," January 31, 1912, in the unclassified archive of Emmanouil Lambadarios, *Elliniko Logotekhniko kai Istoriko Archeio* (Hellenic Literary and Historical Archive), ELIA.

the curing of an infectious disease, compliance with the minimum recovery period and cooperation between the patient's family and the teacher. Having collated information on time and location of the first occurrences, the head of the School Hygiene Service was able to identify the sites of infection and stem the tide by removing the prime suspects. As was the case with other school hygiene issues, the Greek Medical Service aligned itself with the French model, which stressed the establishment of a network of communication between the family, doctor and school.[25]

The circulars issued between 1911 and 1914 on the means of combatting infectious diseases point to the importance the head of the School Hygiene Service attached to the school in spreading diseases. For example, the emphasis he laid on trachoma, TB, smallpox, scarlet fever and diphtheria must be linked to the high incidence of these diseases among the school population. After 1915, the fight against TB and trachoma became the subject of independent campaigns. From the first years of its operation, the School Hygiene Service assigned the task of disease prevention to teachers. Detailed instructions for the recognition of symptoms, nature of germs, means of transmission, potential risks, and means of treatment were passed out in illustrated leaflets that popularized medical knowledge, testifying the importance the head of the School Hygiene Service attributed to the teachers and doctors' collaboration.

Apart from the publication of the circulars individually, Lambadarios also published the book *Instructions to Protect Schoolchildren Against Infectious Diseases* (Odigiai pros Profylaxin ton eis ta Skholeia Foitonton apo ton Loimodon Noson meta ton Skhetikon Egkyklion) through the Ministry of Education in two different editions in 1913 and 1920 respectively. This material provided concise information about the nature of the diseases and preventative measures against them, as well as personal hygiene regulations that teachers should impose. The 1913 edition also included information on protection against the plague and cholera, epidemics that had hit Greek regions during the Balkan Wars. Instructions were given on the vaccination of students and the means of decontaminating the buildings. The latter should be undertaken "as soon as any case of diphtheria, scar-

---

25   Dr. Stackler, "Project du règlement sur la prophylaxie scolaire des maladies transmissibles," *L'Hygiène scolaire* no. 1 (January 10, 1912): 4.

let fever, epidemic meningitis, typhoid fever or smallpox occurs among the school population."[26]

In the early twentieth century, the decontamination of spaces and objects was considered essential to undercutting the spread of infectious diseases. In Athens, following the establishment of the Public Decontaminating Service (Dimosion Apolymantirion) in 1905, the houses of the sick were disinfected at the request of the patient's relatives, either by employees of the Public Decontaminating Service or by voluntary members of sanitation associations, such as the Union of Greek Women, the Patriotic League of Greek Women and the Hygiene Society. Fear of infectious diseases spreading through schools led the School Hygiene Service to collaborate with teachers, instructing them on how to prepare solutions and decontaminate furniture, walls and floors. The school was disinfected using either formalin vapor or antiseptic fluid.

Some questions were raised concerning the extent of teachers' authority over others' personal hygiene. Instructions given by the Ministry of Education at the time indicated that the teachers were responsible for daily inspection of the students, not only of the cleanliness of their clothing and footwear, but also the "systematic inspection of the cleanliness of face, neck, hair, teeth, hands, nails, feet and underwear, demanding rigorous cleaning of the mouth and punishment of dirty children, sending them home to their parents and informing them of the reason for their child's expulsion."[27]

3.2.2 *"Dirty" and "Undisciplined":*
The Role of Schoolchildren in the Popularization of Hygiene

Hygiene education was a crucial step in the success of the state's public health initiatives although it was fraught with difficulties. Teaching hygiene rules and disseminating popularized medical knowledge through school were part of the information campaign launched at the end of the nineteenth century by medical and charitable associations, such as the Union of Greek Women, the Anti-Malaria League and the Pan-Hellenic Association Against TB, in an effort to protect the public against contagious diseases.

---

26 Emmanouil Lambadarios, *Odigiai pros Profylaxin ton eis ta Skholeia Foitonton apo ton Loimodon Noson meta ton Skhetikon Egkyklion* (Athens: Ypourgeion ton Ekklisiastikon kai tis Dimosias Ekpaidefseos, 1920), 32–3.
27 Lambadarios, *Odigiai pros Profylaxin ton eis ta Skholeia Foitonton*, 11.

The Pan-Hellenic Association against TB demonstrated remarkable activity in this field. Following the techniques used by voluntary organizations in Europe in similar campaigns, a competition for the writing of popularized books on protection against TB was launched. The translation of the work of the German Sigard Adolphus Knopf in 1906, *Tuberculosis as a Disease of the Masses and how to Combat it,*[28] marked the beginning of a series of popular publications on the fight against TB, which intensified during the 1920s.[29] Simultaneously, hundreds of copies of guidelines were printed and distributed, such as "The Ten Commandments against Spitting," while signs, put up in public places, carrying the prohibition "do not spit on the ground" alerted dwellers of the dangers they were exposing themselves to should they breach the prohibitions. The school became the prime location for the dissemination of knowledge. In 1915, shortly after the appointment of the first school doctors, the President of the Pan-Hellenic Association against TB, Vassilios Patrikios, asked the Minister of Education to support the fight against TB by recommending that local school doctors inform the students and the public in their regions about "the risk posed by the disease and its threat to the race itself, in terms of politics, economy and ethics."[30] The Ministry of Education supported these efforts, facilitating the distribution of the Association's leaflets to high school teachers and students.

In early 1910, the Lyceum of Greek Women disseminated 3,000 leaflets to primary schools and to the Charity Organization for the Relief of the Poor for distribution to poor women. Taking into account the role of female teachers in the fight against TB, special lectures were organized for them and posters on the Anti-TB campaign were given to them to be put up at their schools. In addition, lectures were organized at primary schools with the permission of the Ministry of Education. Mothers of female students were invited to attend. On the initiative of women volunteers, priests in Sunday schools were also asked to perform an Anti-TB catechism instead of a strictly religious one.

28 It was translated by Miltiades Thalis under the title *I Phymatiosis os Nosos tou Laou* and was published by the Society for the Dissemination of Beneficial Books (Syndesmos pros Diadosin Ofelimon Vivlion) in 1906.

29 Popular publications included *Pos na Profylagometha apo ti Phymatiosi*, a translation of Mark Zakero's work by Konstantinos Melas published in 1925, Panagiotis Pamboukis's, *O Agon kata tis Pthiseos* (Athens: 1927) and the 1930 publication by the Ministry of Hygiene of the book *Pos Prepei na Ziseis gia na Therapefteis*. All three books were circulated in pocket size editions.

30 See the letter of Vasilios Patrikios to the Minister of Education (April 9, 1915), in the unclassified archive of Emmanouil Lambadarios, ELIA.

Moreover, the Athens Hygiene Society (Etaireia Ygieinis Athinon) founded in 1916 to improve the "plight for public and personal hygiene in Greece," sought, among other things, to educate the masses on hygiene issues, through lectures and publication of low-priced, popular booklets.[31] These publications, published from 1916–18, demonstrate the importance the Society attached to the dissemination of personal hygiene habits. Mass vaccinations carried out by the members of the Society in the winter of 1916, when a smallpox epidemic hit Athens and caused many deaths, revealed a dismal picture of the level of personal hygiene. In terms of bodily cleanliness, the public was at a totally primitive level, "uneducated and undisciplined, they lacked the instinctive feeling about the goodness and benefit of bodily cleanliness, due to inadequate teaching and lack of appropriate guidance."[32] According to the doctors of the Athens Hygiene Society, apart from the lack of cheap public baths in major cities, there was also a lack of systematic information. The school and the army barracks were proclaimed the ideal—as well as the most populated—sites for the dissemination of new personal and domestic hygiene habits. During the same period, proposals were made by hygiene associations for the priming of "hygiene indoctrinators," usually workers, who would be taught by doctors in order to inform fellow workers about the means of protection against infectious diseases. These proposals, however, were rather fruitless.

The displacement of populations and the arrival of refugees between 1912 and 1922 contributed to the spread of infectious diseases. Moreover, the arrival of refugees made health education imperative. Greece had experienced two outbreaks of typhus fever, linked to contemporary military events and the subsequent concentration of populations in adverse hygiene conditions. The typhus epidemic that broke out in 1913 during the Balkan Wars in Thessaloniki's refugee camps was not as significant as that of the years 1918–1920, when two further outbreaks claimed many lives: the typhus epidemic that broke out in the autumn of 1918 in east Macedonia, where repatriated hostages returning from exile in Bulgaria had settled; and the epidemic in the summer of 1919 which was spread by refugees from Caucasus

---

31 Georgios Karafyllis, *Dialexis peri Profylaxeos tis Dimosias Ygeias apo ton Loimodon Noson*, Etaireia Ygieinis Athinon (Athens: 1916–1917), 7–8.
32 Karafyllis, *Dialexis peri Profylaxeos tis Dimosias Ygeias*, 17.

and contaminated ports of southern Russia.[33] The quarantine camps set up in various parts of Thessaloniki from July 1919 to March 1920, which were built to carry out decontamination and delousing, prevented the spread of the disease throughout the population. Nevertheless, the number of victims reached several hundred, since, apart from typhus fever, refugees from the Caucasus reached northern Greece exhausted from hunger and deprivation and as a result succumbed to other diseases, such as malaria, dysentery and respiratory diseases. The majority of the victims who died in the quarantine camps were children under the age of ten.

The high percentage of children in the total mortality rates might have alarmed the School Hygiene Service. As personal hygiene played a crucial role in the transmission of diseases, instruction leaflets handed out to schoolchildren demonstrate the extent to which health inspection entered people's private lives, not only of the pupils but also of their families. In order to deal with typhus fever and influenza, the Ministry of Education published leaflets in 1918 and 1919, so as to advise schoolchildren, and by extension their families, to change underwear regularly, keep their hair cut, bathe with vinegar or coat themselves with camphor oil or turpentine, and wash their bodies regularly with warm water and soap. Heating clothes in the oven or boiling them was suggested in cases where the patient was very poor and had no means of replacing them. School doctors and teachers were obliged to report any information "relating to the occurrence of any certain or suspicious cases among pupils or their families" to the police.[34] Moreover, from May 1921, private doctors were obliged to declare any cases of typhoid fever, dysentery, scarlet fever, diphtheria, intermittent fever, rabies, leprosy and influenza to medical authorities.

The great influenza epidemic that struck Europe in 1918 and turned into a pandemic was also addressed by issuing strict instructions to schoolchildren. The School Hygiene Service drew the students' attention to personal hygiene and to avoiding promiscuity with many people. In 1918, the isolation of the sick was still considered the best precautionary measure.[35] School students were forbidden to hang out in places "where people of dif-

33 Fokion Kopanaris, *I Dimosia Ygeia en Elladi* (Athens: 1933), 25.

34 "Circular peri Profylaxeos ton eis to Skholeion Foitonton apo tou Exanthimatikou Tyfou," *Deltion tou Ypourgeiou ton Ekklisiastikon kai tis Dimosias Ekpaidefseos*, no. 2 (February 1919): 4–5.

35 "Odigiai pros Profylaxin ton Mathiton apo tis Epidimikis Grippis," *Deltion tou Ypourgeiou ton Ekklisiastikon kai tis Dimosias Ekpaidefseos*, no. 1 (January 1919): 11–2.

ferent origin and varying degrees of health were concentrated, in particular in dark and badly ventilated areas," and were recommended to rinse their mouth 3–4 times a day with a variety of antiseptic liquids. Instructions were provided on how to prepare them.[36]

Considering all of these new responsibilities, it is evident that the role of the teacher grew to encompass being proponent of good health, and an assistant to the school doctor, while the school itself emerged as the prime means by which new health habits were to reach the lower classes.

3.2.3 Hygiene Textbooks

In the same vein, efforts were made during this period to introduce the study of hygiene to schools' curriculum. With the exception of female schools, where hygiene had been taught since at least 1880, the first references to teaching hygiene can be found in the 1906 curriculum: hygiene was to be taught in the second year of high school (Gymnasium) as part of natural history, which included the teaching of natural science.[37] The influence of school hygiene on education became more apparent in 1914, when it was referred to for the first time in the curriculum of Greek Schools as "Nature and Hygiene." It was taught in the third grade under the title "Hygiene Elements," and in the fourth year of high school where hygiene was a separate subject, incorporating knowledge from general hygiene manuals (concepts and benefits of hygiene, air, water, foodstuff, house, care of the body, exercise and rest, health awareness, knowledge of infectious diseases).[38] These books also demonstrate the influence of the French model. Hygiene lessons were taught in the last term by the school doctor, his assistant, or by a doctor appointed by the Ministry of Education on the recommendation of the headmaster, or the physics teacher, as part of the physics class. Nevertheless, it seems that the lesson was somewhat marginalized.

At the same time, proposals were made for the introduction of the basics of hygiene to primary schools. In an article entitled "On the teaching of hygiene at all levels of education" published in the Ministry Bulletin in

---

36 "Odigiai pros Profylaxin ton Mathiton apo tis Epidimikis Grippis," 12.
37 Vasiliko Diatagma, "Peri Kanonismou tou Programmatos ton en tois Ellinkois Skholiois kai Gymnasiois Didakteon Mathimaton," Efimeris tis Kiverniseos, A´, no. 244 (October 28, 1906) : 998–1004.
38 "Peri Programmatos ton Mathimaton tou Ellinikou Skholeiou kai tou Gymnasiou," Programma 1914, in David Antoniou, Ta Programmata tis Mesis Ekpaidefsis (1833–1929), 611 and 622.

1920, Lambadarios recommended hygiene be taught in a practical way, as a supplement to the natural sciences.[39] Descriptions of flies and other insects could be combined with the ways in which infectious diseases could be transmitted, "particularly the most malignant (typhoid, malaria, intermittent fever, plague)."[40] In grades five and six of primary school, the chapter of the physics textbook on fermentation could lend itself to teaching students alcohol abstinence, while chapters on boiling could teach decontamination and germ killing. Lambadarios recommended in his article that hygiene be enriched and taught by the school doctor in high schools, while in teacher training colleges, knowledge should be more systematic, as the students would have to teach the discipline themselves in primary schools. Particular emphasis was placed upon the material taught in female teacher training colleges, with the addition of nursing and paedological knowledge.

Lambadarios attached particular importance to the teaching of hygiene and paedology in teacher training colleges. He also recommended the organization of a paedological laboratory and the training of teachers in body measurements and psychometrics. The importance attached to knowledge of hygiene is also evidenced by the introduction of paedology and school hygiene subjects into the curriculum of the Secondary Teacher Training College, founded in 1920.

The publications circulated at the end of the nineteenth century lead us to the conclusion that the subject of hygiene must have been introduced into teacher training colleges at least since 1880. Publications were also in evidence, at middle school level, from the 1880s. In the 1910s and 1920s, the circulation of hygiene manuals increased, now authored by school doctors. Some of these circulated with the approval of the Ministry of Education. The best known among these were: *Basic and School Hygiene* by Kostis Kharitakis, published in 1914; *Children's Health (from Birth to School-leaving Age)*, by Theodoros Nikolaidis in 1916; *Health and Treatment* by Anna Katsigra in 1918; and *Hygiene Lessons*, by school doctor Panayotis Khristopoulos in 1919. Spreading hygiene principles among schoolchildren, which would later be mediated by them to their parents, was expected to change the attitude of middle and lower class families, not only towards disease but also towards hygiene habits.

---

39 Emmanouil Lambadarios, "Peri tis Didaskalias tis Ygieinis eis ta Skholeia Pantos Vathmou," *Deltion tou Ypourgeiou ton Ekklisiastikon kai tis Dimosias Ekpaidefeos* no. 13 (January 1920): 44–6 and 70–1.

40 Lambadarios, "Peri tis Didaskalias tis Ygieinis eis ta Skholeia Pantos Vathmou," 44.

4. The Work of the School Hygiene Service before 1920

4.1 The Duties of School Doctors and Nurses

Protection against contagious diseases was addressed more systematically from 1914, when Law no. 240 "on the administration of Primary and Secondary School Education" provided for the organization of school health and hygiene services.[41] This law delegated the health and hygiene inspection of schools and students to school doctors and their assistants. A school doctor was appointed in every educational district and was responsible for the inspections, compiling reports on the state of their health, and submitting them to the general inspector. The state continued passing legislation gradually up until 1920 so as to delineate the work of the School Hygiene Service in detail. In 1914 some posts of school doctors opened up. These posts would be taken up by prospective applicants following a competitive process in front of a committee comprising university professors of Hygiene and Ophthalmology, the head of the School Hygiene Service and an educational consultant.[42] Apart from written examinations on pediatrics and school hygiene, competition for the post involved the applicant writing a report on the hygiene conditions of a school building in Athens in front of the committee directly after visiting the school. Regular monitoring of the sanitary conditions of school facilities was one of the duties the school doctors and their assistants should perform. School doctors, apart from supervising the sanitary construction and operation of school facilities, were entrusted with the main tasks of school health and hygiene, such as mandatory vaccination of students, monitoring their physical and mental health, teaching teachers the basics of health and hygiene, and dealing with emergencies. Assistants to school doctors were required to travel across their assigned province, inspecting schools and teaching health and hygiene classes in high schools and teacher-training colleges.

Legislative amendments before 1920 improved the operation of the external School Hygiene Service. There were two categories of health and hy-

---

41 See the article no. 18 of the law no. 240, "Peri Dioikiseos tis Dimotikis kai Mesis Ekpaidefseos," *Efimeris tis Kiverniseos*, A', no. 97 (April 26, 1914): 505–12, and the article no. 7 of the law no. 567 "Peri Tropopoiiseos tou Nomou 240 peri Dioikiseos tis Dimotikis kai Mesis Ekpaidefseos," *Efimeris tis Kiverniseos*, A' no. 15 (January 12, 1915): 107–8.

42 "Mémorandum sur le Service Hellénique de l'Hygiène Scolaire," typescript in the unclassified archive of Emmanouil Lambadarios, Hellenic Literary and Historical Archive (ELIA).

giene staff in schools: health inspectors and school doctors. The qualifications of school doctors gradually grew, their numbers increased and their responsibilities expanded.[43] Initially, private doctors were appointed as school doctors, one in each inspectorate. From 1925 onwards, a certification in school hygiene was an essential qualification for such appointments. Health inspectors devised a schedule of regular visits by school doctors to schools in their areas. Health inspection in schools took place once or twice a month, and additionally in cases of emergency such as epidemics, or by order of the health inspector. The findings of these inspections were recorded in the school doctor's special register, held by the headteacher. Information about the sanitation conditions of the building was entered on special forms, while the results of pupils' medical examinations were recorded in individual medical cards. The 1917 Royal Decree defined the way medical reports should be compiled by the health inspector on a monthly basis.[44] The December report included the results of vaccinations, the March report included the results of individual medical examinations together with proposals for any changes required to school facilities or grounds, and the June report included a more detailed picture of the overall work carried out by each school doctor. Information on the number of schools inspected, the number of outbreaks of infectious diseases, and the table of examined pupils for whom medical cards had been issued was entered in the June report. Finally, school doctors were responsible for granting convalescent leave to teachers, whose care would be supported by a teachers' fund.

The appointment of approximately 60 school doctors and 12 health inspectors raised hopes that health and hygiene measures in schools might be efficiently implemented, since previous practices had not been successful. In the early years, the head of the School Hygiene Service placed emphasis on treatment of infectious diseases, detection and removal of suspects during epidemics and prompt decontamination of the school, replacing teachers in this role. During the 1920s, school doctors played an important role in planning social and hygiene welfare in schools.

The head of the School Hygiene Service suggested school nurses be appointed to aid medical inspection services in schools. The school nurse, a

---

43 Health inspectors were appointed on a competitive basis while school doctors should hold a certificate awarded after an examination.

44 Vasiliko Diatagma "Peri Kanonismou tis Ygeionomikis Epitheoriseos ton Skholeion," *Efimeris tis Kiverniseos,* A', no. 62 (April 7, 1917): 199–202.

position begun in America at the end of the nineteenth century, had started to gain ground in Europe in the 1910s, mainly through the Junior Red Cross. Following the model of the visiting nurse introduced in the U.S.A. as part of the struggle against TB and promoted by the Rockefeller Foundation, the school nurse would become the main assistant of the school doctor.[45] Her role was significant in that she would inspect schoolchildren for cleanliness, detect suspected cases of illness, treat skin diseases like pediculosis, and carry out measurements of students' bodies.

Her main role, however, would be outside the school. She would visit absent students in their homes and therefore be able to determine the cause of their absence, suggest precautionary measures for the future, take stock of the family environment, living conditions and cleanliness of the house, as well as instruct parents on hygiene standards.[46] As a "disciple" of public health, the school nurse could gain intimacy with the mother, a relationship that permitted her to effectively instill the appropriate precautionary measures and to check whether they were really implemented. Her role as "the eye of the doctor in the house of the poor," was associated primarily with the protection of children from TB. This more hands-on hygiene educator was expected to eradicate popular superstitions that prevented the doctor's advice from reaching the home of the poor.

In Greece, the introduction of this "institution" was associated mainly with the activities of American health organizations following the arrival of refugees in 1919; however, many of Lambadarios's publications from 1912 onwards emphasized the value of the school nurse in bridging the gap between the doctor and the family. His efforts to introduce school nurses to Greece bore fruit in 1920, when the first school nurse was transferred from the American Red Cross to the School Hygiene Service. Eleni Inglezaki, educated in Boston, supervised three primary schools in Athens and, according to the schedule drawn up by Lambadarios himself, was responsible for measuring and immunizing schoolchildren, inspecting cleanliness and hygiene, both at school and at home, communicating practical hygiene knowl-

---

45 Emmanouil Lambadarios, "I Ygieini ton Skholeion en Agglia," *Deltion tis Paidiatrikis Etaireias Athinon*, 1934. For the role of the visiting nurse, see Yvette Knibielhler, "La 'lutte antituberculeuse', instrument de la médicalisation des classes populaires (1870–1930)," *Annales de Bretagne et des pays de l'Ouest* 86, no. 3 (1979): 321–34.

46 For the role and the duties of the school nurse, see Emmanouil Lambadarios, *Skholiki Ygieini meta Stoikheion Paidologiaς* (Athens: 1934), 405.

edge, inspecting homes and guiding parents in their hygienic duties. Despite Lambadarios's efforts to have school nurses appointed, their number remained low until World War II.

4.2 Systematic Vaccination

School doctors also played a crucial role in the systematic vaccination of students, which began to be carried out in a more orderly fashion.[47] The high proportion of unvaccinated students—in some areas as high as 30%—reported by school doctors on their first visits to schools in their districts, revealed the extent of the problem and led to coordinated efforts to raise awareness, both among parents and headteachers. Vaccination was made compulsory by law for all children up to the age of ten. The school doctor was obliged to check if the student's body was clean before performing vaccination. In case he found that the arms or the inside of the clothing were unclean, the doctor dismissed the child to go and get washed, and change clothes. The doctor also had to visit vaccinated children and check whether the vaccination was successful, as well as compile lists of the vaccinated and submit them to the Ministry of Education.

After 1914, these health checks became more systematic. The Ministry expected the registration of vaccinated schoolchildren to help identify irresponsible parents. The keeping of vaccination registers, begun in 1915, where the school doctor entered the names and ages of the vaccinated children, the date of vaccination or revaccination and the result, was considered to be an effective monitoring tool. Should a student be transferred to another school, the headteacher was required to supply him with a certification of vaccination. In addition, according to Law no. 2457/1920, parents were obliged to keep the vaccination certificates of their children; those who failed to do so were fined 50–100 drachmae.[48]

Through these measures, the School Hygiene Service expected to reduce the spread of infectious diseases among children. At the same time, the introduction of vaccination registers in schools marked the launch of a

---

47 Law no. 2457 "Peri Tropopoiiseos tou Nomou 1242 (240, 567, 1069) peri Ygeionomikis Ypiresias ton Skholeion," *Efimeris tis Kiverniseos*, A', no. 172 (August 1, 1920): 1701–3, provided for mandatory vaccination.

48 Law no. 2457, 1702.

network to monitor the health of schoolchildren. According to information compiled by the School Hygiene Service from the school doctors' reports between 1917 and 1920, some 150,000 schoolchildren were vaccinated.[49]

Decontamination also became more systematic, extending into the homes of "germ-carrying" schoolchildren despite difficulties emanating from their family environment. The results of these scientific precautions implemented in schools were attested in the reduction of infant mortality, from 34.2% in 1915 to 23% in 1920.[50]

4.3 The Codification of Information

The organization of health inspection in 12 districts in 1914 and the statutes on the School Hygiene Service which passed in 1917 resulted in more effective supervision of school hygiene. The Ministry of Education issued special forms in an attempt to codify the information, expecting a more complete picture of the hygiene conditions of both school buildings and students. The codification of information on public health was instrumental in shaping health policy in the twentieth century. Emphasis was laid upon a quantitative survey of health conditions. The school doctor described the hygienic conditions of each school building: its location, size, number of classrooms, dimensions of windows, ventilation and lighting in the classrooms, lavatories and school yard, desks and space allotted to each pupil. This codified description, which constituted a kind of identity of the building, highlighted deficiencies and the gap between the condition of the school and the hygiene standards set by the School Hygiene Service. Based on this information, the school doctor ranked the schools in his district in one of the following three categories: healthy, reasonably healthy and unhealthy. The collection of these forms enabled the Ministry of Education to gain a comprehensive picture of educational facilities throughout the country, in order to plan the construction of new school buildings and define educational infrastructure policy on the basis of objective data.

Medical inspection of pupils included examination of their health "in general and individually." The school doctor examined, in the first instance,

---

49 According to information from the typed notes of Lambadarios entitled "Lessons of School Hygiene." See unclassified archive of Emmanouil Lambadarios, ELIA.
50 Emmanouil Lambadarios, *Skholiki Ygieini meta Stoikheion Paidologias*, 249.

any pupils that the school director suspected of illness, as well as those in convalescence from an infectious disease. The school doctor also had to report "the unclean and those suffering from skin, eye and contagious or other diseases in general," and specify the necessary precautions to be taken. He was also expected, with assistance from the school director, to register the indigent students who were absent due to illness on the day of his visit. The doctor had to expel students suffering from infectious diseases and notify their parents in writing. In the letter, he would state the reasons why the student was expelled from school as well as specify the terms of his return. The same applied to those whom the doctor found to be suffering from ailments of "the mouth, the teeth, the eyes, the ears, scalp hair or skin." Furthermore, a "special document" was issued for the children who were in need of "special vigilance and care," due to their general state of health, "in order to enlighten the[ir] family."[51] However, the school doctor was not permitted to take action that might interfere with the work of the family doctor.

As far as the state of the students' health was concerned, the School Hygiene Service was interested in identifying the number of students found to be inflicted with specific infectious diseases on the day of the doctor's visit, the number of absent students and the reason for their absence, potential epidemics, as well as whether improvements were necessary.[52] In the 1910s, scabies, achora, pediculosis, impetigo, stomatitis, acute conjunctivitis, trachoma, TB and scrofula were the diseases expected to be recorded in the school doctor's register. The collection of medical cards, in combination with the annual reports compiled by school doctors that described in detail the health condition of schoolchildren in their area, enabled the central service to determine with accuracy the health of the student population at any given time, the sites of infection and the possible need for emergency measures. In districts where the number of school doctors was inadequate, hygiene supervision was assigned to teachers. The health inspector was even able to impose a fine, "up to 25 drachmae, on those infringing hygiene regulations or demonstrating laxity in the implementation of instructions." According to a circular issued in 1918, the school doctor, or the school director in case there was no doctor, was obliged to submit a list of students

---

51 Vasiliko Diatagma "Peri Kanonismou tis Ygeionomikis Epitheoriseos ton Skholeion," 201.
52 "Vivlion Skholikou Iatrou," see unclassified archive of Emmanouil Lambadarios, ELIA.

suffering from infectious diseases to the School Hygiene Service. The table, in addition to the names of the students, recorded class he/she was attending, the type of disease, the date of onset and the outcome, as well as his/her address.[53]

4.4 The Health Inspectors' Reports

The annual reports submitted by the first school doctors speak of the problems the School Hygiene Service faced during its first steps. The hygienic picture of the school was not far from the accounts of the paediatricians who had carried out research on the student population in 1908. According to the school doctors' reports, in 1916 most school buildings were either unhygienic or only moderately hygienic. For instance, in the first educational district out of a total of 237 schools only 67 were characterized as hygienic, 84 moderately hygienic and the remainder 86 unhygienic.

The presence of too many students in classrooms, the unwillingness of the proprietors who rented property to carry out the necessary changes, and the rise in the prices of building materials due to warfare, all contributed to this unhygienic picture. The number of students per classroom topped 100 in certain cases, for instance in the first primary school of Syros, the number of students per classroom exceeded 205.

In some schools there were no student desks at all. In 1923, out of a total of 22,000 students in Athens and Piraeus 5,000 students either stood up or sat on chairs, brought from their homes, during classes.[54] According to a school doctor report in 1920, due to overcrowding the unhygienic condition of many school buildings and the unsuitability of desks, "the picture of the Greek school was bleak, totally incommensurate to the dignity of the state." As a result, students paid scant attention to their classes.

A host of horrors inflicted on the student population included trachoma, scrofula and malaria, which had the highest incidence, while whooping cough, diphtheria and smallpox ran rampant from time to time. The whooping cough epidemics "swept" across the child population for three consecu-

---

53 Emmanouil Lambadarios, *Odigiai pros Profylaxin ton eis ta Skholeia Foitonton*, 53.
54 See, for instance, the report submitted by the school inspector Khristos Georgakopoulos, *Etisia Ekthesi tou Ygeionomikou Epitheoriti D' Ekpaideftikis Periphereias, Skholiko Etos 1923–1924*, in the unclassified archive of Emmanouil Lambadarios, ELIA.

tive years from 1910 to 1912. Although the disease subsided in the following years, it still remained the most deadly killer among students. Diphtheria also claimed many victims among students, especially in certain Athenian neighborhoods. In 1915, the student population of Athens, Piraeus and the nearby islands was affected mainly by epidemics of scarlet fever, measles, diphtheria and smallpox.

School doctors paid particular attention to trachoma, a contagious eye disease, which in certain cases led to loss of sight. The virus was transmitted from the eyes through hands, handkerchiefs, towels and even insects. School doctors attributed this disease to uncleanliness and tried to raise the awareness of the disease among students and their families. Instructions issued by the department of School Hygiene laid great emphasis upon isolation and observance of hygiene rules. Sufficient food and compliance with individual sanitation rules were considered indispensable: body cleanliness—especially clean underwear—regular nail clipping, regular face and hand washing, airing out the house, avoiding contact with affected people and not sharing personal items such as towels, handkerchiefs and pillows.[55] Timely diagnosis and therapy were believed to play a crucial role in reducing the number of victims. It was recommended that patients suffering from trachoma undergo treatment "firstly, so as to save their eyes and avoid loss of sight and secondly, [...] not to be dangerous for others."[56]

Instructions on how to deal with eye-pain, the training of teachers in implementing therapeutic measures, and the isolating of infected students—who had to be seated further away from their healthy peers—were the first means employed to contend with trachoma. The diligence of some teachers who took it upon themselves to treat the diseased seems to have borne fruit; yet, as trachoma was raging in the classroom, more radical steps were called for. The circulation of leaflets with simplified instructions given out to the families of the students reveals the doctors' anxiety to appeal to working classes. They advised students to swat flies with every available means so as to avoid catching the disease "because flies are attracted to squalor and filthiness," and to pay particular attention to the cleanliness of their homes and bodies. Also, while at school, students were advised to avoid contact with

---

55 See the circular of the Ministry of Education, "Odigiai peri Profylaxeos apo tou Trakhomatos (dia to Koinon)," in the unclassified archive of Emmanouil Lambadarios, ELIA.

56 "Odigiai Peri Profylaxeos apo tou Trakhomatos."

pens, pencils and books of fellow students, "since these might be tainted by anyone suffering from trachoma."[57]

Scrofula was also part and parcel of the welfare notion; the term scrofula signified the state of general weakness of the child constitution. Since doctors had drawn certain connections between scrofula and TB, its prompt detection was considered an indispensable deterrent to possible contamination. The need to detect pre-tubercular students led to school doctors registering students who suffered from glandular fever (adenopathy), tonsillitis, anemia and general weakness. In 1915, a circular of the Ministry of Education on how to stamp out TB encouraged school doctors to intensify their attempts to detect suspicious cases, encouraging them to take steps such as supplying weak students with nutritious food, sending them to summer camps or building school baths, to strengthen their constitutions.[58] Since many students developed symptoms of general weakness, scrofula topped statistics of student morbidity. In addition, in some areas, there were high rates of malaria that could be attributed to geomorphological conditions particular to each region. In the 1920s malaria affected 65% of the student population in the districts of Arta and Patras, while in other areas it reached less than 3%.

Between 1915 and 1920, the School Hygiene Service spent 166,980 to 215,840 drachmae per annum. This expenditure covered the salaries of twelve school hygiene inspectors and sixty school doctors as well as travel expenses.[59] The institution of the school doctor, as described above, was implemented in this form in most cities and provinces until 1925; at that time Theodoros Pangalos's dictatorship began to transfer its responsibilities to municipalities and the institution withered away as a result of cutbacks in public spending. During this period, despite the adverse war conditions, school doctors were proclaimed the most effective means for protecting student health. Favored by Venizelos's politics, the institution of student health supervision was unmistakably connected with the modernization of education.

---

57 Lambadarios, *Kodix Skholikis Ygieinis*, 262.
58 See the circular of the Ministry of Education, May 15, 1915, "Peri Katapolemiseos tis Pthiseos," in the unclassified archive of Emmanouil Lambadarios, ELIA.
59 "Mémorandum sur le Service Hellénique de l'Hygiène Scolaire," in the unclassified archive of Emmanouil Lambadarios, ELIA.

5. Growth Indices

5.1 The Student Personal Health Card

Since the inception of the School Hygiene Service, Lambadarios, aware of the importance of data codification to drawing hygiene policies, was deeply concerned with the accumulation of statistics on the hygienic condition of buildings and students. The "table of the cases of contagious student diseases," filled in by teachers during the early years of the School Hygiene Service, was a tool for observing the spread of contagious diseases. After 1914, the systematization of the School Hygiene Service allowed for the adoption of more modern means for the observation of the students' physical and mental development. The most important means, already in use in other countries, were the student's personal health card and statistics on student morbidity.

The student's personal health card constituted a "mirror" where his/her health was reflected. It was filled in accordance with paedometric tables on the increase of weight, height and thorax circumference and outlined the student's physical condition. Apart from the afore-mentioned indices, the measurements carried out by the school doctor or the school nurse included hearing, eyesight, the dimensions of the head, and strength; in certain cases intelligence was also measured. Special terms were coined for these measurements such as cephalometrics, thoracometry, dynamometria and special devices were invented ranging from the very simple—height measuring board (anastimometro) and weighing scales—to the more elaborate ergometers, cephalometers, spirometers. These advances indicated the degree of specialization that had been accomplished in measuring children's bodies. Analyzing and recording these indices made it possible for the school doctor to determine with mathematical accuracy the relation of the dimensions that implied a disease or detect an aberration. In many European and American cities, the student's personal health card or health booklet (livret scolaire de santé) was used by the administration of the School Hygiene since its inception; the findings of the student's medical examination were regularly entered in it.[60] This novelty drew its origin from military practice since

---

60 Bernard Harris, *The Health of the Schoolchild: A History of the School Medical Service in England and Wales* (Buckingham: Open University Press, 1995), 27–8.

a similar card was used for the examination of conscripts. In general, the numericalization of body measurements dates back to nineteenth century. In 1870 the Belgian mathematician and demographer Adolphe Quetelet applied biometric statistics to the measurements of children to draw conclusions about the biological and moral characteristics of the average human.[61]

In the nineteenth century paedological measurements were systematized under the umbrella of school hygiene. Different opinions about the scientific accuracy of the measurements and the means of determining the indices were expressed at the 1907 London International Congress on School Hygiene. The means of measuring thorax circumference had been a thorny question among paedologists. Since this index was connected with the volume of the lungs and in consequence with the possibility of illness, it was considered important for predicting the occurrence of TB. Breathing exercises were believed to play a crucial role. It was found that this index was higher in children that exercised breathing, i.e., children who were knowledgeable about the mechanisms of inhalation and exhalation. Also, the oxygenation of the blood was better in children who regularly exercised. The latter, then, were less at risk of contracting TB.

The "coefficient of robustness," also derived from military practice, was the most important index, combining weight, height and thorax circumference into a single table that functioned as a kind of health identity. The coefficient of robustness allowed for the categorization of bodies into five health categories as well as the isolation of the weaker constitutions. This index was lower in TB suspects and as such served as unmistakable evidence for distinguishing the healthy from the ones likely to come down with TB. This data was considered valuable for the construction of two tools; the morbidity statistics on student population and statistics on the physical development of the students.

The value of these tools becomes all the more apparent in the light of auxology—coined by Paul Godin—a new field at the time that demonstrates the medical profession's interest in observing the rate of students' physical development.[62] Auxology aimed at determining the type of child growth, a formula resulting from the ratio of the thorax's growth to that of the head

---

61 For the origin of the student's personal health card, see E. Mazoyer, "Le fichier sanitaire scolaire," *La médecine scolaire* 5, no. 10 (October 10, 1913): 329–42.

62 Paul Godin, *Manuel d'anthropologie* (Paris: 1921).

and the limbs. In addition, paedologists were interested in determining the relationship between physical and mental development, a relationship considered especially useful for approaching student's learning difficulties.

According to Lambadarios, the school doctor had to be knowledgeable about the general course the child's development took, i.e., to observe if it followed the progress expected at each developmental stage in order to distinguish "the normally developed child" from deviant types at both ends of the continuum. Lambadarios pigeonholed children into five categories: "the prematurely developed," "the exceptionally able," "the child above average," "the mentally and physically retarded" and the "idiotic" child.[63] The findings of the paedometric examination made it possible to categorise each child, following comparison of the findings with the average included in special charts. For instance, according to the information entered into the personal health card of a twelve-year old male student (height, 125 cm; weight, 28kg; chest expansion, 6 cm; spirometer, 1,950 cub. cm; and ergometer, 20 kg), he lagged two years behind the average Greek child in height and one year behind in weight. Yet, he surpassed the average Greek child in lung volume and power (a full year ahead). He was therefore rather short but quite strong.[64]

The personal health card for students was introduced to Greece in 1911 by Aikaterini Varouxaki at the Arsakeio School, a women's college. A few years later, in 1917, a royal decree laid down the regulations for the individual examination of all students during their first year of studies. The exam results were entered in the personal health card and the exam was repeated in the fourth, sixth and eighth year of their schooling. However, individual examinations of students were not carried out until 1917 due to the small number of health inspectors, reservations towards the introduction of new medical institutions, and lack of the teacher's knowledge.

The findings of the medical exam allowed school doctors to draw teachers' attention to student illnesses and take appropriate steps to combat disease: instructing head teachers on how to deal with "mentally retarded" students; selecting pre-tubercular students who needed to be put in summer camps or open-air schools; and informing parents whose children were

---

63 Emmanouil Lambadarios, "I Somatiki Anaptyxis tou Paidiou," *Paidologia*, no. 6 (October 1920): 186.

64 Emmanouil Lambadarios, "I Somatiki Anaptyxis tou Paidiou (kai idia tou Ellinos Mathitou)," *Paidologia*, no. 9 (September 1921): 2–5.

at risk of infection. It is worth noting that this was the first time special care was taken to detect pre-tubercular and mentally "mentally retarded" students.

Student personal health cards, modelled on the health card already in use in France, were introduced on Lambadarios's proposal. The findings of the medical exam were entered in it, which included information on the eyes, ears, pharynx, lymphoid system, skeleton—especially the spine—skin, hair of the scalp, heart, lungs and the nervous system. The school doctors also had to observe the development of the stature, weight and thorax circumference of students and compile their observations into a special chart. Students' personal medical history with contagious diseases since preschool were also on the health card, as well as what vaccines they had been given.

The personal health card was a powerful tool in the hands of school doctors and evidenced the degree of state modernization in the field of children's health. As such, it was possible to draw both horizontal and vertical comparisons at the national and local level. Children's development could be compared to the average of his or her 'race' and to their own projected development. School doctors were also able to draw comparisons between urban, rural, wealthy, working-class, and foreign children based on the indices of physical development recorded on their health cards.

These personal health cards, drawn by Lambadarios according to European models, reveal a trend to measure student bodies with mathematical accuracy, prevalent among hygienists at the beginning of the twentieth century. This positivist approach could not be contested and was thought to ensure the scientific recognition of hygiene while at the same time corroborating doctors' arguments for the adoption of public health measures. However, objections were raised against the introduction of these measures. In France, for instance, filling in the personal health card highlighted the doctor's right to intervene, replacing the family, in the name of public health. It was argued that the personal health card violated patient-doctor confidentiality and paternal power since it made personal health data—possibly containing family secrets—public.[65] For this reason, in order to en-

---

65   In France, democratic French tradition and Roman law on paternal power deterred doctors from free action. For the discussion about the adoption of the personal health card in France and the objections raised, see Louis Dufestel, "La fiche sanitaire des élèves des écoles de Paris," *Le médecine scolaire* 5, no. 3 (March 10, 1913): 98–101, and also by the same author, "L'Examen médical des ecoliers et les droits du père de famille," *Le médecine scolaire* 2, no. 10 (October 10, 1909): 253–58.

sure confidentiality, precautions were taken for the circulation of this kind of information. Some doctors also expressed fears that the medical health card would evolve into a means of social control as it would follow the individual for their entire lives as a form of identity. For instance, information could pass from school to work place, leading to the isolation of syphilitic or tubercular persons. However, advocates of the personal health card emphasized its importance for the development of a healthy youth, an important asset for the future of the nation. In Germany, Belgium, England, the USA and Scandinavia, where the personal health card was introduced by law, the right of the state to observe the physical and mental development of the student was incontestable. At a time when eugenics had not yet been widely accepted, the right of the state to control citizens' bodies for means of racial improvement was met with reservations.

In Greece, it was made clear that the information entered in the personal health card was a professional secret and as such it had to be protected. As a result, it was protected through specific means, attesting once again to the influence of the French model on Greek medical thought.[66] The information derived from the personal health card was used in drawing up the statistics of student morbidity as well as the annual reports on the health condition of the students submitted by the school doctor of each district. Somatometric research conducted by Lambadarios himself in 1920 based on a sample of 3,521 male and female students aged 6–20 from different social classes resulted in the first comparative studies on Greek children and their counterparts from other countries.[67] According to the evidence of his research, the development of height of the Greek student was similar to that of its Italian counterpart, especially the one from South Italy. Compared to English, German, Swedish and American counterparts, Greek students were on average inferior in height (5–8 cm) and superior in comparison with their French and Belgian counterparts (1,5–3 cm). Lambadarios reached the same conclusions with regard to weight. Based on the evidence

---

66   It was stated that the personal card should be kept only by the doctor "with all the commitment this ensued for the protection of the professional secret." Parents could file an application so as the doctor to reveal part or all the information included in the card. In case the student was registered to another school, the doctor sent the card to his colleague. See the layout of the personal health card published in the journal *Paidologia*, no. 8 (November 1920): 279.

67   For this research, see Emmanouil Lambadarios, *Skholiki Ygieini meta Stoikheion Paidologias*, 167–73 and also by the same author "I Somatiki Anaptyxis tou Paidiou," *Paidologia*, no. 5–8 (May-August, 1921): 129–39.

of these measurements, he drew up diagrams that depicted the curve of the physical development of the Greek children as to their weight, height and thorax circumference. Since these diagrams determined the biological type of the physical development expected from the children of each nation, they immensely contributed to the standardization of racial differences.

5.2 Morbidity Statistics

In January 1917, Dimitrios Digas, Minister of Education, addressed a circular to head teachers and asked them to complete and submit quarterly census returns of student morbidity to the school doctors in their district. These census returns included information on the kind of contagious diseases that affected students in their school, the number of ill students, their age, sex, grade, address, date of illness, recovery, and the outcome of the disease.[68] Evidence was compiled from 60 urban centers and a number of small towns. The circular underlined the fact that the compilation of these census returns would serve the state's best interests, hinting at the difficulties the collaboration between head teachers and school doctors was met with.

Statistics was considered an indispensable tool in the hands of doctors for the implementation of public health policies; yet, the service of morbidity statistics had not been established before 1923. Moreover, the lack of an educational statistical service combined with teachers' complete ignorance of special precautions necessitated its establishment. During the same period, circulars on the prevention of trachoma, typhoid, smallpox etc., addressed to teachers and school doctors, became more frequent, with a peak during the Great War. However, the teachers' indifference to filling in the cards forced the authorities in 1919 to stress once more how important this measure was for the implementation of health policies and to check whoever did not comply with the regulations. Publication of the first census returns on student morbidity at the beginning of 1920 testifies to the fact that the measure had begun to take effect.

Based on student morbidity statistics and the reports of district hygiene inspectors, certain conclusions can be drawn with regard to the diseases

---

68   See circular no. 2.500/January 8, 1917 "Peri Katartismou Statistikis tis Mathitikis Nosirotitas ton Megaleiteron Poleon tis Ellados" in Emmanouil Lambadarios, *Odigiai pros Profylaxin ton eis ta Skholeia Foitonton*, 51–2.

that hit the student population during the 1910s and 1920s. These statistics reveal the importance of some diseases such as malaria, trachoma and TB as well as the extent of epidemic child diseases, in particular diphtheria and scarlet fever. Statistics provided a general account of the students' health at any given time and at the same time constituted an objective criterion for future changes in children health policies. As a tool for the betterment of school hygiene, it could detect not only the weaknesses in the School Hygiene Service, but also its accomplishments.

In 1920, in the preamble of the bill "On the modification of the School Medical Service," which had been based on the Service's statistics, the Minister of Education reported the infant and child mortality rates and ascribed their cause to the peak in contagious diseases. According to those statistics and to the information acquired from the School Hygiene Service, it was estimated that over half of child deaths (aged 5–15) were caused by contagious diseases—scarlet fever, diphtheria, measles, meningitis, TB etc.—in other words, by diseases that science could certainly have protected children from.[69] These findings laid bare the relation between the symptoms of general weakness (weak constitution, starvation, lyphatism, adenopathy etc.) and the possibility of TB occurrence. Based on objective criteria, the school statistics, thus, could contribute to the detection of students who were in need of care. Similarly, the spread of TB among teachers made the adoption of decisive measures imperative. During the school year of 1917–1918, thirty-nine teachers afflicted with TB were off duty.[70] The morbidity statistics, along with statistics on school's hygienic conditions and on vaccination, became a tool for monitoring the health of the student population and highlighted the role the state ought to play in the welfare of children.

Between 1917 and 1920 Lambadarios paved the way for the introduction of legislation on student health. It is worth noting that his rally coincided with significant changes in the legislative framework of education under the influence of pioneering advocates of the demotic language (Greek proper). The high percentage of pre-tubercular children led to the enactment of the first measures for the strengthening of their constitution.

69 Dimitrios Digas, "Oi Proodoi tou Thesmou tis Skholikis Ygieinis en Elladi," *Paidologia*, no. 2 (May 1920): 62–7.

70 Statistiki Phymatioseos Didaskalon: "Pinax ton logo Oxeias Phymatioseos Apomakrynthenton tis Ypiresias Leitourgon tis Ekpaidefseos kata to Etos 1917–1918," *Deltion tou Ypourgeiou ton Ekklisiastikon kai tis Dimosias Ekpaidefseos* no. 1 (January 1919): 17.

The bills on the establishment of summer camps and the teaching of hygiene were passed in 1920; yet, the political juncture postponed their materialization for the following years.

The statistics on pre-tubercular children were also used for educational changes. Lambadarios's proposals on a series of issues were connected with the impact the school curriculum had on student mental distress—for instance, the reduction in school material, the abolition of afternoon lessons, the reduction in teaching hours, the opening time of school according to the students' age and the designing of class schedules by the difficulty of the subjects taught—were based on the high rates of weak student constitutions that appeared in the morbidity statistics.[71]

In addition, the statistics on trachoma compiled since 1917 revealed the extent of this disease. In the primary schools in Piraeus, trachoma affected 15% of the students while in certain areas this percentage reached 30%.[72] In 1920, in order to contain the disease, a bill on the establishment of special anti-trachoma schools and dispensaries was put forward. The compilation of morbidity statistics, then, contributed to the launching of the anti-TB and anti-trachoma campaigns in schools.

As seen from the census returns of the student morbidity for the year 1919–1920, collated by the School Hygiene Service from 60 towns, primary school student morbidity accounted for 27.1% of the students while mortality ranged from 2 to 4%. These rates were lower for secondary school students, only 17.4%.[73] Comparison of these rates with the reports of the health inspectors for the same year reveals some divergence. In the same year it was reported that 42% of the students were affected by various diseases; malaria reached 40% and contagious diseases 8%. The latter were in order of importance the following: measles, chicken-pox, parotitis, flu, scarlet fever, diphtheria, typhus, whooping cough, dysentery and skin diseases (pediculosis capitis, scabies, streptococcus of the scalp, eczema).[74] In this statistics, cited by Lambadarios, there was no mention whatsoever of eye-diseases and

---

71 For these proposals, see Emmanouil Lambadarios, "Peri tou Anthifthysikou Agonos kata tin Paidikin Ilikian," *Paidologia* no. 4 (August 1920): 116–23.

72 See the notes under the title "Idrysis kai Exelixis tis Ypiresias Skholikis Ygieinis par' Imin," in the unclassified archive of Emmanouil Lambadarios, ELIA, 11–2.

73 See the tables entitled "Exelixis tis Mathitikis Nosirotitos" and "Diagramma Iatrikis Exetaseos ton Mathiton," in the unclassified archive of Emmanouil Lambadarios, ELIA.

74 See the notes entitled "Idrysis kai Exelixis tis Ypiresias Skholikis Ygieinis par' Imin," 12.

scrofula, which the school doctors had been concerned with during the following years. Nevertheless, the general rate of primary school student morbidity was lower than that for the school year 1915–16 when it reached 34.2%.

Looking at the student mortality tables in Athens from August until December 1919 compiled by the School Hygiene Service, we come to the conclusion that an average of twenty students died monthly. Typhoid fever, meningitis, TB and respiratory diseases, and intestinal disorders were cited as the most frequent killers.[75]

Despite the adverse political conditions and resource constraints, the 1910s were crucial for the improvement of students' health. The institution of the School Hygiene Service and student supervision by school doctors, both ventures undertaken by the Venizelos's governments, supplemented the legislation on education and testified to the emergence of state interest in the control of student morbidity and its reduction. The improvement of student health indices was attributed to the work accomplished by the School Hygiene Service and mostly to the efforts undertaken by its fervently active head, Emmanuil Lambadarios.

75 "Pinakes Thnisimotitos Mathiton kai Daskalon en Athinais ton Minon Avgoustou, Septemvriou, Oktovriou, Noemvriou kai Dekemvriou 1919," *Deltion tou Ypourgeiou ton Ekklisiastikon kai tis Dimosias Ekpaidefeos* no. 14 (February 1920): 29–30.

CHAPTER IV

MODERNITY AND WELFARE INSTITUTIONS FOR CHILD HEALTH

1. VOLUNTARY ASSOCIATIONS AND SOCIAL HYGIENE FOR STUDENTS

Although indices of student morbidity due to contagious diseases dropped around 1920, as seen from hygiene statistics, the high numbers of students aged 9–16 that showed symptoms of trachoma, malaria and general weakness underline the difficulties the School Hygiene Service faced in setting up welfare infrastructure. Indeed, at the beginning of 1920, according to the statistics of the Ministry of Education, children's infectious diseases—scarlet fever, smallpox and diphtheria—were on the decline while the so called social scourges were on the increase. In 1928, according to the death rates published by the National Statistics Service, most deaths of children aged 5–14 were caused by malaria and respiratory problems (TB, pneumonia, bronchitis, etc.).[1] Without treatment and health care infrastructure, these diseases remained a thorny problem for most destitute families. Advice from the school doctor, then, was a dead letter. However, institutions of child welfare that had already been established in many European cities provided the model for the emergence of a similar movement in Greece. Distributing school meals and establishing open-air camps and schoolchildren polyclinics was the solution most often adopted by municipalities, voluntary organizations and education authorities in order to alleviate destitute and sick students.

---

1   At the beginning of the twentieth century these rates were as follows: malaria amounted to 70% in 100,000 deaths while the respiratory diseases in total (TB of the respiratory system, acute and chronic bronchitis, pneumonia and other respiratory ailments) topped 69,7%. See Agapoula Kotsi, *Nosologia ton Paidikon Ilikion kai tis Neotitas (20os Aionas)* (Athens: IAEN/EIE, 2008), 299.

Although similar ventures were mostly privately funded, at least until the 1920s, the extent of these diseases got the attention of many high-ranking functionaries who realized the need for state intervention. The limited appropriations allotted to the School Hygiene Service allowed no optimism for the possibility of state intervention. It was not accidental, then, when Lambadarios turned to the private sector to secure funds for the establishment of children's welfare infrastructure. The long tradition of charity in Greece, the plethora of educational and social institutions run on donations from wealthy Greeks, in particular those in the Diaspora, throughout the nineteenth century made some optimistic about this reversal.

1.1 The Patriotic League of Greek Women:
Practical Philanthropy and Social Work for Children and Mothers

The Patriotic League of Greek Women (Patriotikos Syndesmos ton Ellinidon) established by Queen Sofia and some middle class ladies in 1914, in the aftermath of the Balkan wars (1912–1913), as a typical women's philanthropic association, gradually evolved during the interwar period into the main institution that implemented social policy on motherhood and childhood.[2] The League was the first to attempt to provide medical care for children and prospective mothers and the first to disseminate hygiene principles to working-class mothers. As an association combining voluntary participation along with expertise and state surveillance, the Patriotic League of Greek Women stands as a characteristic example of "mixed economy welfare." During its long run, its relation with the state, volunteer networks, and status as an institution underwent numerous changes. We can discern in the history of the League three stages: the voluntary stage until 1922; the 'semi-state' stage from 1922 until 1940, when part of the action, as opposed to voluntary action, had been undertaken by the Ministry of Health and Welfare; and finally, the postwar period when the League was absorbed by the state.[3] The stages were due to changing discussion over whether or not working-class welfare should be state-dependent and due to internal politics.

---

2 *Katastatikon tou Patriotikou Syndesmou ton Ellinidon, Anegnorismenou Somateiou Idrythentos ti Ypsili Protovoulia tis A.M. tis Vasilissis kai Proedrevomenou par'aftis.* B' Kanonismoi ton Tmimaton, Athens 1915.

3 For a brief history of the League, see Anonymos, "Idrysis kai Istorikon tou PIPP," *To Paidi,* no. 23 (January–February 1934): 35–9.

The National Schism which left its mark on Greek political history for the first half of the twentieth century also had an impact on the League. The frequent changes in its administrative board, altered goals, and name change from 1917 until 1929 testify to this impact. The term Patriotic League of Greek Women was in use during the "royal" phases, while it was renamed to the Patriotic Foundation of Welfare by anti-royalist liberal governments. Although the League began operating in 1914 as a volunteer movement headed by the Queen, it was dissolved three years later and re-established as a welfare foundation associated with the Ministry of Welfare, a new department introduced by Venizelos's government.

According to its constitution, the aim of the Patriotic League of Greek Women was to organize women's philanthropy more methodically, adopting new principles of the so-called "practical" social policy. Behind these general declarations, an ambitious aid plan could be discerned. This plan was based on the well-known nineteenth century schemata of women's philanthropy as well as on the experience women had gained as volunteer nurses during the Balkan Wars. The establishment of the League a few months after the outbreak of World War I highlighted the patriotic character women's philanthropy had gained during the war. The frequent drafts during the 1910s made evident the lack of state services for the welfare of conscripts and their families.

This kind of organization depended mainly on volunteer work of active women who worked under the aegis of the royal family. Most of these women came from renowned urban class families. Many were wives or daughters of businessmen and politicians and were experienced philanthropists. Male members were mostly politicians, businessmen and jurists. Later on, doctors and high-ranking state officials were brought in as experts.

The journal issued by the League (Deltion tou Patriotikou Syndesmoy ton Ellinidon) attempted to communicate a different notion of welfare, highlighting the preventive and corrective character of voluntary intervention, as well as the deadlock philanthropy had reached at the beginning of the twentieth century. Modernization focused on the introduction of social work, organized on the basis of scientific methods.[4] The role of women

---

4   Spyros Loverdos, "I Koinoniki Allilengii," *Deltion tou Patriotikou Syndesmou ton Ellinidon*, no. 1 (April 1916): 2–4.

was linked to hygiene in that it could contribute to the preparation of a robust young generation.[5] The League aimed at "transforming this human capital—children suffering from rachitis and ill-kept children of the working class—to healthy mothers of healthy children who would constitute the wealth of the nation."[6] The volunteers' aim when intervening in the lives of the working class was to impart knowledge and practical help, attempting to solve the problems they faced at their source rather than simply providing financial aid. For instance, female League volunteers made health inspections of working-class families' aiming to both disseminate practical hygiene advice to women and to inform the authorities about the prevalence of contagious diseases such as TB.[7]

Aid to the poor, however, was not out of the question. It came as medical care or the distribution of food, provided that the real needs of the family had been properly assessed. The foundation of hospitals, the establishment of employment agencies and the providing of wholesome food to workers were methods thought to go hand-in-hand with the new mentality of philanthropic aid and its principles of solidarity. In times of peace, the League's hygiene division worked systematically to fight diseases; raise youth in better conditions, i.e., founding nurseries, kindergartens and open-air schools; and prepare working-class woman to better cope with the harsh difficulties of their lives.

The League's aims were two-fold. On the one hand, it aimed to meet urgent war needs such as the preparation of hospital clothing, the instruction of nurses and the treatment of wounded soldiers. The League was expecting to assist the Red Cross in these respects.[8] On the other hand, it also aimed to cover chronic shortages. The League was expected to take even wider action in peace times. League members would cover a wide spectrum of needs, not only related to welfare but also at the education of the work-

5   *Deltion tou Patriotikou Syndesmou ton Ellinidon*, no.1 (April 1916): 1.

6   Eleni Logothetopoulou, "I Koinoniki Simasia tis Gynaikeias Ergasias," *Deltion tou Patriotikou Syndesmou ton Ellinidon*, no. 1 (April 1916): 4–7.

7   The institution of the female inspector was widely spread at the beginning of the twentieth century in Germany and France, where she was considered an invaluable assistant to the doctor in so far that she helped him eradicate superstition. See Yvette Knibielhler, "La 'lutte antituberculeuse,' instrument de médicalization des classes populaires (1870–1930)," *Annales de Bretagne et des pays de l'Ouest* 86 no. 3 (1979): 320–35.

8   For the aims of the Patriotic League, see *Deltion tou Patriotikou Syndesmou ton Ellinidon*, no. 1 (April 1916): 1.

ing-class. During this period the protection of the poor was frequently mor-
alized through campaigns against "alcohol and other harmful substances"
and the "protection of the unprotected young ladies in big urban centers."
The most active of the so-called "departments of peace" dealt with the organization of soup kitchens in various Athenian neighborhoods, the provision
of work opportunities to poor women, the establishment of medical consultation stations for mothers and children, and the spread of hygiene principles among working-class families.

1.2 Political Changes and Priorities during and after the Great War

After the Allied naval blockade in November 1916, the League intensified
its efforts to combat disease and nutrition deficits, in order to contain acute
social problems such as unemployment, rising prices, and lack of food and
fuel. During the same period the League began collaborating with international charity organizations. The League took emergency measures to
strengthen people's weak constitutions, providing more soup kitchens and
dry milk powder for infants. The League carried out mass vaccinations in
Athens to stamp out the smallpox epidemic and offered additional medical care for infants, expecting that these efforts would combat the epidemics that had broken out during the war. In order to confront the financial
problems of the working-class families during this rough period, the League
distributed ration coupons for bread and "the automatic cooking pots"—a
type of wooden crate coated with straw where the cooking pot was placed—
which were suggested by the League's housekeeping division and designed
to save women's time and energy. Because many fathers were fighting at
the front, mothers had to work to make ends meet. A kindergarten was established in Athens to answer the problem of children's daily care that this
change caused.

Between 1916 and 1922, successive political changes affected the League.
Royalist administrative boards and boards leaning towards Venizelos suc-
ceeded one another in League's leadership. In 1917, when Venizelos was in
power, the League dissolved and the Patriotic Foundation of Welfare (Pa-
triotikon Idrima Perithalpseos) was set up in its place. The Foundation was
transformed from a voluntary society under the Queen's supervision into a
semi-state organization that combined state welfare with private initiative.

The Foundation, which now operated under the auspices of the Ministry of Social Relief, was directed by a board affiliated with Venizelos's party appointed by the Minister himself.

The Foundation's efforts intensified during the Great War, when special war divisions were set up. The problems that the war brought about affected the families of the conscripts and became indelibly imprinted on the Foundation's aims. The mission of the newly established Foundation was to provide relief to the conscripts and their families, natural disaster victims, the destitute and the sick, and unprotected women and children. Many of its old divisions were maintained, such as the division for the poor and the soup kitchen division, and were extended to various Athenian slums. Apart from food distribution—mainly rice, pasta and Nestlé condensed milk—the division for the poor distributed clothes and stipends, provided medical care in special dispensaries that ran in the capital, and gave free hospitalization to the poor. The soup kitchen division ran three kitchens in central areas in Athens and had seven distribution points in Athenian neighborhoods that offered either low-price or free meals to working-class families, provided they had special permission. Special care was taken for destitute breast-feeding mothers who were given meals free of charge in the Foundation's restaurants according to lists drawn up by its medical board.

During this period, the organization of soup kitchens for children became more systematic. Providing healthy food, "specially prepared for weak or sickly children, who could not afford a special diet," offering free medical care and medication, establishing a sun-therapy clinic at the schoolchildren's polyclinic, and open-air schools, were all efforts that very vividly illustrate the new Hygiene Division administration's interest in strengthening weak children's constitutions. The Foundation was orientated towards the welfare of childhood, especially infancy. Its establishment of the first nursery with the support of the American Red Cross, two kindergartens, and a children's asylum where poor working mothers could leave their children testify to that fact.

The Foundation also attempted to provide welfare services to children outside of Greece, namely in parts of the Ottoman Empire where there was a strong Greek presence. The favorable outcome for Greece at the end of the Great War seems to have led to the decision to extend welfare provisions to the areas of the Eastern Thrace and Asia Minor that the Greeks believed—

as they had been assured by the Allies—would come under Greek dominion. Officials, urban class ladies from Athens and the doctor Apostolos Doxiadis went to Constantinople, Eastern Thrace and Pontus from April 19 to May 20, 1919. They intended to examine the problems of Greeks in those areas and recommend steps for the relief of orphans, the repatriation of the expatriated inhabitants of Thrace and Pontus, and the distribution of aid to the poor.

While they were in Constantinople, the Central Foundation of Relief was established to carry out social relief work for children, particularly orphans. This new Foundation would serve not only humanitarian aims, but also contribute to solidifying national bonds with Greeks living in areas that were to be annexed to Greece. In 1920, Apostolos Doxiadis, who was in charge of the hygiene organization in Constantinople, petitioned the city's Chief Commander to establish welfare institutions in Thrace. A very active doctor and politician who played an important role in Greece's hygiene policies in the interwar period, Doxiadis believed that the objective of social policy for public health was not only the fight against the disease but also the emergence of a future generation "able to carry out its victorious cultural cause."

Political changes affected once more the course of the Patriotic Foundation of Welfare and the type of relief it offered. Its means of operation changed following the defeat of Venizelos in the national elections of November 1920. In August 1921, the Patriotic Foundation of Welfare was abolished and the Patriotic League of Greek Women was reinstated. The replacement of the administration board with royalists testifies to the interconnectedness of welfare institutions with politics. This time, however, the League was generously subsidized by the state, a fact that further strengthened the semi-state character the old charity organization had already taken on since the last Venizelos's government. Because the Asia Minor expedition in 1920 prolonged warfare, the League laid emphasis upon the relief of reserves and their families and hygiene care for infants.

2. Novelties and Institutions for Children

Among the works undertaken by the League, hygiene education was the most important and was attempted through lectures on hygiene and the publication of leaflets on preventing contagious diseases. Apart from these pedagogical efforts, the Department of Hygiene collaborated with the School Hygiene Service of the Ministry of Education to provide welfare services that the state was unable to offer. They collaborated to establish a polyclinic for schoolchildren in Athens, summer camps and an open air school for pre-tubercular children.

2.1 Schoolchildren's Polyclinics

In November 1915, due to the efforts of Lambadarios and funding from the League, a polyclinic for school children began operation in the center of Athens.[9] Schoolchildren's polyclinics were already operating in certain European capitals for the treatment of poor students with funding from state or the local municipalities.[10] The schoolchildren's polyclinic in Lucerne might have provided a model for the schoolchildren's polyclinic in Athens, as Lambadarios was likely to have become familiar with this polyclinic when he was studying in Switzerland.[11]

The schoolchildren's polyclinic in Athens was comprised of five clinics: General Pathology, Surgery, Ophthalmology, Dentistry and Orthopedics clinics. The polyclinic was open two hours a day and was supervised by the director of the Hygiene Department. The polyclinic admitted destitute students, who either attended school in Athens and were sent there for treatment by their head teacher or school doctor, or were out-patient students from the provinces. Apart from treatment and medical supervision provided free of charge or for very little money, poor students were eligible for free medication, special bandages, glasses and toothbrushes as well.[12]

The doctor of each clinic had to keep registers of cured patients with students' name and age, as well as the occupation of their parents, dwelling place, grade, school, and case-history. Head teachers were prompted to refer

---

9   For the organization of the schoolchildren polyclinic, see *Patriotikos Syndesmos ton Ellinidon, Ekthesis ton Pepragmenon ypo tou Tmimatos tis Ygieinis 1915* (Athens: 1916) and for the results of the anti-trachoma cause during this period see Emmanouil Lambadarios, *Skholiki Ygieini meta Stoikheion Paidologias*, 312–14.

10 For the evolution of the schoolchildren polyclinic institution in England and the debate on its cost, see J. David Hirst, "The Growth of Treatment through the School Medical Service, 1908–18," *Medical History* no. 33 (1989): 318–42.

11 *Patriotikos Syndesmos ton Ellinidon, Ekthesis ton Pepragmenon ypo tou Tmimatos tis Ygieinis, 1915* (Athens: 1916), 9.

12 See *Organismos tis Mathitikis Polyklinikis Athinon* (Athens: 1915), 4 in the unclassified archive of Emmanouil Lambadarios, ELIA.

to doctors only the students who were certified as poor. Lambadarios, the leading spirit of this venture, was appointed director of the polyclinic and undertook its organization during the first period of its operation from 1915 to 1921. Well-known doctors and school doctors staffed the various clinics such as Ioannis Fassanelis in charge of the ophthalmological clinic, Apostolos Doxiadis in charge of the GP clinic, and Mikhail Khryssafis in charge of the orthopedic clinic. The polyclinic system was expanded to other cities as well. A similar polyclinic for students opened in Piraeus in 1918, initially comprising two clinics—GP and ophthalmological—while a third one with six clinics was founded in Smyrna in June 1919 at the expense of the Patriotic League, following the landing of the Greek army in Smyrna. The work of the Patriotic League on hygiene issues was supplemented with vaccinations and welfare work for weak students, and lectures on popular medicine organized by the doctors of the clinics.

Lambadarios's annual reports for the period 1915–1921 shed light on the way schoolchildren polyclinics operated. According to these reports, schoolchildren's polyclinics were invaluable in that they fought certain diseases and offered financial support to poor families in Athens and Piraeus at the beginning of the twentieth century. They also made it possible for Lambadarios to supplement the work of the School Hygiene Service by attempting to implement for the very first time systematic provision of medical care to students based on their parents' income. The fight against trachoma, the providing of orthopedic equipment, the examination and selection of weak children sent to summer camps, the supply of substantial amounts of food, dental care and the treatment of myopia were important forms of aid for the families of students who were unable to afford the cost of treatment. The rate at which the public responded to the polyclinics reveals the extent of financial problems the students' families faced; their success rendered them undoubtedly exemplary of their kind.[13]

From November to December of 1915, 1,316 students visited the Athens polyclinic. Tonic medication, milk and meat were distributed to strengthen weak and pre-tubercular children admitted to the GP clinic during this pe-

---

13 "Our country is able to be proud because thanks to the institution of the school doctor it acquired the well-run schoolchildren polyclinics from very early on; among them, the schoolchildren polyclinic in Athens is a model polyclinic" in Lambadarios, *Stoikheia Skholikis Ygieinis*, 357.

riod.[14] Moreover, quinine injections were administered systematically to fifteen students suffering from malaria and one hundred and fifty arsenic injections were given to those with TB symptoms. The latter were also given special instructions on the improvement of their diet. As stressed by the polyclinic's annual report for the year 1915, the clinic's primary aim was the fight against TB through the detection of pre-tubercular children and the prevention of the spread of the disease.

In the following years the clientele of the polyclinic increased and the student clinics became better organized. Between 1915 and 1920, a total of 11,577 students were provided medical care between the three polyclinics. During the school year of 1919–1920, 1,421 students visited the Athens polyclinic, another 1,233 the Piraeus polyclinic while the polyclinic in Smyrna admitted 5,305 children irrespective of race and religion.[15] According to the annual report for the year 1920, the patients admitted to the polyclinic in Athens were mostly students aged 5–16, with some poor teachers and working women and quite a few male and female students of the Teacher Training College (Didaskaleion). Apart from medication and instructions, foodstuff—rice, milk and spaghetti—and soap were distributed to many young patients. In 1919, no serious epidemic disease hit the student population while in the previous year flu had run rampant among students. However, Lambadarios considered malaria, trachoma and various adenopathies, due to their extent, the most alarming phenomena.

In 1916 and 1917, malaria turned into a pandemic due to the settlement of the refugees and the movement of the population, especially in Macedonia, claiming many victims among students. Around 1920, the average mortality rate due to malaria was 9.4% per 10,000 inhabitants while in other European countries it ranged between 0.7% and 1.58%. In certain areas of Epirus, Thessaly and Attica these rates were alarming because the disease debilitated child constitutions, making them susceptible to other ailments.[16] In 1919, according to the director of the polyclinic, half to two thirds of the sick children admitted during the first three months afflicted with malaria, the majority of whom resided in the neighborhoods surrounding the Ilis-

14 *Patriotikos Syndesmos ton Ellinidon*, 5.
15 Emmanouil Lambadarios, "I Kinisis ton Mathitikon Polyklinikon Athinon, Pireos, Smyrnis tou Patriotikou Idrymatos Perithalpseos: A' Ekthesis peri ton Ergasion tis Mathitikis Polyklinikis kata to Skholikon Etos 1919–1920," *Paidologia* no. 6 (August 1920): 141–43.
16 Fokion Kopanaris, *I Dimosia Ygeia en Elladi* (Athens, 1933), 200–5.

sos river. For their treatment 27,671 quinine pills, quinine and tonic injections were administered. Generally, malaria, which affected 41% of the sick students in the 1920s, was dealt with quinine and ample advice. Doctors drew the attention of people inhabiting marshy areas or in areas with large amounts of stagnant water to the use of simple means for individual and general prophylaxis. In the instructions issued by Kardamatis in 1919, he mentions the cleansing of stagnant waters and the use of mosquito-nets "as an effective means, which was used in Macedonia by the Allied forces during the Great War."[17]

The highest percentage of students who visited the ophthalmological clinic suffered from trachoma, a disease which, as shown from the statistics, was rampant and in certain districts afflicted 3/5 of the students.[18] Out of 1,233 students who were admitted in the ophthalmological clinic in Piraeus 844 (70%) suffered from trachoma. In some areas of Attica, the percentage of students suffering from the disease amounted to 25–28%, causing alarm that the contagion might spread to the capital.[19] People's defiance of personal hygiene in every way, poorly educated parents, wretched living conditions and the difficulty of isolating students with trachoma in school, all contributed to the increase of affected cases. The high rates of soldiers who were relieved of duty due to trachoma, which ran from 40–55%, are indicative of the state's indifference to the disease.

Therefore, the main reason for the establishment of the ophthalmological clinic was the treatment of students afflicted with trachoma who were excluded from school and hung about in the streets, unable to receive systematic treatment due to poverty. The indifference of their parents, who did not see that their children needed systematic treatment, aggravated the students' condition, which could even result in loss of sight.[20] For parents, their children's temporary exclusion from school due to illness meant that they could drop out of school permanently and get jobs in shops, factories and

17 Lambadarios, *Kodix Skholikis Ygieinis*, 305–11.

18 In certain schools "no student was delivered from them," see Savvas, "Peri Idryseos Ypourgeiou Ygeias kai Koinonikis Pronoias," 70.

19 Ioannis Fassanelis, *Ta Pepragmena kata to Skholikon Etos 1914–1915*, 10–11.

20 Lambadarios felt somewhat bitter about the attitude of parents of students who suffered from trachoma; these parents were pleased because they managed to circumvent mandatory education and therefore gain some income from the work of their afflicted children. See "Odigiai peri Prophylaxeos apo tou Trakhomatos (dia to Koinon)," in the unclassified archive of Emmanouil Lambadarios, *Hellenic Literary and Historical Archive* (ELIA).

offices. Children did do this, and mingling with other persons in the work place then contributed to the proliferation of the disease. The treatment administered to these children once admitted to the polyclinics led to a reduction in the number of victims. However, there were cases of patients who discontinued treatment, causing the disease to spread.

Since its inception the School Hygiene Service issued special instructions for the diagnosis, protection and isolation of students affected by trachoma, which were addressed to teachers and proposed that these students be segregated in a special classroom. Entrance to this classroom "as well as to the taps, lavatories and gym equipment for students with trachoma"[21] had to be different from the ones used by unaffected students. Since 1915, the Ophthalmological Clinic at the schoolchildren's polyclinic had undertaken the treatment of hundreds of destitute students. The polyclinic decreased the number of students affected by trachoma: in its first year 35% of the patients admitted to the ophthalmological surgery were students with trachoma, while in the second year it was only 19%, and in the third year the percentage came down to 10%. Trachoma was in decline around 1920, however, upon the arrival of the refugees it ran rampant again, this time among students living in refugee slums.

2.2 TB: the Scourge of Children

The operation of the schoolchildren's polyclinic was invaluable for the prevention of the third, and most important, school scourge: TB. One of the aims of the GP clinic had been the detection of suspected TB cases. The high rate of tubercular teachers and children made TB one of the greatest, yet invisible adversaries of childhood. The resistance of bacillus, the lack of hygienic living conditions and, most importantly, the lack of sanitary conditions at school combined with the defiance of hygiene rules by the majority of tubercular patients maximized the possibility of youths being infected. Research, which had been carried out by the Department of School Hygiene according to Pirquet method of skin-reaction among school students in Athens in 1917, showed that the percentage of students with positive reaction to TB bacillus ranged from 24.5% for children aged 6–5 to

---

21 Lambadarios, *Stoikheia Skholikis Ygieinis*, 313.

89.95% for adolescents aged 16–18.[22] At the beginning of the twentieth century, the medical press frequently featured articles confirming the spread of disease among children as they grew older. Popular lectures, organized by various voluntary societies, and articles in the daily press underlined the insidious manner in which TB developed "in the tender constitutions of children" due to overcrowding in the classroom and atrocious living conditions.

The factors that favored the transmission of the virus in classrooms could not be controlled by the means the doctors had at their disposal at the time, and treatment of the disease was rarely successful once the disease reached advanced stage. As already noted, the anti-TB campaign at schools put emphasis on prevention, detection of the suspects and isolation of the diseased. The proposal of the French TB specialist, Jacques-Joseph Grancher, to "save the seed," namely the future generation, was adopted as a slogan by Greek school doctors.[23] Grancher's Greek counterparts often highlighted the influential research he had done on TB among French students.

One of the primary aims of the Pan-Hellenic Association since 1912 was to rescue tubercular children. The idea of founding a "seaside health convalescent home" appeared frequently in their annual reports on TB since 1907. In 1919, thanks to the donation of Lady Gramvill [24] the Asclepius convalescent home (Asklipeiion Paidon), was set up in the seaside area of Voula close to Athens, where destitute children afflicted with skeletal TB were hospitalized.[25] An improvised hospital was set up in a building lot allotted by the Church Fund; three prefabricated wooden sheds, used by the English Military Authorities in Macedonia during the Great War, made up the hospital building. Children afflicted with bone TB were admitted in the Asclepius convalescent home with preference given to soldiers' children, provided the latter's financial state permitted it. The Pan-Hellenic League against TB, which supervised the operation of the Asclepius convalescent home, had a sun infirmary installed and hired a doctor and a nurse to deal specifically

---

22 Lambadarios, *Stoikheia Skholikis Ygieinis*, 305.

23 Lambadarios invoked Grancher's view who proposed that children living in a tubercular family environment be removed and sent to the countryside; there they could be accommodated in peasant families. Lambadarios was also one of the very first doctors that applied BCG vaccination to newborns; See Emmanouil Lambadarios, "I en Elladi Efarmogi tou Antiphymatikou Emvoliou BCG en Elladi,"*Praktika tou Synedriou gia tin Prostasia tis Paidikis Ilikias kai tis Mitrotitas* (Athens: 1930), 358–85.

24 Wife to the English ambassador in Athens at the time.

25 For the foundation of the Asclepius Convalescent Home, see Panellinios Syndesmos kata tis Phymatioseos, *Ta ypo tou Syndesmou Pepragmena* (January 1–December 31, 1919) (Athens: 1920), 4–5.

with the treatment of operative TB cases. Every year seventy to eighty children in average were hospitalized in the Asclepius convalescent home. Between 1920 and 1922, 19% of the children died, and 20% were cured, while the condition of the remainder was stagnant. Unable to cover the cost, the League transferred the Asclepius convalescent home to the Red Cross.

As only a small percentage of tubercular children were cured, the medical interest turned to fixing children's susceptible constitutions that were prone to the disease, namely general weakness, lephatism, adenopathy and scrofula. Statistics compiled at the beginning of the twentieth century show high numbers of children with these illnesses. In 1919, out of 1,038 Athenian students who visited the GP clinic at the schoolchildren polyclinic, 23% were categorized as having a "weak constitution," i.e., they suffered from general weakness, chronic malaria, lephatism, starvation, scrofula, etc. Another 10% were found to suffer from adenopathy and another 12% from anaemia. Their cases were indicative of the deficient nutrition and adverse living conditions the students had.

School doctors underlined the social causes that led to the weakening of the constitution. Their concern is evident in the relevant documents they completed. Statistics on student morbidity and the health cards filled in by the doctors of the polyclinic included a certain column where information about social parameters such as the hygienic condition of the student's residence, the family's finances, father's occupation and the number of rooms in their home was entered. According to the reports of some government functionaries, the hygienic conditions of the student's residence in combination with poor personal hygiene and deficient nutrition were responsible for the spread of diseases.

At the beginning of the twentieth century the relationship between disease and living conditions was becoming commonplace not only in the writings of social thinkers but also in the language of bureaucracy. Nutrition and residence were two of the indices that recurred in the study of the living conditions of the working-class living, which were examined in correlation with income. During the 1910s, the health inspectors highlighted in their reports the connection between working-class people's high morbidity and mortality rates and their nutrient deficient diet. The working-class's insufficient income caused malnutrition. Consumption of poor quality bread and legumes plus limited consumption of luxury goods like meat, fish, milk and sugar left their constitutions vulnerable to TB.

The housing problem in urban centers—mainly in Athens and Piraeus—which had already been aggravated before the refugees' influx from Asia Minor, further worsened people's living conditions. Because of internal migration and population displacement during the Balkan Wars and the Great War, the number of available residences could not meet the demand. According to primary sources, a considerable number of large families were packed in one-room dwellings already in 1914. "Down with the holes" became a recurrent slogan in many contemporary publications.

In a 1913 report a work superintendent underlined the terrible hygienic condition of the sunless, underground homes of the working-class in industrial centers as well as the relationship of this type of residence to contagious diseases.[26] Doctors of the Pan-Hellenic Association against TB, who visited patients' houses only to find out that many tubercular parents shared the same bed with their children, reached similar conclusions.[27] In 1921, according to a research by a work superintendent, more than 75% of the working class homes in Athens only had one room, 20% two rooms and the rest three rooms. Similar statistics were found in Piraeus. These one-room houses accommodated four to five people in average. 40% of these houses were found unhygienic and therefore unsuitable for habitation, many had just one window and very few had a kitchen. Moreover, many of these houses were old and dilapidated.

Diet and residence were the central concerns of the Pan-Hellenic Association against TB. Apart from information leaflets, its members had been distributing foodstuff since 1913 and defraying poor tubercular families' rents. Mingling of many people in the same place was considered one of the reasons for TB transmission and since many had not been convinced of the contagiousness of TB, the isolation of patients was thought to be a deterrent to the disease's spread. The foundation of a "sanatorium for the destitute tubercular" in a pine forest near Piraeus in April 1906 was an attempt to undercut the "rapid spread of the horrid disease due to the mingling of the healthy with the tubercular in the same room."[28] In addition, many people refused

---

26 "Genikai Ektheseis ton Epitheoriton Ergasias tou Etous 1913," *Deltion tou Ypourgeiou Ethnikis Oikonomias* 4 (December 1914): 178, in Mikhalis Riginos, *Paragogikes Domes kai Ergatika Imeromisthia stin Ellada, 1909–1936*, 248.

27 Panellinios Syndesmos kata tis Phymatioseos (Phthyseos), *Ta ypo tou Syndesmou Pepragmena* (January 1–December 31, 1916), (Athens: 1917), 4.

28 "Idrysis Apomonotiriou dia tous Phthisiontas en Peiraiei," *Akropolis* April 27, 1916, 3.

to follow doctors' suggestions, neither destroying the clothes of tubercular patients nor disinfecting their houses.

The high rate of TB and scrofula among students and young people generally, among those who visited the surgery of the Pan-Hellenic Association against TB between 1906 and 1926, justified the concern of many members of the medical community over the health of youth. In 1915, the Minister of Education Kharalambos Bozikis wrote a letter to school doctors and educators, attempting to make them aware of the measures that were "the first and most important stage of the scientific defense against TB." These measures involved "providing supplementary nutritional food to needy students; distributing school meals; sending the suspects of coming down with TB to children's colonies."[29]

2.3 The First Trips of Children to Countryside

The School Hygiene Service tried to secure the necessary means to prevent disease by defending people's constitutions, such as plenty of good quality food, rest and clean air. The removal of children with weak constitutions from the germ-infested environment of the town to the countryside was the central idea not only to rescue children's health but also for the community's protection from disease. Influenced by Grancher, doctors advocated for the removal of pre-tubercular children from the unsanitary conditions of the city by sending them to seaside asylums, prevantoriums, summer camps, and open-air schools, ideas that had been tested in other countries. In the 1910s, the idea of sending children to the countryside gained ground in the medical community. The various charity societies that had launched the anti-TB campaign and Greek doctors who had participated in congresses on the study of TB favored the same idea.

Lambadarios was a fervent advocate of the "mountainous or seaside dwellings," children's colonies and open-air schools. Despite the meagre financial means of the Ministry of Education, he attempted to build them with support from women's charities. The first summer camps began in Vouliagmeni in 1911 by Sofia Schliemann, the wife of the renowned archaeologist Heinrich Schliemann, with financial support from the "Association for the

---

29   Panellinios Syndesmos kata tis Phymatioseos (Phthiseos), *Logodosia 1915* (Athens: 1916), 17.

Protection of Children." Earlier, in 1905, Schliemann had financed the construction of the first sanatorium (Sotiria Sanatorium) in a countryside suburb in Athens. Sending sickly children to the countryside was necessary to provide them with "sun, air, meals and sea-therapy."[30] The 212 children aged 8–12, chosen by Lambadarios among the Athenian students for the sanatorium, bore symptoms of malnutrition, weakness, and anaemia, as well as thorax, limb and spine deformities. These children spent twenty-one days in the countryside, an amount of time considered necessary for their recovery according to paedologists in the Geneva Congress. Prolonging their stay in the countryside might have affected negatively the morale of the little "colonists," since they lacked their parents' emotional support there.

Two simple sheds were constructed to accommodate the children. They were able to take strolls in the countryside, play, exercise and bath in the sea. The bathing, sunbathing, and exercise were regulated by a schedule enforced with whistles, which had been drawn up by doctors in order to strengthen the children's constitution. The children's stay in the countryside, however, was not entirely free from education. Apart from learning how to swim, they also learned outdoors botany and physics, which were taught in a simple, easy to understand language.

The children's diet, designed by Lambadarios, attempted to provide them with nutritional food. It included meat three times a week and plenty of carbohydrates and fruit.[31] Before their departure from the camp, children were examined by the doctor and the results were entered in personal cards. The successful increase in their weight, height and thorax circumference provided good reasons to build more such camps. The students' height increased by twelve centimeters on average (as compared to the standard for their age which was five centimeters), while their weight increase ranged from 620 to 938 grams for the majority of children (90.1% of the children).[32]

---

30 For the positive results of this first child mission, see Emmanouil Lambadarios, *Organosis ton Paidikon Exokhon Vouliagmenis kata tin 4etian 1911–1914* (Athens: 1915). In 1912, during the second Pan-Hellenic congress against TB, which took place in Volos, Lambadarios underlined the therapeutic results of the first open-air camp. See "Organosis kai Therapeftika Apotelesmata tis A' Ellinikis en Vouliagmeni Paidikis Exokhis," *Praktika tou B' Ellinikou Synedriou kata tis Phymatioseos, en Volo 20–23 Maiou 1912* (Volos: 1912), 243–60.

31 Emmanouil Lambadarios, "Organosis kai Therapeftika Apotelesmata," 253.

32 Lambadarios, "Organosis kai Therapeftika Apotelesmata," 257–58.

A similar venture to the camp was undertaken by the Patriotic League of Greek Women in 1920. It was not the first time that the League took interest in children. Already in 1915 the League attempted to strengthen destitute "pre-tubercular" students in Athens by distributing meat and milk.[33] In 1920 the League set up a summer camp at the Faliros Delta, a seaside area near Athens.[34] The facilities of the camp were portable. Every morning children rode the bus to the camp grounds where they rest, played, exercised, swam, ate and then returned to the city center in the afternoon. According to the organizers, following this system, education, entertainment and medical treatment were successfully combined. During the children's stay at the camp doctors inspected them. The weight, height and thorax circumference of the campers were entered in personal cards as was the case with the open-air camp in Vouliagmeni, with measurements taken before and after holidays had started.

Due to their small number and their temporary and private funding, the camps could not have permanent therapeutic results against TB. In the 1920s, the head of the School Hygiene Service insisted on establishing permanent infrastructure for student welfare with state funding. These plans saw materialization a few years later under Venizelos's liberal government.

2.4 The First Open-air School

At the beginning of the twentieth century, the institution of open-air schools, established for children suffering from TB, combining medical supervision with special pedagogy, was becoming wide spread in many European cities. In Greece, open-air schools were put forward as a solution for TB for the very first time in 1912 by Dimitrios Saratsis, a doctor with socialist leanings, in the second Pan-Hellenic Congress on TB.[35] Three years later Lambadarios submitted a proposal to the Patriotic League of Greek Women for the foundation of an open-air school, in Patisia, on the outskirts of Athens. He presented this institution as the most important method to help children who were already in the early stages of the disease.[36] He had the chance to study the way open-air schools when he visited some in other

---

33 Patriotikos Syndesmos Ellinidon, *Ekthesis ton Pepragmenon ypo tou Tmimatos tis Ygieinis, 1915* (Athens: 1916), 5.
34 Patriotikos Syndesmos Ellinidon, *I Paidiki Exokhi Falirou, Theros 1921* (Athens: 1922), 3.
35 Dimitris Saratsis, "O dia tou Skholeiou Agon kata tis Phthiseos: Ipaithria Skholeia," 110–41.
36 Emmanouil Lambadarios, *Ipaithria Skholeia* (Athens: 1923), 42.

European countries in 1912.[37] This visit, together with the experience he acquired from organizing the open-air camps, enabled him to later publish a study on open-air schools.[38] Supported by the Ministry of Education, the members of the League decided to run an open-air school on a trial basis during the summer of 1916.

The open-air school opened in May 16, 1916 in an "enclosed orchard," in the area of Patisia on municipal or "Nomikou" property. The area met the requirements of having a healthy climate, clean water and being a short distance from the city. The student's had easy access to the suburb of Patisia, away from the dust and bustle of the city. Students could reach Patisia by tram, with no need to travel long distances or cross city streets filled with dust, dirt and noise, straining their lungs and nervous system. The fruit-bearing trees, the pine trees and the plants offered a tranquil and pleasant environment, similar to the school in Mylhouse, which Lambadarios had visited in 1912 and possibly was a model for his own venture.

Lambadarios chose fifty male and female students himself from the primary schools of Athens to spend time in this flowering and shadowy orchard, from 7.00 a.m. to 7.00 p.m., complying with sanitation rules. The school required to complicated buildings. Wooden benches and big umbrellas were placed in the pine wood. Certain prerequisites for the open-air school, like sheds for the children to take shelter in case it rained and showers were not adopted for financial reasons. It is worth noting that this open-air school was the first to implement mixed gender schooling in Greece.

In this special school, ran in the shade of trees by two teachers and a doctor, teaching hours were no more than three per day. The doctors considered avoiding mental strain crucial to improve the children's physical condition. They took care to attune the school's programme to "the natural laws the development of the child brain follows." Students were divided in groups according to age and were taught in the open air following the principles of the object lesson. Teachers put great emphasis upon subjects that allowed movement and pleasure, such as singing and gym classes, subjects thought

---

37 Together with his professor at the University of Basel H. Griesbach had attended the operation of such a school in Mulhouse, Emmanouil Lambadarios, *Ipaithria Skholeia*, 10.

38 Emmanouil Lambadarios, *Ta Pepragmena tis Mathitikis Polyklinikis gia to Etos 1916*, in the unclassified archive of Emmanouil Lambadarios, ELIA. The task of publishing this study was assigned to him by Queen Sofia. As seen from his written notes, found in his personal records, Lambadarios completed his study on the open-air schools in 1918. It was finally brought out in 1923.

to improve children's health through increased blood circulation and exercise of the lungs.

At Lambadarios suggestion, great attention was given to the menu since food was one of the most important remedial factors. Five meals were distributed from 8.00 a.m. until 6.30 p.m. and included among other things pasta, meat, vegetables, legumes, fruit, bread and cheese. The doctor who was responsible for the organization of the school meals also decided on individual children's diet when occasion arose. In the afternoon children spent their time resting. This light educational programme, which according to the press was received with enthusiasm by the children, was supplemented with work in the garden and excursions.

Despite the encouraging results—an average increase of 2.3 kg in the children's weight in a period of two months—the school shut down in July.[39] A heat wave and sudden weather changes did not permit teaching outdoors any longer. The school did not resume work although the Queen's architect had been commissioned to construct special sheds, based on the model of the open school in Rome. Abrupt rise in prices of essentials[40] might have contributed to the cancellation, but it was mainly the political upheaval caused by the Great War that led to the National Split and the naval blockade of Piraeus. The Ministry's plan to set up more open-air schools running round the year, often mentioned in the press,[41] also did not materialize. During the winter of 1916–1917, the increase in prices of essentials due to the blockade and the lack of basic foodstuffs, even of bread, worsened many delicate children's health.

In spite of the adverse political circumstances, plans for the foundation of a permanent open-air school that would operate in the same grounds were not abandoned, at least by Lambadarios. Together with Dimitris Glinos and Alexander Delmouzos, he laid down the charter of the Open-air School. The experience Lambadarios had gained from the two-month operation of the open-air school at Patisia played an important role in drawing the charter. Although it is not precisely clear when the charter was drawn, it can be assumed to have been between 1917–1920. At this time, the archi-

---

39 Lambadarios, *Skholiki Ygieini meta Stoicheion Paidologia*s, 386.
40 On July, 1 1916 prices of the basic foodstuffs–meat, milk and fish–went up. See "Akriveia,"*Ethnos*, July 1,1916, 1.
41 "Ta Ipaithria Skholeia," *Athens*, June 23, 1916, 2 and "Ta Ipaithria," *Ethnos*, June 24, 1916, 2.

tects of the educational reform served in the Ministry of Education; Glinos as General Secretary and Delmouzos as Supreme Inspector of Education in the Ministry of Education.

Support for the open air-school venture from the advocates of the demotic language Dimitris Glinos and Alexander Delmouzos poses the question of their relationship to the open-air school movement. Both of them studied pedagogics in Germany when reform trends were at their peak. During his studies at the University of Jena, Glinos attended experimental pedagogy lectures by W. Rein. In June 1909 he visited the open-air school set up in the woods in Haubinda by Hermann Lietz,[42] Rein's student.[43] Alexander Delmouzos might have also attended classes by Rein during his stay in Jena[44] and have visited the open-air school "Schloss Bieberstein" run by Lietz.[45] Lambadarios and Glinos knew each other since 1913, when both of them worked in the teacher training college. Their relationship might have become stronger when Glinos, Delmouzos, and Lambadarios collaborated as high-ranking functionaries in the Ministry of Education during their creative period from 1917–1920. Other Greek pedagogues influenced by the New Education movement seem to have been informed about these innovative schools founded by Hermann Lietz. Michael Papamavros had worked in the open-air school in Haubinda for eight months in 1918.[46] Miltos Kountouras also spent time in the open-air schools of Hermann Lietz during his trip to Germany in 1925.[47]

The open-air school remained under the jurisdiction and surveillance of the Hygiene Division of the Patriotic Foundation and the supervision of the Ministry of Education and was a full-time primary school. According to the school's charter, the programme of the school was modified to be in tune with the method of the open-air school, which better provided for the distribution of mental work. Some changes, though, signified a new

---

42 Ralf Koerrenz, *Hermann Lietz: Einführung mit zentralen Texten* (Paderborn: Verlag Ferdinand Schöningh, 2011).

43 Dimitris Glinos, *Apanta*, vol. 1: 1890–1910 (Athens: Themelio, 1983), 486–8 and 598. In his notes entitled "A Trip to Landerziehungsheime" (Taxidi sta Landerziehungsheime), he recounted his experience from his short stay in this innovative school.

44 Kharalambos Kharitos, *To Parthenagogeio tou Volou*, vol. 1 (Athens: IAEN, 1989), 238. Ralf Koerrenz, *Hermann Lietz*.

45 As seen from a letter sent to the journal *Noumas*, no. 261 (September 16, 1907): 5–6.

46 He outlined his experience in an article entitled "Dr. Leitz and his work." See Mikhalis Papamavros, *Deltio tou Ekpaideftikou Omilou*, no. 8 (1920): 100–15.

47 Miltos Kountouras, *Kliste ta Skholeia: Ekpaideftika Apanta*, vol. 2 (Athens: Gnosi, 1985), 641.

more sensitive attitude to the social aspects of the disease. The issues with the working-class's housing and nutrition, which certain members of the medical profession had started associating with the spread of disease, were taken into account when Lambadarios, Glinos and Delmouzos drew the charter. Apart from weak students, students who were recovering from acute disease or living in deplorable conditions were also admitted to the open-air school. It was forbidden to admit children that were in the first or second stage of the disease and as such posed the risk of infection. The school's expenses were covered by parents. In case parents were unable to do so, expense were covered by school funds. Parental rights were specified in detail. Parents did not have the right to accompany their child to school or to visit him/her at any given time outside of visiting hours, which were laid down by the supervisory committee. Parents also signed a weaver stating that they would not hold the school responsible "in case of a disease or unfortunate event (i.e., death of the child)."

However, despite the support offered by wider groups of pedagogues, the plan for the open-air school fell through. Venizelos's defeat in the national elections in November 1920, along with financial problems that the state faced after the arrival of refugees from Asia Minor put an end to the education reform. Discussions for the establishment of open-air schools had to be put off until the late 1920s.

3. ACCOMPLISHMENTS AND PROSPECTS IN PUBLIC HEALTH CIRCA 1920

As was the case with other European countries during the Great War, the prolonged warfare contributed to the worse morbidity rates in Greece and raised the pressing question of how the state would organized health services. Around 1920, the social and political conditions favored the establishment of a ministry of health and social welfare. This shift was evident in the preamble of a bill tabled in Parliament a few months after the Sèvres Treaty and just before the defeat of the Liberals in the national elections of November 1920. The preamble included once again the issues raised by high-ranking health officers during the last thirty years. Konstantinos Savvas, one of the introducers of the bill, referred to "the deplorable condition of the public health in all respects" and pinpointed three elements characteristic of the low standard of public health: the high mortality rates due to common diseases; the frequent epidemics of typhus, dysentery, smallpox and scarletina, etc.; and the high numbers of young men who were unable to serve in the army.[48] The preamble highlighted the relationship between the deterioration of youth and the inability to participate in war and work, or have children.

Following the international treaties after the Great War, Greece's population rise due to the annexation of new areas brought forward issues with the physical condition of the people and their value in war. The same preamble dealt with social and health problems on a common basis and included many references to the importance of health as an economic and military asset. The available sources point out that this had been the first time that a law included references to the notion of race in terms of biological capital. As stressed in the text, if the state was unable to equal the "miracle" that had been accomplished in foreign affairs, the Greek people, plagued by various diseases, would languish.

The foundation of the Ministry of Health and Welfare was the very first attempt to unify the various health services, which until then had been run by semi-state organizations and charity foundations. This reorganization included the protection of children and mothers. Indeed, this was the first attempt to organize systematic relief and hygiene care for children from infancy to adolescence. It included birth-related protection (pregnancy, labor, puerperium), the protection of newborns and infants (foundling homes, nurseries, kindergartens), and the protection of students through school meals, open-air schools, student clinics, and the protection of adolescents.

Although ultimately the refugee influx did not permit the establishment, it could be considered the capstone of efforts undertaken to improve child health at the beginning of the twentieth century. Despite meagre funding during the 1910s, the Venizelos government fervently supported the idea of the state taking over children's hygiene. In this light, history of medical supervision and children's care must be approached in the context not only of the social policies employed by the Liberal Party but also of the intended educational reform.

---

48 Savvas, "Ypomnima peri Ydriseos Ypourgeiou Ygeias kai Koinonikis Pronoias," 69.

4. The Greek Paedology Society and the Journal *Paidologia* (Paedology)

The involvement of doctors, sociologists and pedagogues in establishing the Greek Paedology Society and the journal Παιδολογία in 1920 attest to the gradually increasing interest in children's health. The term paedology was first used in Greece in 1912 by Lambadarios when he taught a course at the in-service secondary teacher training college in Athens. As outlined in the Articles of the Society, this wide scientific field included paediatrics, pedagogy, child physiology, child experimental psychology, school hygiene, child criminology, and baby care. According to the editors of the journal, the term paedology denoted the science that examined "all knowledge referring to the child and its development."[49]

The Society's main aim was to raise awareness among Greeks about the significant advances in child sciences in Europe, America and Japan; promote paedological sciences through lectures, lessons and conferences; publish a scientific journal; establish a paedological laboratory and museum; and communicate with respective foreign societies. In addition, the Society would set up model schools and advise the state services, responsible for these schools, to keep up with scientific standards.

The board of the Society directors and the editorial committee of the journal comprised pioneering pediatricians and pedagogues. Christos Malandrinos, professor of pediatrics and rector at the University of Athens, served as president of the board of directors. Emmanouil Lambadarios held the post of vice-president. The pediatrician Kostis Kharitakis was secretary general and the school doctor Ioannis Fassanelis was special secretary. Renowned pedagogues like Aikaterini Varouxaki, Alexandros Delmouzos, Mirsini Kleanthous and doctors such as Marios Geroulanos, Apostolos Doxiadis, Ioannis Khryssafis and George Makkas all served as directors of the board. The journal, though short-lived, served as a forum where its editors presented their views on the New Education movement, school hygiene, and pediatrics. All of them were important members of the Greek intelligentsia who took up state official posts and played leading roles in the promotion of social hygiene for children during the interwar.

---

49 Anonymos, "O Skopos tis Ellinikis Paidologikis Etaireias," *Paidologia* no. 2 (May 1920): 73.

PART II
From Moralization to the Social Turn in Medical Concern
(1922–1935)

CHAPTER V

HEALTH AS A PUBLIC GOOD DURING THE INTERWAR PERIOD

According to Roger Cooter and John Pickstone,[1] the history of public health in interwar Europe reflects wider social changes and is indicative of the level of political development and state efficiency.[2] During the 1920s and 1930s health was gradually becoming a public issue not only because it was linked to major social changes, but because the right of citizens to state welfare was now recognized. Although there had been various suggestions for how to reform public health systems, it is generally argued that citizens' health was a major issue for states in the wake of World War I, affecting the formation of the family and their lives as well as the establishment of communities and nations. In this context, social policy on motherhood and childhood took on a new meaning and new forms that bore the stamp of state intervention and international collaboration. New institutions were begun to face the humanitarian crisis that affected children during the war and to draw new national population policies. During the interwar period, the state attached new value to motherhood and childhood. Demographic concerns and political and social tensions gradually led to the reform of public health systems. At the same time, the discussion of future generations' natural reproduction affected the way citizens' health, welfare and private life were signified. In order to grasp this new political phase and the family's relation to the state, one should consider the changes European

1   Roger Cooter, John Pickstone, "Introduction," in *Companion to Medicine in the Twentieth Century*, ed. Roger Cooter, John Pickstone (London–New York: Taylor & Francis, 2003), xiii.
2   Iris Borowy, Wolf D. Gruner, "Introduction," to *Facing Illness in Troubled Times, 1918–1939*, eds. I. Borowy, Wolf D. Gruner (Peter Lang: Frankfurt am Main, 2005), 1.

healthcare systems underwent as well as the action taken for the protection of children at the national and international levels.

The bad state of health and living conditions during World War I intensified during the interwar period. Smallpox occurrence in Central and Eastern European countries, the rise in the cases of plague in many Mediterranean ports and the spread of typhus, among other epidemics, hit European populations during the early interwar period. The main reasons for the spread of contagious diseases–which had been localized during the war in just a few areas–was population movement, namely the release of army conscripts, the return of war prisoners and war hostages, and, most of all, migration.

Spanish influenza—the worst pandemic of the twentieth century—had a great impact not only on social conditions but also on the political developments and decisions of the war itself, since many of the leaders that participated in the Treaty of Versailles were themselves victims of the pandemic. At the same time, TB and malaria rates were on the rise because of general hardship. The additional financial exhaustion of the belligerent countries and the subsequent social crisis in some of them paints a paralytic picture of state health services at the end of the war. During the interwar period the health crisis was double-faceted: a time of severe economic instability that resulted in dramatic salary cuts, and high rates of morbidity and mortality.

In the early 1920s, initiatives were taken in various political regimes (Weimar Germany, Sweden, the Soviet Union and the USA) to develop and promote public health welfare.[3] Fears over national dwindling and racial degeneration led to various state welfare services and as a result state intervention was reinforced. Medical action was gradually transferred from charity to the state. Governments across the political spectrum altered their social policies, launching new hygiene institutions (consultation stations, hospitals and health exhibitions), while taking measures to decrease children's mortality and protect mothers. States accepted that health was now the main function of the state given that citizens' health constituted an indicator of state efficiency; this indicator was determined in direct relation to the performance of the workers' body and social security systems. However,

---

3   Iris Borowy, "Crisis as Opportunity: International Health Work during the Economic Depression," *Dynamis*, no. 28 (2008): 29–53.

the timing of when countries actually expressed interest in this and acted on it varied. In general, the establishment of Ministries of Health and Social Welfare in Europe dates back from 1918–1922. Given that the interwar period saw the spread of ecumenical values and the expansion of human and social rights—among them welfare and social security—health was not interpreted as a private issue. Instead, it was approached as an issue of public interest and state policy. This change was due to the action of state agencies and international health organizations that highlighted the nation-state's responsibility for its citizens.[4]

During this period, two issues necessitated a different approach to public health problems: firstly, the millions of casualties, wounded and disabled from the war; and secondly, the "epidemiologic turn," the transition from contagious to chronic diseases as reflected in morbidity and mortality statistics.[5] As European states modernized, the value of the scientific approach to health was stressed.[6] At the same time, it was highlighted that the state's investment in citizens' health was worthwhile. Science was used to plan and legitimize public health decisions. Based on the firm belief that poverty and disease could be scientifically measured, controlled and limited, experimental approaches to intervention were developed. Mortality statistics were prepared while research was carried out on various diseases. Hygiene institutes were set up and the farmers' health and nutrition attracted great interest.[7] Sports and other activities took on a special value for health experts "to reform life," which in itself testified that care for one's body had become an important concept across Europe. At the same time, state action focused on the citizens' private and sexual life so as to raise hygienic standards.

---

4   Norman Howard-Jones, *International Public Health between the Two World Wars—The Organizational Problems* (Geneva: World Health Organization 1978); Paul Weindling, ed., *International Health Organizations and Movements, 1928–1939* (Cambridge: Cambridge University Press. 1995); Milton I. Roemer, "Internationalism in Medicine and Public Health," in *Companion Encyclopedia of the History of Medicine*, ed. W.F. Bynum, Roy Porter (London–New York: Routledge, 1997), vol. 2, 1417–1435.

5   The term was introduced in the 1970s by A.R. Omran so as to describe the trends in the variation of the morbidity rates during the various phases of the demographic transition. See A. R. Omran, "The Epidemiologic Transition. A Theory of the Epidemiology of Population Chang," *Milbank Memorial Fund Quarterly* 49, no. 4 (1971): 509–38.

6   "Die Verwissenschaftilichung des Sozialen als methodische und konzeptionelle Herausforderung fuer eine Sozialgeschichte des 20. Jahrhunderts," *Geschichte und Gesellschaft*, no. 22 (1996): 165–93.

7   Paul Weindling, "The League of Nations, the Rockefeller Foundation and Public Health in Europe in the Interwar Period," in *Dimosia Ygeia kai Koinoniki Politiki: o Eleftherios Venizelos kai I Epokhi tou*, ed. Giannis Kyriopoulos (Athens: Papazisis, 2008), 79–96.

However, the emergence of the welfare state raised expectations for healthy, loyal and obedient bodies and allowed the state's greater intrusion into the private life of its citizens. More often than not, the reinforcement of welfare systems went hand-in-hand with an increase in authoritarian behavior.[8] As a result, medicine became a tool of control and exploitation, especially where racial and authoritarian ideas flourished, as was the case with Germany. There "the adoration of health and beauty" was used as a means of controlling people's fortunes.[9] Physical beauty was interpreted as an organic expression of the harmonious interaction between the body and the mind.[10]

1. The Emergence of Social Hygiene and the Role of Social Medicine

In the aftermath of the Great War, the sociological turn in medical thought replaced the moralistic interpretation for the causes of illness, which held that responsibility for their condition lay with the patient. Since the end of the nineteenth century, the German physician and biologist Rudolf Virchow (1821–1902), known as the father of social medicine, had argued for a sociological approach to the study of health. This turn in medical thought became more clearly articulated at the beginning of the twentieth century in academia, where it was maintained that the social role of medicine should form an integral part of prospective doctors' training by creating a new academic branch, that of social medicine. The same period saw an intensification of efforts to establish social hygiene services for children. The turn of doctors' interest to the social and economic conditions as causes for the spread of diseases played a crucial role in their new demands. Within certain medical circles, the role of social hygiene was stressed and the repercus-

---

8   Weindling, "Health and Medicine in Interwar Europe," in *Companion to Medicine in the Twentieth Century* eds. R. Cooter, J. Pickstone, 39–50.

9   Michael Hau, *The Cult of Health and Beauty in Germany. A Social History, 1890–1930* (Chicago–London: University of Chicago Press, 2003).

10 Of special interest is the movement that developed between 1890 and 1930 in conjunction with a bourgeois culture, wherein a considerable number of Germans started to discipline their body, serving a utopian aim: to secure perfect health and beauty. In this context, some adopted a vegetarian diet, others became nudists, whereas other worked out systematically or turned to alternative forms of health care. All these were part of the Weimar "culture of the free body" (*Freikörperkultur*), the pursuit of authenticity and the "community of people" that surfaced during the same period.

sions low living standards could have on personal and public health were highlighted all the more frequently in the course of the century.

Although social hygiene remains a concept with ambiguous content–used in different political regimes and interchangeably with the term social medicine–its main characteristic had been the critical approach to medical care with an emphasis on the social factors that led to disease.

The conviction that without social policy no improvement would be achieved in hygiene became a point of convergence between the doctors influenced by socialist ideology and the hygienists of the League of Nations (LN). Two medical authorities, the Belgian René Sand (1877–1953) and the Croatian Andrija Štampar (1888–1958), contributed immensely to the social medicine movement in the interwar period. As advocates of social medicine, they both maintained that diseases had to be fought with social measures and played an important role in configuring national and international programmes that aimed at providing healthcare.

In the 1930s, medical and statistical research focused on factors such as housing, nutrition, hygiene conditions and water. Building hygienic houses, improving diet and working conditions, and sanitizing cities became a common argument. As the sociological understanding of health gain momentum, state action to improve and centrally control children's health intensified. Summer camps, soup kitchens for students, schools for special groups of people, family benefits, and the accumulation of biological data, were all forms of systemization brought about through state policymakers in the public sphere.

Inspired by the experiments of social medicine and social hygiene in revolutionary Soviet society in the 1920s, interwar reformers on both sides of the Atlantic believed that the sociopolitical role of medicine could be achieved through its elevation to a social science.[11] There were three models of health care organization at this time: the social model in the West; the popular model in Central and Eastern Europe, and the socialist model in Soviet Union. Although the concept of social medicine was approached from different ideological angles, the end goals for what hygienic living should look like were similar. Social medicine was widely disseminated in Eastern

---

11   Dorothy Porter, "How Did Social Medicine Evolve, and Where Is It Heading?" *PLoS Med* 3, no. 10: (October 2006): 1667–72.

Europe through a policy that combined health programmes with agricultural reform. Public health doctors dealt with the impact the environment had on the spread of diseases, especially malaria and TB.

In Southern Europe in the 1920s, health reformers in Greece, Bulgaria, Romania and Yugoslavia, promoted active state reorganization on the basis of modern hygiene models to improve the health of the population. This development was brought about by dramatic territorial changes, the movement of the general population and of ethnic minorities, and the dominant agricultural character of the population. Developments in health and hygiene reconstruction in the Balkan countries were also dictated by high rates of child mortality, the difficulty in combatting contagious diseases, the inadequate local health infrastructure and the lack of substantial and effective cooperation. Dependence on international organizations and imitation of Western European medical and hygiene models, combined with national competition, created a new scene in health and gave rise to multiple hygiene movements.[12] However, the imitation did not exclude the emergence of local models of social hygiene and public health. Case in point are the theories of agricultural biology or the agricultural universities set up in Yugoslavia and Romania. In the 1920s, novelty aspects of hygiene in rural life like the concept of the ideal national village and the reinforcement of a set of values and traditions contributed on the implementation of new public health policies.[13] Stampar's work had a great impact on the Balkan context, especially on the Greek medical circles, regarding how public health changes were promoted.[14] For Stampar, collaboration with the farmers was one of the ten rules of social medicine—the ten commandments of his medical "religion." For him, improvements in health and hygiene had to focus first and foremost on the life of farmers.

According to Marius Turda, institutionalization of public health in South-Eastern Europe went through two phases: firstly, a legislative, educational and social phase during which emphasis was placed on health and hygiene education, the establishment of healthcare networks, the prepara-

---

12   Marius Turda, "Public Health and Social Politics in Southeast Europe in the 1920s," in *Dimosia Ygeia kai Koinoniki Politiki: o Eleftherios Venizelos kai I Epokhi tou*, ed. Giannis Kyriopoulos (Athens: Papazisis, 2008), 517–22.

13   Turda, "Public Health and Social Politics," 519.

14   His influence was increased as Greek doctors pursued further training in public health issues in various European cities, Zagreb among them.

tion of specialized staff and the foundation of agencies in urban and rural settings; and secondly, an organizational-institutional phase during which agencies, services and health institutes were set up.[15] During this period, various centers and health institutes were started in most Balkan capitals: the Hygiene and Bacteriology Institute in Athens (1923), the School of Hygiene (1929) and the School of Nurses (1931) in Belgrade, the Central Institute of Hygiene (1926) in Zagreb, the Institute of Hygiene and the School of Public Health (1927) in Sofia, the Institute of Public Health (1927) in Bucharest, the Institute of Hygiene and Public Health (1930) in Iasi, and the Institute of Hygiene and Social Hygiene in Cluj (1919). At the same time legislation on health was passed: The National Popular Educational Law on Health in Yugoslavia in 1928, the Law on Public Health in Bulgaria in 1929, the Law on Health in Romania in 1930, and the reform in public health in Greece in 1929. Both phases ran in parallel and were promoted thanks to external support and funding. International organizations such as the Rockefeller Foundation, the Health Committee of the League of Nations and the American Red Cross, which had already taken action in the field of public health, provided more health protection in the form of social hygiene and public health programmes. The involvement of international organizations led to the dissemination of supranational ideals, the promotion of novelties, and the organization and systematization of aid, but also to the imposition of certain models of health that reveal an intent to infiltrate and dominate citizenry as well as to designate fields of power and interests.

Furthermore, during the same period more complex procedures of scientific reconstruction and knowledge transfer between European countries took place. Finally, the notion of national community and linking medical concerns with nationalism had been characteristic of the medical thought and the organization of public health systems in South-Eastern Europe since the end of the nineteenth century. Health and hygiene were the main components of a wider bio-political agenda concerned with the creation of a racially healthy nation through eugenics. It was an agenda even oppositional political and ideological camps tended to agree on.[16]

---

15 Turda, "Public Health and Social Politics" 518.
16 Christian Promitzer, Sevasti Trubeta and Marius Turda, eds., *Health, Hygiene and Eugenics in Southeastern Europe to 1945* (Budapest: Central European University Press, 2011), 14.

2. International Organizations, Preventive Medicine and Health Reconstruction

The interwar period could be characterized as a period of internationalization[17] in public health: formal and informal international bodies were set up to develop and promote new means of preventing and combatting diseases beyond the confines of national borders; concepts and experiences were exchanged on the axis of an international ideal while an international community made its debut.[18] This community wanted to provide more equitable healthcare and contribute to social progress by improving the health of the people and raising their living standards.[19] In addition, the international health and hygiene congresses, and the international conventions on health aimed to help build a modern health ethos.

This international collaboration dates back to the beginning of the twentieth century when efforts were undertaken in many European and North and South American countries to develop an organized network of health services to combat disease and epidemics.[20] The International Sanitary Bureau (1902), the statistics service established in Geneva (1907), the International Bureau of Public Hygiene (Office International d'Hygiene Publique) (1908), the Rockefeller Foundation (1913) and the Inter-Allied Sanitary Committee (1917) exemplify the tradition of health services that emerged before 1920.

The Red Cross, founded in Geneva in 1863 to protect the sick and the wounded during wartime, played a leading part as an international body of aid. The Red Cross Societies depended on voluntary workers. The League of Red Cross Societies (LRCS), a confederation of various societies, was founded in May 1919 and supported a constituent of national societies by promoting new programmes and coordinating international ef-

---

17 Susan Gross Solomon, Lion Murard and Patrick Zylberman, eds., *Shifting Boundaries of Public Health: Europe in the Twentieth Century*, vol. 12 (Rochester–New York: University of Rochester Press, 2008).

18 On the international collaboration on public health issues and the procedures that led to the formation of the first international health system, see Katerina Gardika, "I Diethnis Voitheia sti Dimosia Ygeia: Anthropistiki Krisi, Diakinisi Ideon kai Koinoniki Politiki," in *Dimosia Ygeia kai Koinoniki Politiki: o Eleftherios Venizelos kai I Epokhi tou*, 173–84.

19 Bridget Tower, "Red Cross Organizational Politics, 1918–1922: Relations of Dominance and the Influence of the United States," in *International Health Organizations and Movements, 1928–1939*, 36–55.

20 For the role international organizations played in the field of health, see Paul Weindling, "The League of Nations, the Rockefeller Foundation and Public Health in Europe in the Interwar Period," in *Dimosia Ygeia kai Koinoniki Politiki: o Eleftherios Venizelos kai I Epokhi tou*, 79–96.

forts to deal with various problems. It was an organization devoted to the "improvement of health, the prevention of disease and the elimination of pain across the world." The Health Organization of the League of Nations, whose action is described in the following sections, was also founded in 1919. Hoping that health improvement would lead to social stability and international peace, the international organizations promoted the model of preventive medicine, defined biological and nutritional standards, compared innovative forms and promoted good practice in organizing public health systems.[21]

The systematic study of health and the definition of the prerequisites of healthy living allowed better organization of international aid. A boost to international societies' organization and mobilization came in 1920 when the London Conference on Health took place in response to the typhus epidemic moving threateningly towards Eastern Europe. At the same time, new research tools were devised to collect and systematize health information in many countries. The most important tools for health information systems in Europe were devised between 1918 and 1920 in the UK and the USA, after exploring the possibility of extending health infrastructure and practices beyond borders and the relation between the development of a nation or a culture and the health of its population had been thoroughly investigated. A group of public health experts undertook the task of advising governments that sought to reform their public health services with the assistance of international health organizations. Health researchers crossed borders and conducted studies to exchange experiences, perspectives and findings with their colleagues.

In general, international agencies followed four organizational patterns. The first form consisted of the technical services of the LN. These included the medical department of the International Labor Organization and the Section for Women and Children. The second included the new innovative corporate charity bodies–i.e., the Rockefeller Foundation, the Miliband Memorial Fund and the Commonwealth Fund for child guidance–which offered supplementary financial support and advice to the L N and were also able to develop autonomous aid programmes and support health initiatives

---

21   Weindling, "The League of Nations, the Rockefeller Foundation and Public Health in Europe in the Interwar Period," 79.

in Europe. The Rockefeller Foundation[22] provided financial and technical support that was crucial for the internationalization and systematization of public health issues. The Rockefeller Foundation supported the governments with assistance from the LN and set up its own faculties, workshops and institutes staffed by people who had already worked with the Health Committee of the L N. It promoted an American model of public health orientated more towards community than experimental biology.

The third form of organization was based on the role of the International Red Cross Committee and was promoted by the League of the Red Cross Societies. This international network was inspired by a militaristic rationale, the concept of "the positive medicine," and social medicine connected to public health. The last form of organization was used by charities such as the Save the Children Fund, which approached health as an issue of human rights beyond the competence of the nation-state.

After the war, the USA played an important role in funding and planning international health organizations like the League of Nations Health Organization and the League of Red Cross Societies. However, the role the USA played in promoting a network of international relations, especially between 1918 and 1922, remains to be explored in each national case. The interaction between voluntary and state organizations also calls for further research.

3. The Role and Work of the League of Nations

The establishment of the Health Committee of the L N[23] solidified an elite of experts on biomedicine and medicine, and gave rise to an institutionalized international forum for health and health related safety issues. The aim of the committee, established in 1919 by the Versailles Treaty to foster collaboration between nations and safeguard peace and security, was to combat epidemics that broke out in the wake of the Great War. Initially, the Health Committee invested its energies in establishing an epidemiological committee that aimed to stabilize the new Central European States, es-

---

22 For the role of the Rockefeller Foundation and the National Hygiene Institute in Poland see Maria Balinska, "The Rockefeller Foundation and the National Institute of Hygiene, Poland, 1918–1945," *Stud. Hist. Biol. & Biomed. Sci.* 31, no. 3 (2000): 419–32.

23 Ilana Loewy, Patrick Zylberman, "Medicine as a Social Instrument. Rockefeller Foundation, 1913–1945," *Stud. Hist. Phil. Biol. Biomed. Sci.* 31, no. 3 (2000): 4.

pecially Poland and Czechoslovakia. Following a period of provisional operation, the Health Committee of the L N was formally set up in Geneva in 1924 as the League of Nations Health Organization (LNHO). The key post of this organization—the secretariat—was taken from October 1921 to February 1939 by Ludwik Rajchman (1881–1965), an eminent Polish bacteriologist renowned for his imagination, action and abilities. Rajchman, who had studied in Paris, was the founder of the National Hygiene Institute in Warsaw and UNICEF, and the director of the LNHO. As secretary general of the Health Committee, he was involved in various efforts to reform health systems in many countries and create a worldwide database on epidemics, among other things. Rajchman widened the support of the Rockefeller Foundation by establishing its Eastern headquarters, he designated programmes for Latin America and China, contributed to the reconstruction of the administration of public health in Greece, and underlined the importance of rural hygiene and social medicine. He was a visionary who adopted an innovative international perspective on health issues to create new infrastructure for international collaboration.[24] He was an advocate of social humanism and a political activist. His initiatives were worldwide received by health reformers whose ideas collided with the most conservative governments of their respective countries.

As an international organization, the LNHO assumed both a technical and social role, since it supported the analysis of morbidity data in the light of social conditions. It defined biological models that considered people's living conditions and produced medical statistics through a comparative perspective. It also helped diffuse proper hygiene practices by conducting local medical studies. In general, Rajchman considered the study of health an integral part of the modernization of society and the improvement of living conditions.[25] Due to the economic crisis and the critical state of sociopolitical conditions, the LNHO's widened its hygiene programme in the early 1930s to include studies on the social parameters of health such as nutrition, housing, living standards, and working and hygiene conditions.

---

24 Paul Weindling, "From Moral Exhortation to Socialised Primary Care: the New Public Health and the Healthy Life," in *The Politics of the Healthy Life. An International Perspective*, ed. Esteban Rodriguez Ocaña (Sheffield: European Association for the History of Medicine and Health Publications, 2002) 113–30.

25 Paul Weindling, "The League of Nations Health Organization and the Rise of Latin American Participation, 1920–40," *Hist. cienc. Saude-Manguinhos* 13, no. 3 (July-September 2006): 555–70.

4. INTERNATIONAL CONGRESSES ON CHILD PROTECTION

After the end of World War I, problems and inadequacies in children's healthcare became evident, resulting in the increasing conviction that relevant social policies had to be implanted. Public interest in children's health increased across Europe and the USA, and led to organized movements and initiatives both at the state and international levels.

Apart from the sociological turn in health examination and the state's intervention in health issues, explored earlier, another factor played an important role in building public interest in motherhood and childhood. The development of the eugenics movement and the frequent debates on social policies on family, protection of childhood and motherhood emphasized the importance of the health of mothers and children even within different political regimes; yet, their vision and aim were common. The growing interest in children's rights, mainly health, strengthened the medical movement. The interwar concern about "the child at risk" was organized around two axes: firstly, the body of the child in relation to development, school strain, and nutrition; and secondly, the child's mental health. Both axes were related to the idea of normality. These issues led to the mobilization of certain key individuals and voluntary organizations in establishing child protection and child health care societies both within countries individually and in Europe and other parts of the world.

During the Great War, the international aid to children was mainly undertaken by two American organizations: the American Red Cross and the American Relief Administration. The latter was set up by President Herbert Hoover. Although it did not focus primarily on healthcare and the welfare of children, it did promote programmes that aimed to save the lives of many children. Apart from humanitarian motives, there were also ideological purposes in this attempt as President Hoover laid political importance on securing food for children, for fear that starvation ultimately led to the spread of bolshevism in Western societies. He himself purported that *"Civilization marches forward upon the feet of healthy children."*[26] The League of the Red Cross Societies promoted an ambitious programme of fast action

---

26 "Speech of Herbert Hoover to America" May 17, 1946.

on children's health and welfare.[27] The Junior Red Cross was yet another vehicle for the promotion of children's health and care. It began in Canada and later spread to Europe and the USA to help nations educate their youth in the meanings and responsibility of citizenship. Junior Red Cross members had to take care of their health not only for their own sake but also for other people's health. Reinforcing the role of national branches of Junior Red Cross during peace was also one of the League's aims. Leading personalities in children's health, among them Sir Arthur Newsholme from England, professor Adolphe Pinard from France, and doctors Emmert Holt and Samuel McClintock Hamill from the USA laid down the main principles of a well-planned health and welfare programme. Apart from launching systematic campaigns against childhood diseases, these experts supported the establishment of prenatal clinics and infant and children's clinics, encouraged housecalls to expectant mothers and the introduction of hygiene as a subject in the school curricula. The Junior Red Cross avoided more passive instruction through textbooks and instead promoted hygiene through more practical and appealing to children methods. It also promoted solidarity among them. Social and political education was another weapon the Junior Red Cross carried in its arsenal. Student groups were organized in each school and special discussion sessions were held. School correspondence with children from other countries was yet another means. In the USA the Red Cross got the idea of children's "health games" from the National Association against TB. When World War I broke out, the Association organized a modern crusade, based on an elaborate game that informed children of the community rules on health and personal hygiene.[28] Despite problems, it was inconceivable that the Association would abandon European children since its establishment was accompanied by a rhetoric of the development of a new civilization in which peace and international understanding would replace the war and nationalism.

Attempts to create an international organization for the healthy development of children did not materialize until the mid-1920s when the LNHO funded research on child mortality under the supervision of France Robert

---

27 Alexandra Minna Stern, "Responsible Mothers and Normal Children: Eugenics, Nationalism, and Welfare in Post-revolutionary Mexico, 1920–1940," *Journal of Historical Sociology* 12, no. 4 (2002): 369–97.

28 John F. Hutchinson, "The Junior Red Cross Goes to Healthland," *American Journal of Public Health* 87, no. 11 (1997): 1816–23.

Debré in six Western European countries.[29] Two previous attempts to set up an International Association on Child Protection in Brussels in 1907 and 1913 respectively were cancelled despite the significant support given to the project by international congresses on children's health and hygiene. It was only on January 6, 1920 that the International Association on Child Protection was finally set up in Geneva. These organizations were modelled after the Save the Children Fund, a private voluntary organization, set up by the sisters Eglantyne Jebb (1876–1928) and Frances Buxton in England in 1919 to deal with child starvation in post-war Europe. This organization raised funds to aid starving children. It also promoted scientific social work internationally, since its founders believed that national antagonisms or oppositional politics should not be considered when providing welfare in states of emergency. Both sisters believed that people should get help so that they would not have to depend on charity.[30] Dependence was considered to pose a bigger threat on the moral health of European children than the physical diseases threatening their bodies.

The following year the Save the Children Fund became a branch of an international organization based in Geneva. Thanks to the intervention of the Save the Children Fund, the International Save the Children Union[31] was set up in Geneva in 1920. It comprised fifty national organizations for the protection of children and coordinated international aid for children in need.[32] In 1920, the organization supported agencies that did similar work, especially in Vienna and Budapest, as well as in other areas of Central Europe. Over the next few years national branches of the organization were set up in many countries–Greece included–to relieve refugees. Although Jebb's main concern was to provide food, clothes and accommodation in states of emergency, she soon realized that European children needed more than that to lead healthy and productive lives. Therefore, she attempted to mobilize various organizations and unions in order to collectively respond to the problem.

---

29   France Robert Debré (1882–1978) was a leading French paediatrician who worked at Necker-Enfants Malades and lent its name to a paediatric hospital in Paris.

30   Englantyne Jebb, *A Brief Study in Social Questions* (Cambridge: Macmillan and Bowes 1906).

31   For the action of the Organization see Patricia T. Rooke and Rudy L. Schnell, "Uncramping Child Life': International Children's Organizations, 1914–1939," in *International Health Organizations and Movements 1918–1939*, 176–203.

32   Similar purposes served the Comité Suisse de Secours aux Enfants and Comité International de la Croix Rouge.

The Declaration of the Rights of the Child, known also as the Geneva Declaration, expresses a strong commitment to childhood and the concerns of its writers for children's problems. Drawn up by Jebb herself, the declaration was submitted to the convention of the International Union on February 23, 1923, passed by its executive committee in May 1923. The draft was later ratified during the fifth general assembly on February 28, 1924. The declaration was a significant step towards providing medical care to sick children. The declaration defined children's rights and the responsibilities of parents, society and the state to them. The right to good health was formulated explicitly:

We ought to give children the means to develop their body and soul properly; we ought to raise the child who starves and treat those who are ill; we ought to encourage the retarded child and lead the deviant child to the right path; we ought to pick up and help the orphan and the unprotected child. We ought to help the child first in unfavorable conditions; to provide the child with the means to earn its living, feeling that he/she has to put their best abilities to the service of its siblings [...] The best possible conditions should be secured so as the child to develop normally, body and mind alike.[33]

In 1927 the International Save the Children Union launched a contest for primary school students in Europe to illustrate the Geneva Declaration. Winning illustrations were exhibited in many cities. The declaration, however, did not include details on children's health or the means to fight the most important children's diseases.

The Draft Children's Charter, approved by the International Council of Women (ICW) in a committee that took place in the Hague in 1922, was more child-orientated. It included more than fifty references to childhood issues such as prenatal care, health care for mothers and for schoolchildren, children below schooling age, the children of unemployed parents, etc. Some of these references were included in the health programme for children drawn up and promoted by the American Red Cross Committee for Europe.[34]

---

33 The Declaration featured in the first issue of the journal *To Paidi* issued by the Greek Association for the Protection of Children.
34 Edward Fuller, *The Right of the Child: A Chapter in Social History* (London: Countess Mountbatten of Burma, 1951); K. Freeman, *If Any Man Build. The History of the Save the Children Fund* (London: Hodder and Stoughton, 1965). See also Dominique Marshall, "The Construction of Children as an Object of

In the early 1920s, the programmes of the American Red Cross in Europe began to crumble. By that time enthusiasm for international intervention and social improvement had seen a sharp decline. It was clear that few governments were willing to allocate more funds to improve children's health and many cast doubts on the effect of humanitarianism and the stability of the international organizations.[35] In the late 1920s, the American Red Cross decided to promote an extended programme to improve children's health in Europe. According to the initial plan, children's clinics staffed with all necessary doctors and medical auxiliaries would be established in certain parts of Europe, especially in problematic countries.[36] From the beginning, the programme stressed prevention rather than treatment. Despite its initial plans, the American Red Cross decided to give up on the children's health programme only a few months after its promotion due to dwindling public support from the USA. In the end, some funds were allocated to the programme, but they could not support its nutrition programme, efforts to improve European hospitals, or doctor and nurse training programme. Because of this lack of funding, it was preferable to launch a prevention programme using health centers for children to reduce child mortality, put a limit on diseases and decrease hospital insufficiencies. The first of these health centers, mainly for mothers, began in the spring of 1921. In addition, mobile medical units were started in an attempt to cover all districts and boost public interest in children's health, combing training with propaganda. The first portable clinic, which was used as a children's health center, started operation in Poland. The aim of the mobile medical units was to train mothers to raise more healthy children, to introduce school-age children to hygiene principles and to improve children's health in the community. The outcome was considered satisfactory, although recipients of the service were more enthusiastic about the medium rather than the message; in the villages that had been hit hardest by the war, the chance to watch a film or listen to a lecture was in itself both a novelty and an attraction. Thus, the public appetite for entertainment resulted in increased public interest in healthy living.

International Relations: The Declaration of Children's Rights and the Child Welfare Committee of the League of Nations, 1900–1924," *The International Journal of Children's Right* no. 7 (1999): 103–47.

35 John F. Hutchinson, "Promoting Child Health in the 1920s: International Politics and the Limits of Humanitarianism," in *The Politics of the Healthy Life. An International Perspective*, 131–50.

36 Clyde E. Buckingham, *For Humanity's Sake: The Story of the Early Development of the League of Red Cross Societies* (Washington DC: 1964), 153.

From the mid-nineteenth century international congresses on hygiene were organized in Europe and the USA, testifying to early interest in these issues. Congresses were often combined with exhibitions. As Anne Rasmussen noted "the exhibitions reveal, the congresses present, explain and enlighten."[37] Congresses covered issues ranging from social welfare, child labor, children's rights, vagrancy, prostitution, and child delinquency to the means of disciplining children and legal ramifications for criminal children. Delegates of these congresses included mainly doctors, pedagogues and professors of medicine and hygiene as well as engineers, architects and chemists who were concerned with child protection. Countries like Belgium, France and Germany played leading roles organizing these congresses and the majority of delegates also came from these countries. The beginning of the twentieth century saw the spread of international school hygiene congresses (the first one in Nuremberg in 1904; in London in 1907; in Paris in 1910; and in Buffalo, New York in 1913), while their thematic scope gradually broadened, reflecting concerns of national and international scientific associations. Also a turn to a more scientific interpretation of problems in school hygiene and a turn towards the study of the social parameters of school, mental, and moral hygiene are evident in this period.

The first international congress for the protection of children was in 1920. Among its goals were people's education, the dissemination of health principles, raising hygiene awareness and the cultivation of social solidarity. The second congress took place in Geneva in August 1925 and signified the beginning of more systematic work on issues of children's health and protection. This congress was a landmark for the International Union as it was since then that disease prevention was prioritized over treatment with regard to children's health. In 1928, the second international exhibition for the protection of children took place in Brussels, while a few years later in 1933 another congress took place in Paris. Themes discussed in the congress included scoliosis, bio-morphology, pedagogy, methods of medical supervision, detection of TB at school, and overly strenuous student workloads. In 1935 the International Child Conference also took place in Brussels. Congresses on the protection of children took place in the Balkans as well due to

---

37 Anna Rasmussen, "Les Congrès internationaux liés aux expositions universelles de Paris, 1867–1900," *Cahiers Georges Sorel* no. 7 (1989): 26.

the increasing interest there, and the emergence of local approaches to hygiene issues. Various associations for the protection of children and eminent figures participated in these congresses.

CHAPTER VI

THE ARRIVAL OF REFUGEES:
NEW PRIORITIES AND SHIFTING TARGETS

The end of the Great War marked an important milestone in the history of public health and hygiene in Greece, as well as in other European countries. Population movement and increasing numbers of refugees during the prolonged wartime, which for Greece included the Balkan Wars, Great War and the Asia Minor campaign, exacerbated public health problems. Besides, the annexation of new territories forced Greece to assume new public health responsibilities. Political changes, state concerns about the preparation of healthy people, along with the early postwar social crisis, placed public health on a new basis.

Not only did the settlement of a large number of refugees from Asia Minor, Pontus and Eastern Thrace—who surged into Greece in September 1922—bring about financial and social problems, it also generated a public health crisis. The lack of preparation for the refugees' coming and the inability of public health services to accommodate the needs of the refugee influx paralyzed the state. As far as relief, accommodation and workplaces for the refugees—one fifth of the country's total population—were concerned, the resettlement of these refugees was a colossal venture. Greece remained in this emergency state for about a decade and had to seek international aid to overcome it.

During the interwar period, the organization of hygiene and social welfare services for children in Greece went in new directions. Historical developments and the intellectual framework within which child health was now approached, dictated new answers to new problems. The internationalization of the methods used to tackle social problems, in conjunction with the challenges the postwar states had to face, and changes in the approaches to health did not leave the children's health and welfare agencies unaffected in Greece.

In the following sections, we explore the landmark events in the field of children's health and welfare during the interwar period and we trace possible changes in the policies on and understanding of children's health. These changes occurred in three phases: the first, spanning from 1922 to 1924, saw attempts to meet pressing needs, the second (1928–1932) witnessed the radical changes accomplished by the last interwar liberal government, and the third covers the authoritarian regime of Ioannis Metaxas (1936–1940).

The arrival of the refugees disrupted the progress achieved in children's health since health conditions declined, bringing changes in the way social policies were drawn up. The pressing need to accommodate refugees' needs and combat epidemics dictated a readjustment of priorities in public health policy. As a result, the then recently initiated health care institutions for mothers and children were given priority. The political upheaval of the period, characterized by frequent governmental changes, military coups, and acute financial problems, had a strong effect on the health care policy.

Nevertheless, mortality rates due to childhood diseases and contagious diseases were increasing, caused by the deterioration of living conditions and student overcrowding in schools. Under these dire circumstances, children's health care and social welfare services and institutions, had to redefine their goals by resorting to international aid. The deterioration in children's health fed into the discourse of racial decline that characterized the interwar period.

1. The First Measures for the Improvement of Public Health

1.1 Child and General Mortality: the Deterioration of the Indices

That refugees kept relocating between 1913 and 1922, especially in Northern Greece, made it almost impossible to address public health and social welfare problems with the means the Greek state had at hand at the time. These problems intensified after 1922. This chapter traces the developments in children's healthcare during the critical period of 1922–1925 by using primary sources like the records of state health services that have not yet been fully utilized in relevant historical studies. We present the action of old and new philanthropic organizations that tackled the urgent problems of the refugees, as well as the health institutions that had been set up during the previous decade.

At the beginning of the twentieth century, successive Greek governments already had considerable experience organizing services for refugees due to successive war events in the Balkan Peninsula. Greece's participation in the Balkan Wars (1912–1913), the Great War and the Asia Minor Campaign were the main reasons for population movement. These people's situation was becoming more and more precarious due to atrocities and the cleansing operations conducted by the belligerent countries. During the 1910s and 1920s, the most important refugee surges came from Bulgaria and the Ottoman Empire because of the Balkan Wars, the Hellenic-Bulgarian treaty on voluntary migration in 1919 (Peace Treaty of Neuilly-sur-Seine of November 27th, 1919), and the Asia Minor Campaign from 1919 to 1921 when Greeks relocated from areas not under the protection of the Greek army into to Greece.[1] The Russian Revolution was also a contributing factor since 50,000 Greeks in Russia and the Caucasus were repatriated to Greece in 1919. The prolonged involvement of Greece in the ongoing warfare led to an increase in the number of the not bodily able and orphans, and contributed immensely to the sordid poverty of the lower classes. It is estimated that welfare institutions became responsible for around 450,000 persons before 1922.[2]

In 1917, the Ministry of Welfare was established and began to build the first infrastructure to handle the refugee problem. Medical care services, which until then had been handled by the Ministry of Internal Affairs, were transferred to the newly established Ministry of Welfare. However, the state institutions for refugee welfare could not cope with the refugee overflow in 1922. It is estimated that approximately 1,300,000 refugees arrived in Greece from August 1922, following the collapse of the Asia Minor Front, until 1924, when the compulsory population exchange, regulated by the Lausanne Treaty, was completed. The bulk of this population arrived between August and December 1922. The majority of refugees comprised widows, or-

---

1 Kostas Katsapis, "To Prosfygiko Zitima," in *To 1922 kai oi Prosfyges. Mia Nea Matia*, ed. Antonis Liakos (Athens: Nefeli, 2011), 125–69.

2 Katsapis, "To Prosfygiko Zitima," 131.

phans and elderly persons. Most refugees settled in Northern Greece, 52.5% in Macedonia and 8.8% in Thrace.[3] The refugees' arrival cancelled the plans for the country's health reconstruction begun in September 1920 when the Ministry of Hygiene and Social Welfare was set up. Due to important political changes and the work of the Medical Association, the law for the reconstruction of the health service passed two years later, on August 27, 1922, just a few days before the arrival of the refugees[4]. However, on account of the Asia Minor Disaster, the law was not implemented. Instead, a new law "on the establishment of the Hygiene and Social Welfare Ministry" passed.[5] The services that came under the jurisdiction of the 1917 Ministry of Welfare were then incorporated into the newly established ministry.

As expected, the admission of the refugees by the thousands in just a few centers and the subsequent overcrowding posed a risk to public health and order. The fight against the epidemics that broke out during the first surges of refugees necessitated the organization of lazarettos and the reorientation of the government's public health priorities. The newly established ministry's Hygiene Service was set up to handle emergencies by coordinating available hygiene services to avoid unnecessary expenses and to contain the spread of epidemics. Reports filed by the service's officials, contemporary testimonies, and mortality statistics compiled by Fokion Kopanaris, director of the Hygiene Service in Macedonia in 1922–1923, illustrate the conditions of refugees arriving in Greek ports and in refugee settlements during the first months following the collapse of the Asia Minor Front.[6]

Nikolaos Makridis, one of the refugee doctors mobilized to deal with emergencies, outlines the problems the Hygiene Service had to face during the early months of the refugees' arrival. He spoke of the lack of experienced doctors "able to handle the terrible surge of too many migrating souls who are not only mentally but also bodily wretched; besides, they are carriers of far too many contagious diseases." He made extensive reference to lack of hospitals, lazarettos, vaccines, tents, nurses and sufficient funding, as

3   Nikolaos Makridis, *Ai Ypiresiai Ygieinis en Elladi* (Athens, 1933), 41–2.
4   Law 2882 "Peri Metarythmisoes kai Sympliroseos tou Ypourgeiou tis Perithalpseos Metonomazomenou eis Ypourgeion Ygeias kai Koinonikis Pronoias," *Efimeris tis Kiverniseos*, A', no. 122 (July 22 1922): 577–582.
5   Nomothetiko Diatagma, "Peri Metonomasias tou Ypourgeiou Perithalpseos eis Ypourgeion Ygieinis, Pronoias kai Antilipseos," *Efimeris tis Kiverniseos*, A', no.269 (Decenber 22, 1922): 1617–18.
6   Fokion Kopanaris, *I Dimosia Ygeia en Elladi* (Athens, 1933).

well as to the reluctance of private doctors to work in the provinces.[7] This surge in needs called for prompt decisions and actions. Hygiene inspectors were entitled to make on the spot decisions regarding the appointments of doctors and nurses and, in collaboration with authorities and charities, to requisition buildings to accommodate and assist refugees. In the provinces military hospitals were made available to hygiene services, abandoned convents were used to accommodate typhus and smallpox victims, and refugees themselves formed groups of hygiene guards. The worst housing shortages were in Athens and Piraeus; there makeshift refugee hospitals were set up, military hospitals were requisitioned and lazarettos were set up.

The high refugee mortality rate indicates the adverse conditions of their movement, resettlement and living. Refugees died by the hundreds not only during their journey but also upon their arrival in Greece, in quarantine stations and in hospitals where they had been admitted for the treatment of contagious diseases. Starvation, hardships and diseases were the main killers in quarantine stations.[8] Epidemics broke out not only in Northern Greece, where the biggest refugee influx had settled, but also in ports across the country, posing great risk to local people. Typhus, smallpox and dysentery epidemics claimed many victims and malaria and TB led the exhausted refugees gradually to death. The head of the Hygiene Service in Macedonia remarked: "Typhus broke out all over the old Kingdom where refugees had settled, reached epidemic proportions and spread among the native population regardless of social class; even the well-off classes were affected."[9] About half a million of the victims were refugees arriving from the infected ports of Pontus and Asia Minor, however, the number has not been well documented. Among the victims, infants and children under the age of ten made up a high percentage.

In 1923, the worst year for mortality rates, 4,032 cases of typhus were recorded, out of which 893 victims succumbed. In addition, according to formal statistics, 1,507 people suffered from typhoid fever, of which 666 died. However, these statistics cannot be trusted since many cases went unrecorded. In order to fight typhus off, decontamination and frequent delousing were conducted not only on refugees but also on locals in areas where

---

7   Makridis, *Ai Ypiresiai Ygieinis en Elladi*, 41–2.
8   SDN, *L'Établissement des réfugiés en Grèce* (Geneva, 1926) 4 and Antonis Liakos, *Ergasia kai Politiki sta Khronia tou Mesopolemou. To Diethnes Grafeio Ergasias kai I Anadysi ton Koinonikon Thesmon* (Athens: Idryma Erevnas kai Paideias tis Emporikis Trapezas, 1993), 321.
9   Kopanaris, *I Dimosia Ygeia en Elladi*, 40.

refugees had settled, preventing the epidemic from spreading further. The same period also saw a smallpox epidemic. Despite vaccination and revaccination carried out by municipal doctors under the supervision of medical officers, it was not possible to contain this epidemic before 1925. Deaths due to smallpox amounted to 40% of the most severe cases.[10]

The problems of water supply, sewage and hygiene are evident behind the dysentery and typhus epidemics, which very often broke out in the refugee slums, at least before 1928. In 1923 most deaths were caused by dysentery. In refugee settlements in Macedonia, 20% of the refugee population died from diseases caused by contaminated water. During their first years there, destitute living conditions were the main reason for high rates of dysentery deaths. The dysentery and typhus epidemics that hit the refugee population in 1923 also claimed hundreds of children. Trachoma was on the rise among the refugees as well because of the appalling living conditions and overcrowding. Characteristically, every two or three years there was an outbreak of a trachoma.[11]

Despite the aid offered by other countries, starvation and the wretched living conditions accounted for high rates of malaria infection among refugees relocated in the marshy plains of Macedonia and Thrace, ranging from 80 to 100%.[12] From 1921 until 1930, malaria caused 2,402 deaths, while chronic cases amounted to 90% in the prefectures of Kavala, Pella, Rodopi and Thessaloniki. To these victims, one should add death due to flu or other conditions which had a bad effect on people's bodies in the Northern provinces, already affected badly by malaria. In 1930, Greece had reached the highest mortality level due to malaria compared to other European countries. The fact that between 1925 and 1929, the country imported one quarter of the world quinine production is revealing. In 1923, malaria accounted for 70% of deaths among refugees who had settled in the rural areas of Northern Greece.

During the 1920s, circumstances favored TB more than other diseases. In the refugee settlements, TB was rising so rapidly that the contemporary press called these shanties "TB towns."[13] These makeshift dwellings were

---

10 Kopanaris, *I Dimosia Ygeia en Elladi*, 40.

11 Makridis, *Ai Ypirisiai Ygieinis en Elladi*, 41–2.

12 For a detailed presentation of the refugees' health problems and the steps taken by the state, see the article by Kostas Katsapis, "Dimosia Ygeia, Prosfyges kai Kratiki Paremvasi stin Ellada tou Mesopolemou," in *Pera apo tin Katastrophi. Mikrasiates Prosfyges stin Ellada tou Mesopolemou*, ed. Giorgos Tzedopoulos (Athens: Idryma Meizonos Ellinismou, 2003), 41–73.

13 "O Antiphymatikos Agon kai oi Prosfygikoi Synoikismoi," *Prosfygikos Kosmos* (May 20, 1928): 1.

built with inexpensive materials in the outskirts of urban centers. Poor housing, starvation and the lack of basic hygiene along with insufficient health care infrastructure (only four anti-TB dispensaries were set up after 1920) led some doctors to concentrate on the TB problem and to connect the refugees' social conditions with the spread of TB. Their publications, which became more frequent in the 1920s, stressed the necessity of popularizing hygiene rules among the working class and the state's obligation to lead the anti-TB campaign.[14]

The general deterioration in public health went hand in hand with increased mortality rates due to childhood diseases.[15] Lambadarios noted that "at least until 1925, Greece came first among the states that displayed the highest mortality rates for this age group." Between 1922 and 1928 deaths from diphtheria, scarlet fever, measles and whooping cough increased, especially among the rural population. In this latter case, mortality rate was triple that of the urban population, perhaps due to the lower level of hygienic care. In 1924, out of 350 diphtheria victims 300 were infants and children under the age of nine. The case of measles was quite similar. In 1923, 1928 and 1929 measles intensified, accounting for 700 to 1,000 deaths per year. Refugee children were the first victims these epidemics claimed, since morbidity rates due to these diseases in refugee settlements had risen. In 1923 there were 2,171 cases of dysentery resulting in 1,727 deaths, 1,863 cases of measles resulting in 309 deaths and 2,101 cases of smallpox resulting in 687 deaths.[16]

Finally, the societal health crisis was reflected in child birth. There was 3,1% more births than deaths in 1921, while between 1922 and 1924 there was a decrease in births in Athens and Piraeus, fluctuating from 3.2% to 3.8% and from 7.4% to 11.7% respectively. There was a rise in infant mortality, especially in 1923, 1924 and 1927, fluctuating from 91.58 to 100.50 in every thousand births of alive infants.[17] In addition, infant mortality reached 30–33 deaths in every thousand infants, which was six to nine times higher than in Central European countries. It was only in the 1930s that births numbered more than deaths. Although the accuracy of the statistics is un-

14 See, for example, Nikolaos Oikonomopoulos, *I Phymatiosis os Koinoniki Nosos kai ta Endeiknyomena Metra pos Katapolemisin Aftis* (Athens: 1930).

15 Emmanouil Lambadarios, "Prostasia tis Ygeias tou Mathitou," *Praktika tou A' Panelliniou Synedriou Prostasias Mitrotitas kai Paidikon Ilikion* (October 19–26, 1930): 112.

16 See the tables for the years 1923–1931 published by Kopanaris, *I Dimosia Ygeia en Elladi*, 160–61.

17 Agapoula Kotsi, *Nosologia ton Paidikon Ilikion (20os Aionas)* (Athens: IAEN/EIE, 2008), 99.

clear since many deaths went unregistered, other sources confirm the surge in general mortality indices due to the refugee settlement.[18]

1.2. The Fight against Epidemics and the Contribution of International Organizations

The first measures adopted by the Revolutionary Government of the generals who were Venizelos's followers who took office in September 1922, concerned the disinfection of refugees and refugee medical care. Hygiene services focused on preventing the spread of epidemics and contagious diseases. They banned the free circulation of refugees, set up disinfection and delousing stations, while they established lazarettos and hospitals for the treatment of contagious and non-contagious diseases in towns where refugees had settled, organized vaccination campaigns and made attempts to reduce the density of population.

In 1923, the government attempted to organize regional services to prevent epidemics at the local level. This decentralization met with difficulties because of meagre funding from local councils, lack of trained staff and the unstable political situation that lasted until 1928.[19] However, it was the first time that provincial medical care was attempted.[20] The establishment of a hygienic council and the appointment of a hygiene officer were allowed for along with the appointment of communal and municipal doctors. The latter had to provide medical care to destitute citizens, take steps to contain contagious diseases, bring any incidents related to public health to the attention of medical officers, and take preventive hygiene measures in their respective municipalities. However, the financial difficulties faced by local councils prevented this institution from succeeding, at least during its early years. In addition, hospital treatment of the refugees was far from effective. Although sixteen hospitals for refugee patients had been set up in Central and Northern Greece, the limited number of beds meant they could not meet the growing need.

For the refugees' free treatment, the Ministry entered a contract with hospitals and clinics across the country, defraying 15–20 drachmas per per-

18 Kopanaris, *I Dimosia Ygeia en Elladi*, 160–1.
19 Makridis, *Ai Ypiresiai Ygieinis en Elladi* 47–8 and Kopanaris, *I Dimosia Ygeia en Elladi*, 472–73.
20 Khristos Zilidis, "I Epidimiologiki Pragmatikotita stin Ellada tin Periodo tou Mesopolemou kai i Politiki gia tin Organosi ton Ypiresion Ygeias," in *Dimosia Ygeia kai Koinoniki Politiki: o Eleftherios Venizelos kai I Epokhi tou*, ed. Giannis Kyriopoulos (Athens: Papazisis, 2008), 131–49.

son. In addition, the institution of the refugee doctor was introduced. These doctors were in charge of dispensaries in refugee settlements, although these were problematic since the medical staff in them were often inadequately trained. Finally, the Refugee Relief Fund, established in November 1922 in order to allocate money raised through donations for the construction of refugee settlements especially in large urban centers, provided the refugees with bedding, underwear, cooking utensils, firewood and coal. The Fund offered materials and supplies to six hospitals and two lazarettos, distributed medicines and vaccines, and established a contagious disease ward in the Syngrou and Saint Barbara hospitals.

However, the measures against epidemics adopted by the government proved far from adequate. Because of this, the government decided to resort to international health organizations. At the end of 1922, the Greek government appealed to the League of Nations Epidemics Committee, asking for its support in monitoring refugee health. The Epidemics Committee had already offered help to Central European countries such as Poland and Hungary that had faced similar problems after World War I. The members of the Committee stayed in Greece from November 1922 until April 1923, carrying compulsory vaccinations against malaria, smallpox, cholera and typhoid fever on 1,674,585 people. Vaccinations were made possible thanks to the money Fridtjof Nansen offered to the members of the Committee.[21] Although initially the measure was considered enough to keep the situation under control, later on the members of the Committee suggested the vaccinations be extended and the hospitals expanded.

Apart from the League of Nations, it was mostly American international voluntary organizations that had previously worked in the Middle East that assisted the Greek government with refugee relief, particularly children's care. They offered medicine and disinfectants, and trained hygiene staff. Following the Asia Minor Disaster, meetings were held in New York with delegates from philanthropic organizations to send aid to Greece, while a public appeal was made to the American people for help. The American Red Cross and the American Near East Relief were the most active among the

---

21 For the members of the Committee and their action in Greece, see Doxiadis Archive, 256, file 4, The Benaki Mouseum's Historical Archives; Marta Aleksandra Balinska, "Asssistance and not Mere Relief: the Epidemic Commission at the League of Nations 1920–1923," in *International Health Organisations and Movements 1918–1939*, ed. Paul Weindling (Cambridge: CUP, 1995), 81–108.

organizations working in Greece; the former helped refugees while the latter took care of orphans. Both organizations sent skilled staff and social
work volunteers who worked in Athens for at least two years. The Save the
Children Fund, the American Women's Hospital and the Friends of Greece
worked on a smaller scale organizing soup kitchens and building lazarettos.

The contribution of the American Red Cross was important to refugees'
health care. Doctors, nurses and hygienic materials were dispatched to Greece
to meet the urgent need, while the Ministry of Hygiene and Social Welfare supplemented the work of the American Red Cross with healthcare staff and materials. At the same time, from November 1922 until June 30, 1923 the American Red Cross provided food for 600,000 refugees, spending about 3,000,000
dollars.[22] According to the estimations of the organization, each refugee was
allotted 50 cents, offering them a diet of 1,000 calories per day. The American
Red Cross continued working in Greece well after 1923, operating students'
clinics and social hygiene clinics in refugee settlements.

The Near East Foundation had much experience in the relief of orphans
from work it had done in the Near East after World War I. These children were
either war orphans or victims of persecution in Asia Minor. At the end of August 1922, when people from the inland of Asia Minor moved to Smyrna, the
Near East Foundation distributed food and money to each underage person
regardless of ethnic origin. American doctors and nursing staff from Constantinople, where the organization had its headquarters, were also sent to
the islands of Lesvos, Chios, Crete and mainland Greece.[23] The same organization undertook the transport and care of 17,000 orphans—among them
a considerable number of Armenian children—from Asia Minor and Anato-
lia, accommodating them in buildings requisitioned by the Ministry of Welfare, including the Old Palace, the Zappeio, the Mon Repo and the Achilleio
stately homes, the Amaleio orphanage, the Aidipsos and Loutraki hotels, the
barracks in Korinthos, and the abandoned coal-miners' houses on the island
of Thasos.[24] The organization's doctors vaccinated children upon their arrival.

---

22 See the memorandum of the special commissioner of the Ministry of Welfare, B.P. Salmon, to the
    USA, dated December 3, 1923 and entitled "Statement. Regarding the Refugee Situation in Greece,"
    Venizelos's Archive, 173, file 131, The Benaki Mouseum's Historical Archives. This memorandum gives
    an account of his action in America so as to convince charities to continue offering aid to Greece.
23 "I Amerikaniki Organosis Near East Relief eis tin Ellada," *Ellinis* no. 12 (December 1923):13–5.
24 For the work of the organization, see James L. Barton, *Story of Near East Relief* (New York: Macmillan,
    1930), 161–64.

The organization built an orphanage with the help of children in Ermoupolis on the island of Syros to accommodate 4,000 orphans. A preparatory industrial school for both boys and girls was set up in the orphanage. Notably, orphans in Macedonia were trained by the organization's volunteer social workers to undertake hygienic work such as mosquito extermination and drainage of fenland.[25] During the following years, the Near East Foundation continued to fight malaria with the help of the Rockefeller Foundation.

The involvement of the Near East Foundation in refugee relief was considered a means to disseminate American welfare methods in Greece. Training in the principles of self-help, solving everyday practical problems and educating citizens on their hygienic duties were among the issues the members of the Committee came back to time and again. Apart from relief, the organization laid great emphasis on the orphans' elementary education and their preparation for professional life. As a result, this philanthropic organization set the protection of children from contagious diseases and the care of sick and handicapped children among its primary goals. The establishment of a wing for a group of tubercular children in the Sotiria Sanatorium, a school for blind children, a school for hearing-impaired children, the sanitization of an orphanage through the anti-malaria campaign in Korinthos, and the training of nurses were forms of social relief work for children carried out according to the American conception of social work.[26]

By the end of 1923, the work of the philanthropic organizations had been gradually limited, although the problems of the refugees' relief had not yet been dealt with efficiently. The Greek government appealed for the help to be continued, while at the same time attempting to settle the refugee issue.[27] According to the letter-memorandum on public care submitted to the American Government and the philanthropic organizations by the special chargé d'affaires of the Greek Government B. Salmon on December 23rd, 1923, 25% of the refugees had already been integrated in the country's economic life. The destitute amounted to 600,000 and Salmon feared that their condition might deteriorate during the coming winter.

---

25 For the hygienic work undertaken by the organization in rural areas, see John Badeau and Georgiana Stevens, eds., *Bread from Stones: Fifty Years of Technical Assistance* (n.p., 1956).

26 Barton, *Story of Near East Relief*, 165.

27 See the letter by M. Tsamadou, the Greek ambassador to the USA addressed to the Near East Relief, asking them to extend their action to adults. Venizelos's archive, 173/file 131, The Benaki Mouseum's Historical Archives.

In his lecture "The Condition of the Refugees in Greece" delivered in Geneva in August 1924, Apostolos Doxiadis, Minister of Welfare between 1922 and 1924, offered a synopsis of the work accomplished by philanthropic organizations during the early months of the refugees' settlement. According to him, the American Red Cross had provided financial support to 500,000 refugees, the Near East Foundation had accomplished great work in the relief of orphans, the American Hospital of Women had built thirty-three medical stations and hospitals, the Save the Children Fund had distributed about 50,000 rations to children and adults on a daily basis, the Help Committee of Switzerland had supported the female students of a women's orphanage during their first year, and—through the organization The Friends of Greece—the aid of the American people had reached the refugees as food and medicine.[28]

However, meagre funding and lack of welfare planning led the Greek government to seek more systematic solutions to the refugees' relocation. In February 1923, Doxiadis petitioned the financial department of the League of Nations to secure a loan for the refugees' resettlement. As a result, the Refugee Settlement Committee (Epitropi Apokatastaseos Prosfigon) was set up, an autonomous body working under the auspices of the League of Nations to resettle refugees in rural and urban environments.[29] The accomplishments of the committee were very important. During its six years of operation (1924–1930), the Refugee Settlement Committee alloted land holdings and distributed supplies to refugees to enable them to cultivate the land on their own. The committee built refugee settlements especially in the rural areas of Macedonia and Thrace and improved the hygienic condition of their respective populations.

Realistic estimation of the situation along with national aspirations of securing ethnic homogeneity in a frontier area with mixed population dictated the settlement of the bulk of refugees in the rural areas of Macedonia and Thrace. Refugees settled in the agricultural lands of the previous Muslim residents who had to leave. Undertaking large public work efforts to dry Macedonian marshes would contribute to increasing agricultural yield.

---

28 Apostolos Doxiades Dr., "La situation des réfugiés en Grèce," (Genève, 1924) (extrait de la *Revue internationale de la Croix Rouge*, 6me Année, Septembre 1924): 724–34.

29 Elsa Kontogiorgi, "I Apokatastasi. 1922–1930," in *Istoria tou Neou Ellinismou 1770–2000*, ed. Vasilis Panagiotopoulos (Athens: Ellinika Grammata, 2004), vol. 7, 101–18.

In this context, the Refugee Settlement Committee attempted to promote a system of hygienic organization among the rural populations in Macedonia and Thrace. This system would operate in parallel with the Ministry of Hygiene. According to the initial planning, agricultural dispensaries would operate in each refugee village to serve between 500 and 800 refugee families. The inhabitants would be charged with a sum of money for medical and pharmaceutical care, which under certain conditions would be accessible even to destitute patients.[30] This model proposed by the Refugee Settlement Committee was quite efficient as it allowed for the medical care of refugees and the administration of scientifically tested medicines. In 1929, there were fifty-nine rural dispensaries in operation, mostly in refugee villages in Macedonia. The League of Nations public health experts who visited Greece the same year to study the reform of its healthcare system found them satisfactory.[31] When the Refugee Settlement Committee was dissolved, the rural dispensaries came under the jurisdiction of the Ministry of Hygiene, but after 1932 they gradually fell into disuse.

1.3 The Work of Women's and Philanthropic Organizations

During the crucial period 1922–1924, many women's philanthropic associations and aid committees gave food and offered volunteer work to refugees in various parts of the country in parallel with the work of the Ministry of Welfare and the Greek Red Cross.[32] The social work of female volunteers in these efforts, many of whom had previous experience in charity work, should not go unnoticed. Although the efforts of these women were not systematic and their historical narrative is fragmentary since their work was often unrecorded, some sources allow us to outline the general trend.

---

30 Kostas Katsapis, "Dimosia Ygeia, Prosfyges kai Kratiki Paremvasi stin Ellada tou Mesopolemou," 72–3; Elsa Kontogiorgi, "The Rural Settlement of Greek Refugees in Macedonia: 1923–1930." Ph.D. Diss. University of Oxford, Oxford 1996, 234; Vassiliki Theodorou and Despina Karakatsani, "Health Policies in Interwar Greece: the Intervention by the League of Nations Health Organisation," *Dynamis* no. 28 (2008): 53–75.

31 For the list of the dispensaries set up by the Refugee Settlement Committee and transferred under state jurisdiction, see the letter by the Committee's president Charles Eddy to Doxiadis, Doxiadis Archive, 256, file 9, The Benaki Mouseum's Historical Archives.

32 For example, the Aid Committee in Elefsina helped refugees, among other things, by setting up a soup kitchen where 700 refugees could dine on a daily basis. See untitled manuscript, related to the refugees' relief in Doxiadis Archive file 265, The Benaki Mouseum's Historical Archives.

Feminist and philanthropic organizations, as well as private donors, played the leading part in these women's charitable movements; providing medical care to children was part of their work. A central body, the Central Pan-Hellenic Collection Committee was set up in November 1922 to coordinate the activities of the various organisations. Its executive committee established neighborhood committees for rationing and medical care.

During the interwar period, women's organizations focused on securing accommodation, finding job vacancies for women and providing daily childcare. The National Council of Greek Women which published the magazine *Ellinis* (Hellenis, 1921–1940) was one of the two most important women's organizations in the interwar period that arranged for accommodation and distributed essential foodstuffs like sugar, milk, and rice, and primary necessities like soap, cooking utensils, shoes and clothes. In addition to overseeing forty refugee settlements, it also provided relief and accommodation to a number of families distributing clothes, beds and blankets. The organisation also secured jobs for refugee women. It established seamstress, embroidery and book-binding workshops employing roughly two hundred and fifty women. Anna Papadopoulou, an active member of the Council, ran similar workshops in the Old Palace.[33] The Association of Greek Women for the Rights of Women, another equally important women's organization during the interwar period, founded an employment agency for destitute women and an orphanage in Kallithea, the National Shelter, where eighty-five refugee girls lived and received vocational training.[34]

The Greek Red Cross set up in the Army School the "Refugee Orphanage" for the relief of healthy orphans. Sick orphans (about 315 children and babies) from Pontus, were accommodated in wooden shanties in Athens.[35] The Minister of Welfare established the Refugee Hospital in Athens, for sick refugees, while the Greek Red Cross established the "Refugee Shelter" in makeshift shacks behind the hospital to accomodate them. The hospital also annexed a maternity clinic to the hospital; here expectant refugees stayed before and after labor, and were taken care of.

The Greek Red Cross set up a Public Health Nurse School to give refugee women a profession while also providing health organizations with trained

---

33 "Ta Anaktora ton Stenagmon. Ti Ginetai sta Palaia Anaktora," *Ellinis* no. 11 (November 1923): 284.

34 *O Agon tis Gynaikas* no. 3 (October 1923): 5.

35 "I Merimna gia tous Prosfygas," *Ellinis* no. 10 (October 1922): 253.

staff. The school began operating in October 1924 under American social hygiene norms, which treated the visiting nurse as a missionary of public health. Accordingly, the School was supposed to help form a class of visiting nurses who specialized in school hygiene and general hygiene, puericulture and the treatment of TB.[36]

Nurseries and workshops for destitute women opened in 1923 and 1924 with the initiative taken by wealthy urban women. About three hundred refugee children, up to 8 years-old, were provided with shelter, food, education and medical care in the nursery set up by Mrs. Kountourioti with funds from Greek donors in America. Twenty infants were fed, given medical care and looked after during the day in the nursery at the expense of Virginia Benaki in Kifisia and supervised by Penelope Delta, a well-known children's writer. In the workshop set up with her donation, a hundred refugee girls made underwear for other refugees. They accepted commissions from refugee groups as well as from the Greek and the American Red Cross.[37]

2. THE WORK OF THE PATRIOTIC WELFARE FOUNDATION IN THE 1920S: URGENT NEEDS AND NEW DIRECTIONS

The Patriotic Welfare Foundation played the most active role in providing aid to female refugees and children especially. It gradually took on the pressing needs of refugees and formed modern maternity and child protection policies. Although between 1922 and 1924 the emphasis was laid upon the refugees' relief, from 1925 on the Patriotic Welfare Foundation did important work in the field of social hygiene under the influence of modern conceptions of mother and infant protection. The collaboration of the foundation with government officials and liberal scholars, who later played a leading part in establishing the General Society for the Protection of Childhood and Adolescence, lent an international dimension to its work. Finally, between 1925 and 1933, the inspired leadership of Apostolos Doxiadis, a visionary liberal doctor and Venizelos's advisor on health issues, contributed immensely to the renewal of the Foundation's public image and to implementing modern methods for children's health.

---

36 "Skholi Adelfon Nosokomon," *Ygeia* no. 11 (June 1, 1925): 238.
37 "Ta Anaktora ton Stenagmon. Ti Ginetai sta Palaia Anaktora," 285.

Due to political changes, the Foundation underwent changes in its name, structure, orientation and staff in September 1922 for the third time since its inception. One of the very first decisions of the new government formed after the coup of the Revolutionary Troika that leaned towards Venizelos, was to change the laws on the operation of the Welfare Ministry and the Patriotic Foundation. With the legislative decree of September 26, 1922 the Patriotic League of Greek Women was dissolved and the Patriotic Welfare Foundation reinstated itself. As already mentioned, the latter was dissolved in 1921 following the defeat of the Liberal Party in the 1920 election.[38] Its reestablishment was followed by the reorganization of the board of trustees, replacing the royalist members with ones who leaned towards Venizelos. Its organizational structure was similar to that which it had in 1917. Reform affected relief recipients as well; the previous royalist board of trustees had directed its work to the group of reservists, while the new board shifted more to refugees, the majority of whom supported Venizelos. The political strife between Venizelos's followers and the royalists, which marked the Greek political scene during the early twentieth century, did not leave the philanthropic and semi-state institutions unaffected. A case in point was the fact that the general secretary of the Foundation was appointed by the Minister of Welfare—in this case by Apostolos Doxiadis himself.

During the early months after the refugees' arrival, the Foundation reorientated itself to meet the urgent needs of the masses of refugees that streamed into the capital. Among its first steps were the organization of soup kitchens in the capital, the relief of refugees' and finding jobs for refugees. In October 1922, there were only two soup kitchens in the whole capital, centrally located, that prepared about 22,000 servings per day, but during the following months more soup kitchens were organized. In terms of medical care, it seems that the Foundation directed its energies to treating sick refugee children from Pontus, eastern Thrace and Asia Minor in the schoolchildren polyclinics in Athens and Piraeus.[39] It further distributed medicine and food supplies, supervised the dispensary it had previously set up in the Varvakeio Market and made sure sick refugee children were admitted to the

---

38 Nomothetiko Diatagma, "Peri Tropopoiiseos kai Sympliroseos tou Nomou 748 peri Systaseos Ypourgeiou Perithalpseos kai ton Symplirosanton afton Nomon," *Efimeris tis Kiverniseos*, A', no.178 (September 27, 1922): 1093–94.

39 "I Merimna dia tous Prosfygas eis tas Athinas kai ton Pirea," *Ellinis* no. 16 (November 1922): 276.

Saint Sofia hospital. In four months, one hundred and eighty three children were admitted to this hospital. Moreover, the Foundation allotted a considerable amount of money to various hospitals (24,560 drachmas) for the refugees' treatment and dispensed 11,569 prescriptions. Its female volunteers supervised the hygienic condition of the refugees that settled in Athens. To achieve better results, the city was divided into thirty sectors. According to Doxiadis's report, the Foundation offered supplies to 65,000 people during the last three months of 1922.[40] It also secured job posts for young destitute female refugees. The women either entered domestic service or worked as seamstresses in the workshops run by the Foundation where they made army clothes. Through this the Foundation attempted to provide young female refugees with an income indispensable for their survival.

In collaboration with the Ministry of Hygiene and Welfare, the Patriotic Foundation began organizing infant medical care. In the baby nursing center in Varvakeio Market at the center of the capital, doctors and volunteer nurses advised young mothers on cleanness, clothing, food and medical care. The city was divided into six sectors for the better operation of the nursing center. The expansion of this institution to other crowded Athenian neighborhoods testifies to its success. Once registered with the center, expectant mothers were required to visit on certain weekdays according to their place of residence. Specialist doctors examined those who came and kept them under observation until delivery and in the first few days after child birth. The center also supplied mothers with necessities and instructed them how to raise infants. Nursing stations were run through the voluntary contribution of women who had attended public health classes delivered by eminent doctors. As the institution gradually expanded, voluntary work was replaced by paid staff, directed by graduate nurses who had received theoretical and practical training in the School of Nurses of the Greek Red Cross.

Collaboration with foreign philanthropic organizations began in this period and lasted until the mid-1930s. In 1923, the Foundation had already reached prewar work standards. It continued its joint work with the American Red Cross in operating six nursing stations, two nurseries and a children's hospital in Athens, while its division in Thessaloniki undertook the

---

40 Apostolos Doxiadis, "Apologismos tou Prosfygikou Provlimatos," in Doxiadis archive, file 256, no 3. The Benaki Museum's Historical Archives.

gathering and accommodating of thousands of orphans. According to their reports, members of the Foundation gathered refugee children from the city streets, housing them in "temporary shelters" in the Lembet and Harmankioi settlements, and subsequenty placed them in orphanages, schools and adoptive families.

2.1 Steps against Infant Mortality: Control and Education of Mothers

In the 1920s, especially after 1925, the main concern of the Patriotic Foundation was to establish institutions that would contribute to the scientific support of mothers and infants. Starting in 1924, the work of the Foundation was limited to the protection of children. As a result, the departments for the destitute, refugees and employment were dissolved. At the end of 1924, Apostolos Doxiadis became president to the Foundation. Since then, he reoriented the organisation, diverting it from a philanthropic to scientific organisation for social work in children's welfare and hygiene. From 1925–1927, consultation stations for mothers and nursing services increased. In 1927, there were ten such stations in Athens. New branches were set up in the provinces and new institutions begun, like the model dairy-farm in Athens that provided Athenian children with fresh milk and the summer camps in Voula where the city's sickly children were sent. The nursing services in the center of Athens, organized by the American Red Cross, functioned as staff training centers for the respective provincial branches.

In order to encourage mothers involved in the education campaign launched by the Foundation, two modern institutions were initiated in 1925: the Award to Healthy Babies in 1924 and the Children's Week, which was the last week of the year. They were based on American models and presented an opportunity for the Foundation to display its goals and progress, primarily by giving doctors the opportunity to communicate directly with middle-class and working-class mothers. The Foundation invested much in this communicative policy targeted at young mothers.

During the Health Festival, four types of money prizes were awarded to the families of the healthiest and most beautiful babies in the nursing stations. However, the honor of the prize went mostly to mothers "whose application of and obedience to the advice delivered to them by doctors in these stations and visiting nurses was exemplary."[41] The Children's Week included the screening of informative films, popular lectures and distribution of educational leaflets to stress the relationship between the right, healthy upbringing and the duty of the parents to the nation.

The reason for the introduction of these institutions, according to Doxiadis, was not only "to give pleasure to children," but also to systematically and scientifically organize the protection of destitute children to improve the Greek race by instilling the people with a sense of responsibility to children, to support children "in every possible way, in every possible direction, in its every possible manifestation" so as "to secure the physical, social and mental capitals which would allow the nation to perform its role."[42]

Mothers' hygiene education and training in duties related to eugenic concerns were aspects of interwar governmental policy, through which the government tried to recover from the casualties inflicted by World War I and subsequent dramatic fall in childbirth. In the 1920s, the government encouraged women to give birth to more children, while treating the practice of abortion sternly. This ideology of motherhood was a crucial factor in deteriming the "well-being of the nation" and acted as a deterrent to the deterioration of future generations. Since politics during this period were understood mostly in terms of military confrontations and national survival, the physical well-being of mothers and their familiarisation with children's hygiene became increasingly important for the state. The words of an Italian fascist aptly illustrate the national importance attached to natural duty: "motherhood is female patriotism."[43] The collaboration of mothers with state agencies seemed more necessary than ever since the health of mothers was closely associated with children's health, causing the state to try to regulate through childbirth policy the attitude of mothers towards reproduction. Besides, training women in their maternal duties was a fairly easy and inexpensive method to accomplish "the cut of biological losses" and restore family life during the interwar period.[44]

---

41 See characteristically "Apo tin Drasin tou Patriotikou Idrymatos," *To Paidi*, no. 56 (June 1939): 24.

42 In a feminist publication in 1927, the celebration was characterized as the "Little God's Week." See "I Evdomas tou Paidiou," *Ellinis* no. 1 (January 1926): 5–6

43 Mark Mazower, *Skoteini Ipeiros. O Evropaikos Eikostos Aionas*, translated by Kostas Kouremenos (Athens: Alexandreia, 2001) 91. Originally published as *Dark Continent: Europe's Twentieth Century* (New York: Vintage, 2000).

44 Mazower, *Skoteini Ipeiros*, 88.

The decline in childbirth after World War I gave rise to international concerns about the well-being of the nation, though, in the Greek case concerns about women's willingness to respond to their natural reproductive calling sprang from high rates of infant mortality and child abandonment after 1922. This worrying phenomenon was the result of the forced movement and terrible living conditions under which women lived in the refugee settlements. The press and medical journals published between 1923 and 1928 gave three reasons for the imbalance between birth and death rates: high infant mortality, which doubled between 1921 and 1926; the rise in the number of abortions; and the early labor caused by abject poverty and hardships. Doctors classified the "inhumane work of the pregnant mother" into the same risk category as syphilis and alcoholism. Concerns about the repercussions these phenomena would have for the "eugenic progress of the young generation" were expressed in the Third Pan-Refugee Congress organized in Serres in 1925: "Abortions are in the daily agenda. Women's fertility has fallen to such a degree that serious attention to this matter is required and in general the situation is terribly hopeless."[45] Apart from women's sexual exploitation, the hardships many families had to go through were blamed for infanticide and the increase in abandoned children. This rise is also confirmed by the increase in the capacity of hospitals for abandoned children. It was suspected that some mothers, due to their extreme poverty, sought jobs in these hospitals as wet-nurses of their own babies, having already exposed them on purpose.[46] In order to sell their breast-milk, some mothers either abandoned their infant-babies or left them in the maternity clinic. These babies ended up in the Municipal Foundling Home where congestion and deplorable hygiene conditions sooner or later killed them. Around 1925, infant mortality in the Municipal Foundling Home was 90%.

In order to contain this malpractice, the authoritarian regime of Theodoros Pangalos drew the first law on "the protection of the nursing baby" in March 1926.[47] Following the model of the respective Italian law, the state took under its protection babies up to the age of two along with their destitute mothers. It provided for the registration of births and the control of

---

45 "To Trito Pamprosfygikon Synedrion tou Nomou Serron: Pos Emfanizetai I Katastasis ton Prosfygon eis tin Makedonian," *Pamprosfygiki*, February 3, 1926.

46 Athina Gianniou Gaitanou, "To Vrefokomeio Athinon kai I Mitrotita," *Ellinis*, no. 4 (April 1924): 30–1.

47 Nomothetiko Diatagma, "Peri Prostasias tou Thilazontos Vrefous," *Efimeris tis Kiverniseos*, A', no. 137 (April 26, 1926): 1025–26.

mothers working as wet nurses. Doctors and midwives had to register the births they had attended to the nearest police station within 24 hours of the delivery or the state would take their license for a period of time from six months to two years. In practice, this protective but also preventive legislation resulted in the formation of local committees "on the protection of infants." These committees, assisted by the police, would take care of birth registration in their assigned areas, observe the degree of the mothers' poverty, and offer financial aid to the destitute ones. The latter would be given the opportunity to work as wet nurses in the Foundling Home, provided that they would breast-feed other infants, following the "instructions of the Home's authorities."

In a period when the state was in need of births, the registration and medical observation of pregnant women became a national policy tool. The network of professionals involved in child birth was also under supervision. Doctors and midwives were liable for homicide if they failed to register the birth with the police, while private individuals who hired wet nurses without a police certificate were given a fine. The law also gave prison sentences to women who abandoned infants. In order to offer full protection to mothers, the state drafted a law a few months later that provided for the popularization of puericulture knowledge and the establishment of a model nursing station and a Eugenics and Puericulture Museum. The establishment of a puericulture institute would serve all these goals.[48] After the fall of Pangalos's authoritarian regime, these attempts, clearly inspired by the Italian model, did not materialize. However, due to the reform of the last Liberal government, they took on a more systematic and complete form.

During this period, two liberal paediatricians seem to have played a crucial role in these efforts: Kostis Kharitakis, director of the Social Hygiene Department of the Ministry of Hygiene since 1925 and Apostolos Doxiadis. Having paid frequent visits to social hygiene institutions for children in various European countries in the interwar period, these two doctors attempted to import certain European social policies on motherhood to Greece. To some extent, their views contributed to the improvement in the living standards of women and to reinstating the value of motherhood. As such, fem-

---

48 Nomothetiko Diatagma "Peri Organseos Ethnikou Paidokomikou Institoutou,"*Efimeris tis Kiverniseos* A', no.391 (November 6, 1926): 3139–40

inist organisations which considered their views acceptable disseminated them through the interwar feminist magazines.[49]

During the 1920s, the alignment of feminists and doctors on issues of motherhood and eugenics became better articulated in articles in the magazines *Ellinis* (Hellenis) and *O Agonas tis Ginaikas* (The Woman's Struggle) published by the National Union of Greek Women and the Association for the Rights of Women since 1921 and 1923 respectively. Articles on the role of eugenics in the reduction of infant and child mortality written by paediatricians or obstetricians such as Kharitakis, Doxiadis, Angeliki Panagiotatou and Moysidis were published in these two journals to communicate new scientific concepts to women.

During this period active feminists such as Athena Gianniou-Gaitanou, Avra Theodoropoulou and Maria Svolou made frequent references to the protection of mothers and children in light of women's political and legal rights. They believed that knowledge of puericulture and eugenics would help women raise healthy children. In addition, feminists expected that medical care for destitute pregnant women would prevent the birth of mentally deficient children and would secure deliveries in a medical environment.[50] It would also put a limit on infanticide and abortion, which put women's health at risk. Feminists and doctors seem to agree with the French paediatrician and president of the French Eugenics Society, Adolf Pinard who stated that "mothers hold the future of puericulture." For this reason, these two groups worked together to prepare the first congress on children in Thessaloniki in 1925. The hygienic upbringing of children (hygiene, medical care, social welfare and upbringing) and mothers' education (feeding, labor, breast-feeding, scientific organization of nursing stations) were among the themes the congress touched upon.[51]

Among the governmental officials and scholars who were engaged in the mid 1920s in the improvement of hygienic conditions for the benefit of chil-

---

49 See, for example, the articles published between 1924–1928 in the magazine *Ellinis* by Kostis Kharitakis, after he had visited social hygiene institutions in Germany, Italy and Austria. "Koinoniki Ygieini," *Ellinis* 6 no. 11 (November 1927): 233–5; *Ellinis* 6, no. 12 (December 1927): 259–62; *Ellinis* 7, no. 1 (January 1928): 10–12; *Ellinis* 7, no. 2 (February 1928): 40–2; *Ellinis* 7, no. 3 (March 1928): 63–5.

50 Vassiliki Theodorou, "I Prostasia tis Mitrotitas kai tis Paidikis Ilikias ston Mesopolemo: Ethnikes Proteraiotites, Koinoniki Politiki kai Diekdikiseis gyro apo ti Sygkrotisi tis Ennoias tou Physikou Kathikontos ton Gynaikon," in *Logos Gynaikon*, ed. Vassiliki Kontogianni (Athens: ELIA, 2008): 639–56.

51 "Panelladiko Synedrio Thessalonikis," *Ellinis* no. 2 (February 1925): 27. The congress was postponed and took place in 1930.

dren, one should not fail to mention the members of The Society for the Protection of Childhood and Adolescence, which was the local branch of the International Union for the Protection of the Child. Its founding members in 1925 included paediatricians, judges, jurists, psychologists and high-ranking state officials in social welfare services as well as feminists, who had already dealt with children's issues. Many of them had participated in international organizations or congresses and were familiar with the current international literature on childhood issues. The Society aimed, among other things, to improve the financial and social conditions of children's lives, particularly infants, to study issues related to children's social hygiene, to secure the prophylaxis of the child within the family, to put a limit on paternal authority, and to ensure the rights of children born outside wedlock. These issues had also been tackled by feminist organizations during this period. In addition, the society sought to protect and control street children, working children and children with special needs, as well as to introduce novelties like children's courts, reformatories or asylums for abused children, already institutionalized in other countries. The journal *To Paidi* (The Child) began in 1930, with articles related to these issues. The journal also publicised the Foundation's work, since the Society members held the view that the Foundation promoted their aims.

Two main points should be stressed regarding state policy on the protection of motherhood after the arrival of the refugees: firstly, the absence of efficient state social policy for handling the serious financial problems of the working class; and secondly, the fact that voluntary organizations mushroomed. Due to lack of resources, infrastructure and frequent governmental changes, policy on motherhood and childhood was disrupted. The state emphasized birth control and mothers' education on children's hygiene and upbringing. In other words, the state used measures that foregrounded the ignorance and backwardness of the working class and the value of the female body for the nation's strengthening. Apart from the state, voluntary organizations worked to modernize the measures for the protection of children and create networks with international movements. The active role of philanthropic organizations in dealing with social issues in Greece during the nineteenth century might explain the dynamism the interwar voluntary societies exuded.

3. HEALTH CARE MEASURES FOR PUPILS (1922–1928):
FINANCIAL LIMITATIONS AND CONTAINMENT OF THE ATTEMPTS

Since the available sources offer only a fragmentary picture of the situation, it is not easy to answer many of the questions related to how student health problems were dealt with during the period under consideration. Some aspects of these problems are illustrated in the school officers' reports, legislative decrees and the reports of voluntary organizations that collaborated with the School Hygiene Service, attached to the Ministry of Education. These sources highlight mainly two problems: firstly, the deterioration of student health, blamed on classroom congestion that spread contagious diseases; and secondly, the condition of the school building worsening not only due to the increase in the number of students—especially in the areas where refugees had settled—but also due to the requisition of school buildings between 1922 and 1924. A few days after the refugees' arrival, the state requisitioned public school premises, private high school classrooms, tutorial and commercial schools to temporarily accommodate the refugees. Special advisory committees were set up comprising a school inspector, a civil servant from the Ministry of Hygiene and Social Welfare and a school medical officer. Following their investigations, these three-member committees recommended which schools or classrooms should be requisitioned.[52]

Although problems persisted, the funds allotted by the Ministry of Education to the School Hygiene Service were drastically cut down in the mid-twenties as a result of Greece's financial problems and political instability. The collaboration of Lambadarios with voluntary organizations, which adopted modern social work practices, such as the Red Cross, solved the problem partly. However, results were limited only to certain Athenian neighborhoods. Consequently, the attempt to create school hygiene infrastructure, already under way since the previous decade, was disrupted during the period 1922–1928.

---

52 Nomothetiko Diatagma "Peri Epitaxeos tis Khriseos ton Didaktirion Aithouson ton Idiotikon Ekpaideftirion," *Efimeris tis Kiverniseos*, A', no. 22 (January 18, 1923): 149–150. The requisition followed the terms specified in article no. 6 of the Decree "Peri Epitaxeon Akiniton di'Egkatastasin Prosfygon," *Efimeris tis Kiverniseos*, A', no. 237 (November 17, 1922): 1426 on the requisition of buildings. See also *Deltion tou Ypourgeiou ton Ekklisiastikon kai tis Dimosias Ekpaidefseos*, no. 30/31 (January-February 1924): 23.

3.1 The Course of Student Morbidity

During the early years following the refugees' settlement, the School Hygiene Service emphasized containing the most important problems: school supervision, student vaccination, organizing the anti-trachoma and anti-TB fight and the medical examination of students. Statistics on the hygienic condition of the school buildings, published in the *Bulletin of the Ministry of Education*, show that the prefecture of West Macedonia faced the most acute problems with school overcrowding and lack of desks.[53] The area also had the highest percentage of sick students and teachers as well.

From 1922–1925, thirteen hygiene inspectors and seventy school doctors comprised the staff of the School Hygiene Service. As needs skyrocketed from 1923 onwards, temporary school doctors were assigned permanent posts. Unfortunately, the picture we get about the situation is fragmentary since only a part of the reports submitted by school doctors and inspectors has been preserved. However, the reports of Khristos Georgakopoulos, hygiene inspector of the fourth prefecture (north-west Peloponnese), found in the Lambadarios archive, show the deterioration of the situation immediately after the refugees' arrival. For example, in 1924, thirteen schools in Patrai and ten schools in the wider region were occupied by refugees. In addition, between 1923 and 1924, many schools in the villages of Peloponnese were unsuitable low buildings, with no roof or floor, insufficiently lit and aired. 80% of the schools did not have toilets and unhygienic and unsuitable desks were found in 90% of the schools. In general, school doctors blamed "the excessive increase of the refugee students" and the lenient exams teachers gave for the insufficient capacity of schools. Based on the personal cards of the students (male and female) for the years 1923–1924, it is evident that the majority suffered from malaria (approximately 50%), pediculosis, trachoma and adenopathy. Their height and weight had decreased compared to the findings for the years 1918–1919.

Statistics compiled by the Ministry of Education show that between 1924 and 1927 student morbidity went from 27% to 30% and 17.4% to 20% for primary and secondary school students respectively. Compared to the previ-

---

53 *Miniaion Deltion Skholeiatrikis Ypiresias February 1924, Deltion tou Ypourgeiou ton Ekklisiastikon kai tis Dimosias Ekpaidefseos*, no. 34 (May 1924).

ous decade, the deterioration is evident. According to Lambadarios, there had been an increase in the number of students examined in the school clinics, however, the fact that these documents were produced by the director of the School Hygiene Service, and as such stressed the progress accomplished, should not elude us. State expenditure on the School Hygiene Service appearing in the same document tends to increase until 1925. Starting in 1926 there was a fall in state expenses that lasted until 1930.[54]

Year	Estimates in Drachmas
1915–1916	166,980
1919–1920	215,840
1924–1925	738,400
1925–1926	2,069,000
1927–1928	968,360
1928–1929	985,000
1929–1930	1,628,000
1930–1931	1,624,000
1931–1932	1,844,000

Table I: State Expenses on School Hygiene Service (1915–1932)

Cuts in state allotments were not justified by the increased student morbidity rates. During 1925–1926, epidemics of plague, smallpox, typhus, meningitis, typhoid and paratyphoid infections, dysentery, diphtheria, scarlet fever, measles, whooping cough, flu, etc., broke out. In addition, the rates of the students affected by TB, malaria, and trachoma were on the rise. Despite the deterioration of the indices, there were considerable cuts in the School Hygiene Service's expenses that resulted in a decrease in the number of school doctors and even in their redundancy. The year 1926 must have been the worst year in the history of the institution, since almost all school doctor posts were cut out.[55] It was decided that reparations of 500 drachmas should be paid to each school doctor from

---

54   *Mémorandum sur le service hellénique de l'hygiène scolaire. L'Organisation de l'hygiène scolarie en Grèce* (Athens: Pyrsos, 1933), 14.

55   In March 1926, their number came down to eight but from April 1 onwards all school doctor positions were abolished.

municipal or local funds. However, only a few municipalities and local councils were eager to take on the cost. In addition, the institutional regime regarding the appointment of school doctors changed. The legislative decree of October 15, 1927, required a school doctor certificate to secure the relevant appointment. The certificate was awarded following an oral exam in front of a committee composed of university professors of Hygiene and Microbiology, Ophthalmology, Paediatrics, Dermatology as well as the Head of the School Hygiene Service or the professor of Paedology and School Hygiene at the Secondary Teacher Training School.[56] All these changes resulted in the disruption of the School Hygiene Service, but some school doctors continued to work gratis, in the belief that this situation would soon improve.

3.2 The First Social Welfare Centers: Vaccination and Health Propaganda

During this period, Lambadarios stressed the value of mass vaccination and hygiene propaganda at school. On average about 12,000 children were vaccinated every year. Voluntary organizations conducted vaccination in addition to the School Hygiene Service. The establishment of the first social hygiene center for children by the Greek Red Cross in the refugee settlement of Vyronas made possible the medical supervision of children using modern concepts about the organization of social work. Lambadarios must have played an important role in the establishment and operation of the center, as he expected that the center could respond to a series of novelties: the application of the BCG (Bacile Calmette-Guérin) vaccine on newborns, the introduction of school nurses and the detection of pre-tubercular students.

The center played a leading part in the vaccination of students. In October 1927, the Social Hygiene Service conducted a mass diphtheria vaccination for students in the social hygiene clinic. Students from schools in Pagrati and Kaisariani[57] were vaccinated and, on April 14, 1925 in the cen-

---

56 Diatagma, "Peri tou Tropou Apoktiseos tou Endeiktikou Skholiatrou," *Efimeris tis Kiverniseos*, A', no. 226 (October 20, 1927): 1575–76.

57 Emmanouil Lambadarios "Peri tou Antidipheritikou Emvoliasmou eis ta Imetera Skholeia" reprinted from the journal *Kliniki* no. 28 and no. 29 (July 9 and 16, 1932): 8.

ter of social hygiene run by the Greek Red Cross within the premises of the Civilians' Hospital in Athens the BCG vaccine was tested for the first time in Greece. The vaccine, discovered by Albert Calmette, was the introduction of the Coch bacillus into people who had not been affected by TB, i.e., into newborns. Calmette-Guérin first tested the vaccine on children in 1921 in France. In 1925 it had not yet been fully embraced by some members of the medical community. Despite reactions from the Greek medical community, Lambadarios, who must have been in contact with Calmette, was in favor of testing the vaccine.[58] Greece was one the very first countries where this vaccine was applied. Between 1925 and 1930, a team under Lambadarios's supervision, in collaboration with Eleni Vasilopoulou, the head nurse and general inspector of the Red Cross nurse team, vaccinated 2,500 children who came from the poor refugee neighborhoods in Athens. The visiting nurses of the Red Cross had undertaken the detection of family environments suspect of TB.[59] After the vaccination, children were observed by the center of social hygiene in Vyronas as well as by the Patriotic Foundation's Department of the Protection of Childhood. According to the statistics published by Lambadarios, the results were very satisfactory. Between 1925 and 1929, mortality rates of infants who had not been immunized against TB came to 10% of all death cases while mortality rates of inoculated infants amounted to 2,5%, many of whom had been living in a consumptive environment.

Apart from the vaccination station in the center, other departments were gradually added such as ophthalmological, paediatric departments, a school dental clinic and a paedological station. The latter carried out research under the guidance of the staff of the Peadological Laboratory of the Ministry of Education. The school nurse at the center observed the students' hygiene attending the seven schools in the area. Due to full medical care offered to the children and to the center's collaboration with the School Hygiene Service of the Ministry of Education, the center was recognized as a model of social welfare equal to the student polyclinic set up in 1915.

---

58   See Emmanouil Lambadarios letter to Calmette on May 15, 1931, Lambadarios Archive, ELIA.

59   Emmanouil Lambadarios, "I en Elladi Efarmogi tou Antiphymatikou Emvoliou BCG," *Praktika A´ Panelliniou Synedriou Mitrotitas kai Paidikon Ilikion*, 358–85 and Emmanouil Lambadarios, "La Vaccination Préventive des Nouveaux- nés Contre la Tuberculose," *Phtisiologie Medico-sociale* vol. 9 (Octobre 1928): 417–22.

3.3 Trachoma and the Role of the Greek Red Cross

Trachoma was one of the contagious diseases that worsened after 1922. The refugee surge disrupted the progress achieved before then. According to the tables drawn by the School Hygiene Service, during the 1926–1927 school year, 40% of the students suffering from ophthalmological diseases were affected by trachoma. Trachoma cases in the refugee settlements in Athens came up to 5% of the examined students in Vyronas, 10% in Nea Ionia, 15% in Kokkinia and 16.3% in Mesogia of Attica.[60] Research carried out by the School Hygiene Service in 1927 found that in a total of 223,349 children examined across the country, 5,000 suffered from trachoma. Lambadarios estimated that the number of sick children must have been higher than that since many students who suffered from light trachoma were considered either healthy or suffering from epipephycitis.

In order to tackle the problem, Lambadarios drew up a special programme, *The Plan for the Fight against Trachoma at Schools*.[61] This programme envisioned travelling anti-trachoma teams and trachoma schools, along with preventive and therapeutic measures like anti-trachoma clinics, dispensaries and stations in proportion to the population of each area. All these were to be supervised by doctors specializing in the model ophthalmological surgery of the Student Polynclinics in Athens or Piraeus.

However, although trachoma problems became worse, cuts to funding prevented the materialization of the anti-trachoma campaign. Since the financial resources of the Ministry of Education decreased, the Head of the School Hygiene Service resorted to the Greek Red Cross. The Greek Red Cross set up three anti-trachoma clinics at its expense between 1925 and 1927. The first clinic began in Lavrio, the most affected area in Attica, in a building rented by the Ministry of Hygiene to be used as an anti-TB clinic. The anti-trachoma clinic in Lavrio stood as a model for this type of clinic. Yet, it was not possible to register patients affected by trachoma so as to contain the spread of the disease. The doctor in charge of this clinic accused both the locals and the local authorities of indifference, and sought the help of the police to force them to visit the clinic.[62] In 1926, two more special

---

60 Khristopoulos, *Ekthesi Ygieinis Epitheoriseos Skholeion, 1927–28*.
61 Emmanouil Lambadarios, *Diagramma Katapolemiseos tou Trakhomatos eis ta Skholeia* (Athens: 1927).
62 Dimitrios Oikonomopoulos, "O Agon kata ton Trakhomaton. To Antitrakhomatikon Iatreion tou Ellinikou Erythrou Stavrou," *Ygeia* no. 9 (September 1926): 197–99.

clinics were set up in Larisa and Volos. Similar clinics were organised in the refugee hospitals of Athens, Nea Ionia, Kaisariani and Kallithea. These clinics, directed by specialized ophthalmologists, diagnosed and treated children suffering from trachoma.

Since the means to combat contagious diseases were limited, health authorities resorted once more to the more inexpensive and easier method of spreading preventive means. The press stressed the importance of two factors for the popularization of hygiene practices: the use of simple language, without scientific terminology when addressing patients orally or by written means, and the involvement of the school. According to the tenth French Congress on Hygiene in 1925, teaching hygiene should be the number one priority for the national economy. Instilling hygienic habits in the students would improve their health while also indirectly spreading them to their familes, contributing to the cultivation of personal and social hygiene in a wider circle. Therefore, the school could be connected with society through teaching hygiene and play an important role in raising an elementary hygiene awareness.

Following the refugees' arrival, the School Hygiene Service multiplied its publications; leaflets with instructions on various diseases such as scarlet fever and trachoma were published in 1923 to educate the masses.[63] During the same period, miniature posters showing the reasons of infection had been published and they were hung on classroom walls. In order to combat malaria, students were prompted to form groups to fight mosquitoes and larvae, and drain areas of stagnant water. School doctors, who had played an important role in the organization of the School Hygiene Service for national reasons among others, considered it imperative that hygiene be popularized and introduced to school as a compulsory subject. For example, Dimitris Stefanou, who became head of the School Hygiene Service, after the retirement of Lambadarios, in his article featuring in the magazine *Ygeia* (Health) in 1925, stressed that hygiene had already been introduced to the curricula of schools across all levels of education in the neighbouring Balkan countries, Romania, Serbia and Bulgaria. [64]

---

63 See the written instructions by the Ministry, "Odigiai peri tis Nosou Ostrakias kai tis ap' Aftin Profylaxeos" and "Odigies gia tin Prophylaxi apo to Trakhoma," in publication of the Ministry of Education "Peri Prophylaxeos ton eis ta Skholeia Foitonton apo ton Loimodon Noson."

64 Dimitrios Stefanou "[...] Pro Pantos, na Eklaikefthi I Ygieini. Anagki na Eisakhthei eis ola ta Skholeia os Kyrion Mathima," *Ygeia* no. 8 (April 15, 1925): 161–4 and by the same author, "Eklaikefsate tin Ygieinin. Na Eisakhthei Afti eis ta Skholeia mas os Kyrion Mathima," *Ygeia* no. 9 (May 1, 1925): 186–90.

During this period, voluntary organizations such as the Greek Red Cross and the American Near East Relief took up important initiatives to popularise hygiene. Evident in the archive of Lambadarios, around 1925, popular publications addressed to children were modelled on the leaflets published by the American Red Cross. These models imply a rift with tradition due to the use of new communication media, i.e., leaflets, posters, films. In addition, the Greek Red Cross commissioned a series of American educational films on various topics like venereal diseases, TB and malaria. The films were screened in barracks, associations, factories and schools to familiarize the public with similar issues. A popular health magazine of the period commented that these films included scenes derived from real life, mixed with "obscure" scientific knowledge.

In its education campaign the School Hygiene Service collaborated with the Junior Red Cross, a new institution established immediately after the end of the Great War. The Junior Red Cross aimed to help the newly founded states educate their youth to make them aware of their responsibilities as citizens. Since the mid 1920s, the Greek Red Cross distributed free soap, toothbrushes and toothpaste and since 1924 published postcards and a popular magazine, contributing to the dissemination of hygiene principles. It is not known whether the health games *Health Crusade* and *A Trip to Health-land* made by the American Junior Red Cross for American schools were ever introduced in Greece.[65] It seems that some school doctors responded to similar institutions because they were in favour of a more entertaining way of teaching, but also of applying hygiene principles. They wanted to make children pick up hygiene principles in a spirit of noble emulation.

The American influence on the renewal of hygiene dissemination methods is also evident in the call made by the Near East Relief for a children's hygiene textbook. In 1925, along with the School Hygiene Service of the Ministry of Education and the Greek Red Cross, the organization issued a call for the writing of a popular school hygiene textbook intended for C, D, E, and F graders, and their families. The critical committee consisted of both Greeks and Americans: Professor of Hygiene and Microbiology at the University of Athens Konstantinos Savvas representing the Greek Red Cross;

---

65 By 1925, the American Red Cross Library had compiled a list of more than 60 health plays and games available for classroom use. John F. Hutchinson, "The Junior Red Cross Goes to Healthland," *American Journal of Public Health* 87, no. 11 (November 1997): 1816–23.

Emmanouil Lambadarios on behalf of the Ministry of Education; George Wilcox, director of the educational department of the Near East Relief; and George Mikhailidis, professor. The award was funded by Barkley Acseson, the director of the East organisations and was named in honour of the general director of the Near East Relief in Greece Harold C. Jaquith.

First prize was awarded to George Sakellariou, a pedagogue who had studied psychology in Switzerland and the United States, for his book entitled *The Student's Hygiene*. The latter was published at the expense of the Junior Red Cross in 1926. A circular issued by the Minister of Education, Aiginitis, encouraged students to buy it at a low price. The book was written in simple language and amply illustrated. Following modern concepts on hygiene teaching promoted by the American Red Cross, the book emphasized the practical application of acquired knowledge and the cultivation of a sense of hygienic duty. Each chapter concluded with questions to the student and drills with bits and pieces from contemporary games influenced by war. These drills presented health problems as castles, viruses as enemies, etc. An attempt was made to introduce elements of self-government and self-examination. The student had to answer twelve questions by marking in a table which hygiene exercises they did everyday (brushing their teeth, washing their hands, respiratory drills, sleeping with the window open, etc.). These exercises were part of a hygienic model students had to conform with. The more hygienic exercises the students completed, the healthier they were considered.

However, despite the efforts of the voluntary organizations to spread personal hygiene principles and establish social hygiene institutions such as the Vyronas hygiene center, social welfare works for students—a new term in use during this period—were inferior to those in other European countries.

CHAPTER VII

THE LIBERAL GOVERNMENT AND THE PROTECTION OF CHILDHOOD AND MOTHERHOOD: LANDMARKS AND CONTINUITIES (1928–1932)

The Liberal government (1928–1932) was a landmark in the interwar political history of Greece, signifying a period of relative stability following successive government changes, political upheaval and military coups. Social welfare and the protection of children and mothers were some of the challenges the Venizelos government faced. During this four-year period, initiatives were undertaken to solve pressing issues related to internal and external affairs which arose after the arrival of refugees. Interstate agreements for aid and collaboration were signed with neighboring Balkan countries in an attempt to break away from large establishments. In addition, large scale public works were undertaken to curb the problems of refugee integration and urban hygiene.

The interest the Liberal government took in reforming the public health system through international health organizations and the establishment of a social insurance system demonstrate the importance the government attached to solving acute social problems that arose during the interwar period. This reform is evident in the attempts of central and eastern European governments to modernize public health, and the attempt of Venizelos government to rebuild the Greek economy and avoid social unrest. Venizelos, a liberal politician that left an indelible mark on the country's politics during the first half of the twentieth century, attempted during these four years to pass a series of reforms aimed at modernizing social relations. Improvement in the fields of social welfare and health counterbalanced the collective fears of social insurrection fed by leftist ideas mounting up in the 1920s.

1. The Plan for the Reorganization of Public Health: Expectations and Frustration

In October 1928, the Liberal government appealed to the Health Committee of the League of Nations (LN) for the hygienic reconstruction of the country; the appeal was accepted later in December of the same year.[1] Recourse to the Health Committee of the LN was dictated by the weakness of previous governments to deal with public health problems and with the breakout of a dengue fever epidemic. Between October 1927 and July 1928, 1,320,000 persons came down with dengue fever, bringing the economy to a standstill. This epidemic—which Venizelos himself fell victim to—raised awareness of the dangers and brought to the fore the issue of public health services. The Health Committee of the LN accepted the request of the Greek government and sent a group of experts to observe these problems. In spring 1929, a committee comprised of seven hygienists of the LN arrived in Greece; during their four-month field research they visited three major cities, fourteen towns and eighty-two villages. As a result, a hundred and forty-eight reports were filed with the committee's observations and their surprise at the low quality of health services. According to the Geneva experts, Greece was a dangerous country as far as hygiene was concerned. The plan the committee proposed for the country's hygienic reconstruction followed the standards adopted by other Central and South European countries. At the time, Yugoslavia stood as model for the reconstruction for the fight against malaria and TB, and protection of children. In addition, the committee highlighted how important the establishment of public health services were, like water supply, town planning, construction of hygienic houses and schools, creation of drainage system and athletic centers. Preparation of public health staff was of prime importance for the hygienic reconstruction as prevention was lacking. The final proposal submitted by the committee stressed the need to establish a central organization that would coordinate all public and private

---

1   Vassiliki Theodorou and Despina Karakatsani, "Health Policy in Interwar Greece: the Intervention by the League of Nations Health Organisation," *Dynamis*, no. 28 (2008): 53–75.

health services. This organization would be staffed with experts and would lay the foundations of preventive and social medicine in Greece. The establishment of a hygiene school in Athens and the sending of doctors to Europe and America to pursue specializations would fill the gap in the education of hygienists and visiting nurses. At the same time, the operation of health centers across the country would decentralize health services. The reconstruction aimed to consolidate all the widely dispersed hygiene services under the Metropolitan Hygiene Service in Athens-Piraeus. The health center was at the core of this proposal and was responsible for carrying out hygienic checkups throughout the country. Each center included one or more clinics for malaria, TB, children's diseases, groups of visiting doctors, hygiene officers responsible for drainage and water supply issues, a pharmacy and public baths. Aside from this, the health center would offer possibilities to educate the local people on hygiene. This new plan was planned to take effect in 1933, following five years of systematic preparation. During this transition period, all hygiene services attached to various ministries would come under the jurisdiction of the Hygiene Undersecretary. This plan would be piloted in the areas where the LN experts had conducted their research—Athens, Thessaloniki, Ioannina, Chania, Corfu and Macedonia. This pilot programme aimed to convert the bureaucratic system of district hygiene organization into a network of health centers, comprising three to five centers in each area. The Rockefeller Foundation, which supported this venture by sending expert hygienists and offering staff immediate instructions, carried out pilot programmes to counteract malaria in the villages of Macedonia by coordinating the School of Hygiene, the Ministry of Hygiene and its own anti-malaria groups.

The programme was not fully implemented. Only a few of its parts materialized: the School of Hygiene and the sending of experts abroad. The School of Hygiene was one of the first schools in Europe that aimed to further educate hygienists and engineers, hygiene officers and visiting nurses. In 1934, the plan was abandoned due to economic and political reasons, the most important reason of which was the 1929 financial crisis that hit Greece in 1932, driving its economy to a deadlock. As a result, the Greek government declared bankruptcy. Unable to draw funds from the international market, the Liberal government was forced to abandon its plan for hygiene reform and resigned in May 1932. The intense political upheaval, characteristic of interwar politics, was yet another reason for the cancellation of this venture since the succeeding government, supported by the Popular Party, cancelled all reform plans of this otherwise ambitious programme. Finally, the conflict between the members of the Greek medical community and the foreign experts, the confusion of responsibilities between different services and the general animosity of medical circles towards a reform not based on their needs, who feared the undermining of their authority were also responsible for the failure of this venture and the withdrawal of foreign experts in 1935.

During this four-year period attempts to set up a unified social insurance organization in step with the legislation on labor, passed earlier by the Liberals in 1920, were intensified. The directives of the International Labor Organization (ILO) of the LN as well as the collaboration between the staff of the ILO and the delegates of the Ministry of Labor and trade-unionists played a key role in establishing a social insurance system for working-class people.[2] The deliberations, which started on Venizelos's initiative and lasted for a few years, resulted in the passage of Law no. 5733/1932 "on social insurance." However, this law did not come into effect due to political developments; two years later, it was replaced by Law no. 6298, which provided for the establishment of the Social Insurance Foundation.

2. Hygienic and Social Policy on Infants

Curbing infant mortality and protecting children were the main priorities of the Liberal government as can be inferred from the electoral campaign of its leader. Many of the issues that concerned the scientific community and voluntary organizations were regulated by a series of laws. Many of the propositions for improving children's health put forward by high state functionaries, social thinkers, scientists and scholars affiliated with the Liberals were met with responses by Liberal politicians. The establishment of the Sub-ministry of Hygiene in 1928, its subsequent upgrade to become the Ministry of Hygiene the following year, and its eventual evolution to become the Ministry of State Hygiene and Social Welfare are all concrete evidence of the importance the government attached to health is-

---

2   On the issue of social insurance, see Liakos, *Ergasia kai Politiki*.

sues, but also of the discontinuities that characterized government health policy. The most important aims of the Liberal government with regard to hygiene living standards for school-aged children were pursued through a series of works: modern hygienic school buildings, open-air school, schools for special groups of students (blind, deaf and "anomalous"), student summer camps and student soup kitchens, and hygiene as a school subject at all education levels.[3] Within ten months, from August 1928 until June 1929, the Parliament passed seventeen laws protecting children and attempting to decrease infant mortality.

The two most important laws were law no. 4062/1929, which changed the name of the Patriotic Foundation of Welfare into Patriotic Foundation for the Protection of the Child (PFPC), and law no. 4061 "on hygiene and protection of motherhood and childhoods." The latter provided for the transition of the Foundation into a semi-state foundation for the protection of children under the jurisdiction and control of the Sub-ministry of Hygiene. At the same time, the National Council for the Protection of Motherhood and Childhood was established in the Ministry of Hygiene. Its mission was to supervise and instruct institutions that dealt with the hygiene and welfare of infants and pregnant mothers.

Having maintained many of the characteristics of its previously voluntary organization and having secured financial support both from private sources and from the Ministry of Hygiene and Social Welfare, the PFPC became the only state organization that was trying to materialize children's health policies. The transition towards state intervention in child welfare had been evident since 1924. As a result, the PFPC was organized on a more secure basis starting in 1929. Among its goals were the construction of model centers for children's social hygiene in Athens and in the provinces and the proper education of higher and lower technical staff. Calling into action a large group of volunteer middle-class women who worked in various departments under the guidance of doctors, jurists and social thinkers, the Foundation worked to secured food and fresh air for children and instruct young mothers in hygiene principles. The stations run

---

3   For the educational philosophy behind these changes, see Alexis Dimaras, "Kharaktiristika tou Astikou Phileleftherismou sta Ekpaideftika Programmata ton Kyverniseon Venizelou," in *Venizelismos kai Astikos Eksykhronismos* eds. Giorgos Mavrokordatos, Khristos Khatziiosif (Irakleio: University of Crete Press, 1988), 21–32.

by the PFPC, which commenced operation in all major towns (thirty-six branches) since 1924, provided mothers with advice and healthcare. In the departments of expectant mothers, doctors and nurses, assisted by female volunteers, observed and recorded infant development, distributed food to destitute mothers and organized summer camps for weak children. In addition, in the Department for the Protection of Infants, an institution similar to *La Gouttes de lait* operated. The expansion of child protection in the provinces led the Patriotic Foundation to organize two one-year classes for visiting nurses (1931–1932) led by eminent doctors. Yet, the small number of doctors could not efficiently meet the needs of its branches. The publication of popular science leaflets with advice to young mothers, the institution of health awards to the healthiest infants and the celebration of mother's day supplemented the Foundation's policy on lowering infant mortality and on instruction in scientific motherhood.[4]

As president of the PFPC, from 1924 until 1932, Doxiadis, who also served as Undersecretary of Hygiene from 1928 until 1932, played an important role in materializing the PFPC programme. The Sub-ministry took legislative steps for the country's hygienic reconstruction, the fight against contagious diseases and the protection of public health at large. It worked to expand the system of hospitals, establish new sanatoriums and clinics, apply an extensive programme of inoculation, fighting malaria, trachoma, smallpox, and to protect children.[5] It also took steps to curb infectious diseases (typhus and plague) and flu and promoted the anti-TB, anti-trachoma and anti-alcohol campaigns. While Undersecretary of Hygiene, Doxiadis supported imposing taxes on the unmarried, though this remained a dead letter. In collaboration with the Ministry of National Economy and the Ministry of Justice, the PFPC studied issues such as hygiene at the workplace,[6] social insurance, and the hygiene of prisons and prisoners.

---

4   For the relevant laws, see *Efimeris tis Kiverniseos* A', no. 294 (March 9, 1929): 914–18. For the action of the PFPC during this period, see Kostas Saroglou, "I Prostasia tou Paidiou stin Ellada," *To Paidi*, no. 4 (November–December 1930): 59–77.

5   *Logodosia Yfypourgeiou Ygieinis*, September 1, 1928 – February 15, 1929.

6   Lida Papastefanaki, "Apo tin 'Ygieini ton Epitidevmaton' stin 'Ifximenin Nosirotita tis Ergatikis Taxeos': i Epaggelmatiki Ygeia stin Ellada, 1870–1940," in *Dimosia Ygeia kai Koinoniki Politiki: O Eleftherios Venizelos kai I Epokhi tou*, ed. Giannis Kyriopoulos (Athens: Papazisis, 2008), 265–88. Also by the same author "Dimosia Ygeia, Fassanelis kai Epaggelmatiki Pathologia stis Ellinikes Poleis stis Arkhes tou 200u Aiona," in *Eleftherios Venizelos kai Elliniki Poli. Poleodomikes Politikes kai Koinonikopolitikes Anakatatakseis* (Athens: Ethniko Idryma Erevnon kai Meleton Eleftherios K. Venizeos, Skholi Arkhitektonon Mikhanikon, 2005), 155–70.

As president of the PFPC, Doxiadis tried to secure funding from the government.[7] He also visited child protection institutions in Dresden, Berlin and Vienna, and later suggested the adoption of various hygiene measures for children.[8] His articles in the press informed the public about the social welfare system in these countries and compared them to Greece while severely criticizing the lack of funding for healthcare.

On the initiative of the Patriotic Foundation, the first Pan-Hellenic Congress on the Protection of Motherhood and Childhoods took place in Athens (October 19–26, 1930). The congress stressed the necessity of reorganizing the School Hygiene Service and the introduction of personal health cards for children from infancy until the end of adolescence. The congress also emphasized improving hygiene teaching, both in terms of quality and quantity, in schools across the country and the establishment of a teachers' fund for medical care and treatment of teachers. Themes also included rearranging the school timetable according to paedological concerns, support for the Junior Red Cross, the establishment of schools for the disabled, the deaf and the feebleminded, and the creation of a center for the protection of adolescents. The establishment of either special asylums or branches in the existing mental hospitals or psychiatric clinics, the proliferation of reform schools and the creation of a central medico-pedagogical institution with provincial stations were also promoted. The establishment of juvenile courts and the special education of those engaged in their operation were also stressed. In 1930, the tenth anniversary of the National Union for Child Welfare was celebrated in Athens, and in April 1930 the first congress on hygiene took place coinciding with the centenary of the country's independence.

Part of the initiatives for strengthening children's health during this period came from voluntary organizations such as the Greek Red Cross.[9] The School of the Red Cross Nurses, established in 1924, and the School of So-

---

7   Doxiadis Archive 1, 22/256, The Benaki Mouseum's Historical Archives and Kostas Dafnis, *Apostolos Doxiadis. O Agonistis kai o Anthropos* (Athens: 1974).

8   Various articles published in epistolary form by Doxiadis in July 1930 in the newspaper *Elefteron Vima* referred to his visit to the Hygiene Exhibition in Dresden; See "Ti Parekhoun oi Germanoi eis to Aporon Paidi," (July 8, 1930), "I Koinoniki Ygieini gia to Paidi" (July 11, 1930), "Ekthesi Ygieinis tis Dresdis" (July 17, 1930), "I Prostasia ton Polyteknon. To Provlima tou Plithysmou" (August 4, 1930), "Eis to Germanikon Peripteron. Klironomikotis kai Evgonismos" (August 6, 1930).

9   Law no. 371 "Peri Katastatikou Khartou tou Ellinikou Erythrou Stavrou kai Tropopoiiseos tou apo 13 November1927 N.D.," *Efimeris tis Kiverniseos* A', no. 272 (December 23, 1928):2407–2408.

cial Hygiene Visiting Nurses, which operated as a branch of the Hygiene School since 1930, played an important role in protecting infants. In 1932, the Society of the Social Medicine and Hygiene was set up by a group of doctors and pharmacists, with the aim to conduct scientific research, study the conditions of hygiene of the working-class and to improve them. In order to attain this goal, the following means were suggested: educational lectures, both scientific and popular ones, scientific research and appeals to the authorities.

3. School Hygiene and Hygienic Propositions

Between 1928 and 1932, the state attempts to tighten supervision of students' health intensified.[10] The increase in funding for School Hygiene and the incorporation of school doctor salaries in the budget of the Ministry of Education are evidence of the government's interest in strengthening the School Hygiene Service. Better nutrition, the spread of hygiene principles, open-air teaching and summer camps were the main directions the government's social policy on student health took. Although the Liberals' attempts since 1914 to protect children continued, they took on a more systematic character during this period. Among other initiatives, the Liberal government attempted to decentralize hygiene services and focus on the fight against certain diseases. The press and the protagonists of the health reform accentuated the social causes lying behind child malnutrition and morbidity.

The trends in strengthening and protecting children in many European countries after World War I were also evident in Greece. Lowering child mortality, which had reached high levels, lay at the core of the government's agenda. Approximately 150,000–160,000 children died each year.[11] The mortality rate of children under four years old, 31 out of every thousand infants, caused particular concerns. Mortality rates among Greek children were especially frustrating when compared to central European countries and Scandinavia where the respective mortality rates were 7.5‰ and

---

10 For the importance ascribed to child health care, see the article "Apo tin Ygeiav tou Ftokhou Paidiou Exartatai to Mellon tis Ellados," *Elefteron Vima*, December 27, 1928, 1.

11 Emmanouil Lambadarios "To Ygieionomikon Programma," *Ergasia*, no. 28 (July 19, 1930): 21–3 and Solon Veras, "I Prostasia tou Vrefous," *Ergasia* no. 35 (November 1, 1930): 12–3. However, the rate of student morbidity seems to have fallen to 18.6% in 1928–1929, compared to 24.5% for the years 1926–1927.

4‰ respectively. Infant mortality rose in Greece in 1931, reaching the highest levels in Europe.[12] The most important reason for child morbidity and mortality remained the triad of social diseases which took a heavy toll on the working classes: trachoma, malaria and TB. For this reason, the fight against these diseases targeted schoolchildren during this period.

Trachoma[13] kept rising in many areas, such as Athens, Piraeus and Lavrio, where it hit three-fifths of students.[14] In certain Athenian neighborhoods, 40–50% of children suffered from trachoma. School doctors expressed fears that this could reach 100% within thirty years.

As malaria continued to plague certain provinces, especially in Northern Greece, a law passed in 1930 regulated the anti-malaria campaign.[15] The Ministry of Hygiene was given an allotment of 24 million drachmas for its budget. Teachers were also important in the fight against malaria. Their role included: the systematic administration of quinine to the students, their theoretical and practical education about malaria, the establishment of specially instructed student groups to kill mosquitoes and larvae and to drain stagnate water. The students had to begin with the school yard and then sanitize the entire village or neighborhood. Finally, it was expected that the anti-malaria campaign would educate students and the public through film screenings and lectures delivered by properly educated staff. Lambadarios suggested that the first week of June be Anti-malaria Week, during which students would leave the classroom and perform anti-malaria activities.[16] Law no. 5043/1931 established the state monopoly on quinine giving it the exclusive right through the Ministry of Hygiene to import, package, sell and circulate quinine in powder or any other form.

The rise in the number of tubercular students and teachers heightened concerns about the speed with which the disease spread in schools. In order

12 Vasilios Valaoras, "To Provlima tis Thnisimotitas en Elladi," *Praktika Akadimias Athinon*, 7, 15, 1940, 205–18. Khristos Zilidis, "I Epidimiologiki Pragmatikotita stin Ellada tin Periodo tou Mesopolemou kai Politiki gia tin Organosi ton Ypiresion Ygeias," in *Dimosia Ygeia kai Koinoniki Politiki: o Eleftherios Venizelso kai I Epokhi tou*, 131–49.

13 Theodoros Tzanidis, "To Trakhoma, i Megali Pligi tou Ergatikou kai Agrotikou Plithysmou 500.000 Astheneis kai Akhristoi pros Ergasian. Oi Kindynoi tis Afxiseos kai Epektaseos tis Nosou. Ti Prepei na Gini eis ton Mathitikon Kosmon kai eis ton Straton," *Elefteron Vima*, September 28, 1928.

14 Leonidas N. Khristopoulos, *Etisia Ekthesi Pepragmenon tou Ygieionomikou Epitheoritou ton Skholeion tis A' Periphereias. Perilpsis ton Pepragmenon tis Olis Skholeiatrikis Ypiresias*, 1928.

15 Law no. 4555/April 19, 1930.

16 Emmanouil Lambadarios, *Eniafsia Ekthesis peri ton Pepragmenon tis Skholikis Ygieinis, 1930–31*, published by the Ministry of Education.

to counter TB, new sanatoriums were set up in various areas across Greece. In 1930, the sanatorium "Sotiria" was reorganized, including the establishment of a scientific department designated as "Tubercular Center." Moreover, extra funding was allotted for the fight against TB.

Measures taken to protect school children, especially the rise in funding, bore fruit. According to Lambadarios, from 1929 until 1931, student morbidity dropped while the number of vaccinated students rose.[17] Mandatory vaccination and re-vaccination reduced or eliminated certain contagious diseases such as diphtheria.[18] During this period, school doctors and school nurses carried out systematic measurements and entered data concerning weight, height and thorax circumference into health cards.[19] The social clinics set up in some Athenian neighborhoods, despite their low number, contributed to the systematization of measurements and the import of hygiene models from other countries.

4. Teaching Hygiene in School

During the interwar period, debates on the importance of teaching hygiene[20] and cultivating new conceptions of hygiene dictated by eugenic perspectives proliferated in various countries where some doctors and pedagogues expressed their views on this issue.[21]

In 1929, the systematic teaching of hygiene and paedology began in schools across Greece. Hygiene should be promoted both in theory and practice as it had been one of the most effective means for individual development and social reform. The object lesson as a teaching method (tables/blackboards, pictures and illustrated textbooks) was promoted in the lower

---

17 The rate in 1915–1915 amounted to 34.25%, in 1919–1920 to 32.03%, in 1920–1921 to 23%, in 1925–1926 to 22.5%, in 1926–1927 to 24.5%, in 1928–1929 to 18.6% and in 1930–1931 to 18.25%.

18 It was at that time that the anti-diphtheria vaccination was used for the first time due to the aggravation of the disease in refugee neighborhoods.

19 During the first Pan-Hellenic Congress on the Protection of Motherhood and Childhoods, Z. Nafpliotou, head of the tenth Primary School, mentioned that the personal health card had not become common, as was the case with bakery workers, printers and tanners.

20 Dimitris Stefanou, "Eklaikefsate tin Ygieinin. Na Eisakhti Afti eis ta Skholeia mas os Kyrion Mathima," *Ygeia,* no. 9 (May 1 1925): 186–190 and 193; *Ygeia* no. 9 (September 1929): 206.

21 The tenth French Congress on Hygiene in 1924 stressed that hygiene should be the number-one priority in social and national economy; teaching hygiene should be obligatory at all schools; all the institutions had to be equipped with suitable equipment so as to make possible the practical teaching of hygiene (wardrobes, showers and offices).

grades of primary school and the role of the teacher in propagating and adopting new hygiene practices was strengthened. A nurse was also available to offer assistance to this direction.[22] Chapters on hygiene, life needs, nutrition, clothing and housing were included in science textbooks, taught at the upper grades of the primary school. Hygiene continued to be taught in secondary schools following the above system, namely teaching somatology and individual hygiene as part of science lessons. The new curriculum of secondary schools, implemented during the school year 1931–1932, included an hour-long hygiene class in the fourth grade. A doctor or school doctor taught with a special textbook that included the following subjects: somatology and individual hygiene, general hygiene (contagious diseases, on air, water, soil, nutrition, clothing and housing and hygiene according to age and profession), nursing and first aid. In female secondary schools, elements of puericulture were included as well.

Starting in 1925, the School Hygiene Department in the Ministry of Education gave instructions for the introduction of sexual education into secondary schools and secondary teacher training colleges. Law no. 4152 made sexual education a subject taught by the hygiene teacher in these institutions. It seems that sexual hygiene caused great concern not only in Greece but also in other European countries. According to Lambadarios, teaching sexual hygiene started in Belgium in 1920, and was extended to high schools and colleges when the results proved to be promising. This issue was discussed at the medical teaching congress in Brussels in 1923, and the majority of doctors and educators were in favor of teaching this subject. In Germany, Italy (where there were special courses to prepare and further educate secondary school teachers), Switzerland (where the issue was vigorously propagated by the Union for the anti-venereal fight) and Czechoslovakia, sexual education was considered by health experts of utmost importance and was seen as a duty to school youth. Teaching hygiene was accompanied, according to the regulations, with visits to social hygiene museums, hospitals, maternity clinics, public nurseries, the assignment of books and the screening of films which had as their subject sexual education.[23]

---

22 "Peri Programmatos Didaskalias tis Ygieinis eis ta Skholeia tou Kratous," in Antoniou, *Ta Programmata tis Mesis Ekpaidefsis*, 98.

23 Lambadarios in his book *Skholiki Ygieini* cited the following textbooks as extremely interesting with regard to this issue: *Maman dis-moi*, 1927 by Montreuil-Strauss and *Sag'mir die Wahrheit, liebe Mutter* by Mary Wood Allen.

An approved textbook was used in primary and secondary schools while in teacher training colleges hygiene textbooks were used. The textbook *Ygieinai Synitheiai* (Hygienic Habits) by Lambadarios, based on American textbooks and intended for primary school students, is an interesting example. The philosophy that permeated this book was groundbreaking. At the end of each chapter hygiene problems were listed with drawings and hygiene related questions, while its simple form and illustration made the book easy to follow.

Hygiene was taught in a considerable number of secondary schools and practical high schools, and in all seminaries. Here government funding made it possible to grant school doctors who taught hygiene a monthly pay of 250 drachmas. At the rest of the secondary schools, hygiene was taught by teachers of science. Teachers with some background in hygiene taught the subject in primary schools, having graduated from teacher training colleges where they had had a similar course. It was highlighted that it was necessary that prospective doctors, jurists and pedagogues had some background in hygiene and paedology. In 1932, a special seat on "Paedology and School Hygiene" was established at the Medical School to provide expert knowledge to prospective doctors.

Thanks to state appropriations and school funds, special collections of equipment, leaflets and films were made available for teaching. Among the methods of teaching hygiene, "the game of health" is of particular interest. Students wrote down everything they did on a form daily: bathing of the entire body at least once per week, brushing their teeth, sleeping with the window open, drinking of milk, etc. The School Hygiene Service placed emphasis upon educational cinema and its use at school, army and navy and suggested an organization of educational cinema under the auspices of the Ministry of Education be set up in Greece.[24] In the international congresses on Educational Cinematography some decisions were made to facilitate the international exchange of hygiene films, to exempt them from customs du-

---

24 The film archive in Paris, set up in 1925, had taken special action so as to screen films related to hygiene, its popularization, and the practice of its principles. Also, the Rockefeller Foundation had laid great importance on educational propaganda. Mobile propaganda groups played an important role in popular teaching, especially in provincial and rural settings. Many international congresses as well as the LN had looked into this issue; the latter set up in Rome in 1928 the Institute of Educational Cinematography which published a monthly journal especially devoted to cinema as a means of education. Emmanouil Lambadarios, *O Kinimatographos kai I Paidiki Ilikia* (Athens-Alexandreia: Kasigoni, 1928).

ties, and for the International Institute of Educational Cinematography to produce educational films, following scientific, medical and pedagogical standards.[25]

In Greece, the Association for the Development of Cinema for Children set out to do this. The Association was created after the Philological Association of Parnassus, the Lyceum of Greek Women, the National Council of Greek Women and the Patriotic Foundation merged. The School Hygiene Service drafted a bill on educational cinema to have films screened at schools and for film archives to be founded. The government passed the legislative decree on September 10, 1935 establishing the Educational Cinema Office in the Ministry of Education.[26] The company Gaziadis and Bros produced quite a few educational films.

5. Papandreou's Programme on School Buildings

When Venizelos took office in 1928, the problem of school buildings reentered the government's agenda. Due to the refugees' arrival, many school buildings had been requisitioned in order to meet acute accommodation needs. Between 1920 and 1928, 976 new school buildings had been constructed. Funds for their construction came from tuition fees and bequests intended to cover educational needs.[27] Yet, as Lambadarios had often stressed in his papers, these needs were quite serious, especially in the big urban centers—Athens and Piraeus.[28] Out of a total of 7,675 schools across the country, 2.69% were inside other schools, churches or mosques; 133 were in wooden buildings, 747 in brick buildings, and 6,882 in stone buildings.[29] A report for the school year 1930–1931 mentioned that in Athens, a city with around 40,000 students, only two school buildings, intended to accommodate primary schools, had been constructed in the last forty years.

---

25   In the third International Congress on Educational Cinematography in Vienna, Sofia Gedeon and Loula Marketou participated, as at the time they had been studying there.

26   Lambadarios, in response to the request of the president of the International Institute of Educational Cinematography of the LN to present the accomplishments of the Greek educational cinema, wrote that in 1931 there were four to five films on the protection against TB, typhoid fever and malaria, which had been shot by the Patriotic Foundation for the Protection of the Child together with the Greek Red Cross.

27   "I Didaktiriaki Kinisis," *Epetiris Dimotikis Ekpaidefseos* (Athens: Dimitrakos, 1932).

28   A' Panellinion Synedrion Prostasias Mitrotitas kai Paidikon Ilikion (Athens: October 19–26, 1930), 8.

29   Sifis Bouzakis, *Georgios A. Papandreou, 1888–1968. O Politkos tis Paideias, 1888–1932* (Athens: Gutenberg, 1997) vol. A, 37.

By contrast, the suburbs had more new school buildings. In order to compensate for this deficiency, thirty-three primary schools, thirteen junior high schools and two practical senior high schools had to be built in the capital. It was estimated that Greece needed an extra 4,000 school buildings, costing 2,400,000 drachmas.

In 1927, the Architectural Department of the Ministry of Education issued requirements for the construction of school buildings, school building plans, the financial support they needed including state contributions, and repairs that should be carried out. However, according to a 1927 report, the hygienic condition of school buildings was atrocious. Out of the 2,105 schools examined in 1926–1927, only 804 (approximately 1/3) were considered hygienic.[30] The hygienic conditions of the schools in the refugee shanties were especially alarming.

Some observations on the problems of school buildings concerned the need to deal with the teachers' morbidity, which had reached worrying proportions in the 1920s.[31] The reasons that dictated the medical examination and supervision of the teachers' health were not only connected with their performance in their assigned duties, but also with the risk of infecting the students and the rest of the school staff. Since 1928, thorough thorax X-ray had been imposed on prospective students at teacher training colleges.[32] If a teacher came down with TB, it was suggested drastic measures be taken and his/her health be systematically monitored.[33]

5.1 Action, Funding and Architectural Novelties

During Venizelos's second prime ministership, the government planned and carried out a school construction programme in connection with the educational changes accomplished between 1928 and 1932. This programme was designed to meet the needs of the time while implementing innovative ar-

---

30 *Etisia Ekthesis tis Ypiresias tis Skholikis Ygieinis, 1926–1927*, Ministry of Education, Tmima Skholikis Ygieinis (Athens: 1927). The same condition was aptly illustrated in the report filed by Leonidas N. Khristopoulos, *Etisia Ekthesis ton Pepragmenon tou Ygieionomikou Epitheoritou ton Skholeion A´ periphereias*, Ministry of Education and Religious Affairs (September 15, 1928).

31 Circular no. 35377, "Peri Iatrikis Exetaseos ton Ypopsiphion Mathiton ton Didaskaleion."

32 Lambadarios, *Skholiki Ygieini meta Stoicheion Paidologias*, 321–33.

33 Leonidas N. Khristopoulos, *Etisia Ekthesis ton Pepragmenon tou Ygeionomikou Epitheoritou ton Skholeion tis A´ Periphereias*, 1928.

chitectural ideas. The Ministers of Education Konstantinos Gontikas[34] and Georgios Papandreou shared the same views and fervor as each other, and took special interest in school buildings. Before 1929, the Architectural Department had built 1,100 buildings, testifying to the government's interest in moving past neoclassicism, adopted earlier by Kallias's plans. These buildings were built in harmony with nature and rurality.[35] Following this spirit, the Minister of Education, G. Papandreou promoted a plan of mass construction of school buildings. The building of 4,000 new classrooms began with collaboration from the Office of Architectural Studies, set up in 1930 and incorporated in the Architectural Department of the Ministry of Education.[36] The results were visible, but without substantial funding this ambitions project could not be completed. As G. Papandreou noted in 1931, "A serious and efficient attempt to construct school buildings was made. During this current year, we provided aid to 1,500 schools of local communities and we do hope that during the next two years on the loan of one million liras we will solve the problem of school buildings in cities to a great extent. And at this point, I wish to praise and commend the teachers and school officers on their official pride, which was channeled into the construction of as many school buildings as possible."[37]

Until 1929 a policy of limited funding for new buildings was followed so as not to put a strain on state budget.[38] In March 1929, the Minister of Education, K. Gontikas, introduced a bill "on the construction of school buildings" that focused not only on the need for buildings but also on the

---

34 Circular, "Peri Efarmogis Orismenon Ygeionomikon Metron en tois Skholeiois pros Prophylaxin ton Mathiton apo ton Loimodon Noson," (August 29, 1928). This circular was signed by the minister K. Gontikas.

35 Andreas Giakoumatos, *Stoikheia gia ti Neoteri Elliniki Arkhitektoniki. Patroklos Karantinos* (Athens: MIET, 2003) 68.

36 For the programme of the school buildings during the period 1928–1932, see the table published by Alexis Dimaras and Vassiliki Vasilou-Papageorgiou, eds., *Apo to Kontyli ston Ypologisti*. (Athens: Metaikhmio-ELIA, 2007). Theodoros Mikhalopoulos who played an important role in the handling of the programme served as director of the technical services. See Giakoumatos, *Stoikheia gia ti Neoteri Elliniki Arkhitektoniki*, 72.

37 Alexis Dimaras and Vassiliki Vasikou-Papageorgiou, eds., *Apo to Kontyli ston Ypologisti*. George Kalyvas mentioned that the programme provided for the construction of 1,897 schools whose cost came up to 1,500,000 drachmas. He also mentioned that up to that year 1,809 schools were completed and another 178 were under construction. G. Kalyvas, "Ecoles nouvelles en Grèce," *L'Architecture d'Aujourd'hui* no. 2 (1933): 68–70.

38 Eleni Kalafati, *Ta Skholika Ktiria tis Protovathmias Ekpaidefsis 1821–1929* (Athens: IAEN, 1988), 208. Also by the same author "Istoriko ton Skholikon Ktirion tis Dimotikis Ekpaidefseos (1821–1940)," *O Politis* no. 67–68 (1984): 34–40.

means of covering their cost.[39] The government adopted a decentralization rationale in response to this bill. The construction cost moved from
the state budget to local communities and funds. The state was only to provide some financial allocations for the completion of the buildings, allotting 1/5 from the fund of tuition fees in the National Bank. The funds were
enough, since tuition fees were separated from the state budget because of
law no. 3189/1924.[40] In order to construct the new school buildings, Papandreou contracted a loan on June 4, 1930 amounting to 1,000,000 liras
from Aktiebolajet Kreuger and Roll, a Stockholm company. The largest portion of this loan, which was ratified by law, was allotted to the construction
of school buildings, while a smaller part was for the completion of school
buildings already under construction.[41] Between 1928 and 1932, 3,167 new
school buildings were constructed (8,190 classrooms), and by 1938 that
number was 4,000. Out of these buildings, 330 had more than one classroom and were constructed with funds by the Ministry of Education and
the local committees for school buildings.

5.2 Modernity and Hygiene Intervention

In order to respond to the acute need for new school buildings, but with minimum financial means, the Ministry of Education suggested that as many
new school buildings as possible be built without particular requirements for
proper organization and construction. However, the regulations set by the
General Charter of Building Schools in 1930 were followed; particular care
was taken with regard to the dimensions and the orientation of the buildings, the size of the playground and the school yard, lighting, ventilation and
heating, cleanness, water supply, drainage and the suitable placing of toi-

---

39 Konstantinos Svolopoulos, ed., *Konstantions B. Gontikas, 1870–1937. Thesmikes Allages kata ton Mesopolemo* (Athens: 2003), 54.

40 Under law no. 2442/1920, "Peri Idryseos Tameion Ekaipedeftikis Pronoias pros Kataskevin Didaktirion
kath'apan to Kratos kai Promitheian Skholikon Epiplon kai Didaktikon Organon," the foundation of
school welfare funds was accomplished. These funds handled the construction of the school buildings
across the country but also the supply of school furnishing and teaching equipment; they also saw to
the application of a complete decentralization system. See Leonidas Khristopoulos, *Etisia Ekthesis ton
Pepragmenon tou Ygeionomikou Epitheoritou ton Skholeion tis A' Ekpaideftikis Periphereias, os kai Perilipsis
ton Pepragmenon tis Olis Skholeiatrikis Ypiresias* (Athens, September 15, 1928).

41 See the article no. 1 of the Law no. 4799, "Peri Kyroseos tis apo 4 Iouniou 1930 Synaftheiseis Symvaseos
peri Khorigiseos Daneiou 6% L. S. 1.000.000 pros Anegersin ton Skholikon Ktirion tou Kratous,"
Efimeris tis Kiverniseos, A', no. 232 (July 8, 1930): 1961–67.

lets, baths and sinks. These rules specified that the architectural plans for the school buildings should be simple in form and structure, easy to apply and economical, avoid luxury and useless elements, superfluous space and complex architectural forms, and be decorated simply. Special care was also taken for their adjustment to the particular climate conditions of each area. Particular instructions were given for the construction of classrooms and supplementary rooms, but only in some schools. Attention was also paid to the design of baths, dining rooms and separate houses for guards.

In 1930, the Minister of Education and Religion accepted applications from civil engineers and architects for the position of temporary school architects. The same year a service made up of young architects, influenced by Modernism, formed in the Ministry of Education. They revised the form of school buildings and attempted to introduce to Greece the achievements in modern architecture. The French architect Em. Hébrard was contracted to supervise their work. Initially, Mitsakis and Karantinos, and later on K. Panagiotakos, Dimou, G. Zoggolopoulos, B. Douras, Ag. Siagas, K. Laskaris, I. Despotopoulos, Th. Valentis, P. Georkakopoulos, A. Kakkouris, and S. Leggeris participated in the Architectural Department of the Ministry of Education. D. Pikionis and A. Zakhos also collaborated with the service. The civil engineer Panagiotis Soursos and the architects George Pantzaris and Kostas Rousopoulos also played an important role. These young architects were advocates of modern architectural principles: functionalism, speedy and economical construction, attention to soil morphology and subversion of the monumental style.[42] Modernism was an attempt to adapt architecture to technological development and the progress of modern industrial culture. In other words, it used new materials for buildings—concrete, iron, glass and synthetic materials—and new industrial methods, as well as the simple designs. Various construction work like apartment blocks and the social house fall into this architectural movement, which also paid special attention to school buildings and health and welfare facilities. Modernism blended with the general modernizing trend of the Liberals and was evident in the social character of their intervention in the field of hygiene.[43]

42 *Tekhnika Khronika* no. 3 (March 1967): 24–46 (special issue on school buildings) and Dionysis A. Zivas and Maro Kardamitsi-Adami, "Syntomo Istoriko ton Skholikon Ktirion stin Ellada," *Arkhitektonika Themata* 11(1979): 174–83.

43 Andreas Giakoumatos, "I Skholiki Arkhitektoniki kai I Empeiria tou Monternou stin Ellada tou Mesopolemou," *Themata Khorou kai Tekhnon* no. 18 (1987): 50–61.

The school buildings built under Minister of Education, G. Papandreou, included showers,[44] kitchen-restaurants, craft and design classrooms, sheds for physical education, long corridors with aligned windows that allowed plenty of light, quasi-outdoors areas, big staircases, terraces, yards, and even chapels and school gardens. These schools also had special recreation and teaching areas, and in big schools there were also assembly and ceremony halls. The color of the buildings was of great importance, as well as the physical orientation of the classrooms. They had to face southwards, while corridors faced northwards. In certain cases, corridors were open galleries above lower floors. Windows lined classroom walls for even distribution of light. One of the goals of these new buildings was to use stonework and concrete for terraces.[45] Although during the construction of the earliest buildings no special attention had been given to shade, later on this was achieved by adding permanent light shelters. In addition, open corridors in the eastern parts of buildings and bilateral lighting were implemented.

Patroklos Karantinos,[46] Dimitris Mitsakis and Dimitris Pikionis were important architects who contributed immensely to the design and construction of school buildings in the 1930s. They developed a dialectical relation between the school building and outdoor areas, experimenting with new shapes and forms, especially with quasi-outdoor solutions popular during the period.

Two types of school were constructed according to climate: in cold, humid areas with strong winds, the most typical type of school building had north roofed corridors and classrooms facing eastwards. In areas with mild, dry weather, without south winds, school buildings with corridors made up of open verandas or galleries were preferred. Classrooms faced southwards for even distribution of light. The Kharokopou Primary School and the Kallithea Primary School, designed by Karantinos, are interesting examples of these building requirements. The latter was the first to be designed by Karantinos and the first to be inaugurated by Venizelos, as a start for the materialization of its reform plan. The school had six classrooms plus a crafts

---

44 In 1931 municipal baths for children were set up.

45 Giakoumatos, *Stoikheia gia ti Neoteri Elliniki Arkhitektoniki.*

46 He replaced the traditional corridors with a terrace and an open gallery eastwards. The open areas served the circulation, airing and lighting while also functioned as "cells of social life." See Giakoumatos, *Stoikheia gia ti Neoteri Elliniki Arkhitektoniki,* 131. Patroklos Karantinos, *Ta Nea Skholika Ktiria* (Athens: Ekdosis Teknikou Epimelitiriou tis Ellados, 1938).

classroom, offices, a canteen, a gym shed, usable terrace and a huge garden. This educational model was called "the New Acropolis" because of its relationship with residential areas.[47] In 1930, as part of the same reform plan, a complex comprising two six-classroom primary schools "with a crafts classroom, sheds for gym and a big common yard" designed by Dimitrios Klapsis, was built in Volos.

During the school year 1930–1931 (Minister G. Papandreou, director E. Lambadarios), two hundred buildings were constructed following hygiene standards, laid out in the charter of pedagogical, hygiene and technical conditions. The school buildings and complexes of the so-called "Papandreou programme," were admired by the architects of the fourth International Congress on Modern Architecture in Athens in 1933. During his visit to the school complex on Mikhail Vodas street, Le Corbusier did not hide his admiration both for the architectural work itself and its creator, writing a congratulatory note on the school wall. Le Corbusier himself was a source of influence and inspiration for many Greek architects, with Karantinos the first to follow him. The primary school on Kolettis street, designed by Mitsakis, was called one of the most important buildings internationally between 1879 and 1970 by the French journal *Architecture d'Aujourd'hui* in 1971. The 1934 special issue of the same journal, highlighted the austere and functional character of these schools, their limited cost, the organic co-existence in them of different educational levels in the same buildings, their organization of special halls that met new pedagogical perspectives and educational needs, and especially their attempt to adopt elements from local tradition.

However, some critics expressed reservations towards the innovative character of these buildings. They stressed that the pioneering character of this architecture could only be seen in school buildings that had many classrooms, while others bore structural and architectural elements of the period before 1930, i.e., of classicism and "the return to roots" movement.[48] Others supported that the 1930 charter on school buildings[49] retained some of the

47 Giakoumatos, *Stoikheia gia ti Neoteri Elliniki Arkhitektoniki*, 89. *Tekhnika Khronika*, translation of an article for *Arkhitektoniki* from French (August 15, 1934): 731.

48 Kalafati, *Ta Skholika Ktiria tis Protovathmias Ekpaidefsis*, 484 and Katerina Kyriakou, *To Arkheio tis Diefthinsis Tekhnikon Ypiresion tou Ypourgeiou Paideias kai Thriskevmaton*, General State Archive, no. 23, Athens 1992.

49 Manolis Mantoudis, "Les Bâtiments Scolaires en Grèce," *L'Hellénisme Contemporain* no. 7 (1936): 633.

requirements laid out in 1911.[50] Many of the elements put forward in this charter, i.e., the teaching classrooms, the arrangement and use of tables instead of desks, in combination with the principles of the work school (arbeitsschule) do not seem to have been adopted.[51] In addition, baths were also not constructed in the schools, although in certain cases their construction was imperative for the delousing of students and the fight against typhus (as was the case in Macedonia and Thrace).

The existence of corridors in every school irrespective of their size and needs also received negative criticism. Also, although the classrooms had a seating capacity of 30–40 students, in practice classrooms accommodated up to a hundred students, further testifying to the violation of certain new architectural elements due to objective circumstances and financial problems.[52] Furthermore, criticism was levied against the location and use of various facilities; for example, toilets were located in a small building outside the main one and more often than not right next to the shed for gym and baths. Also, the lack of connection between the main building and the toilets, either roofed or open, and the difficulty in properly maintaining these areas due to lack of drains, water pipes and shortages in supervising and cleaning staff were problematic. Despite these problems, this educational model was successful and innovative due to its larger student capacity and architectural and hygienic novelties.

6. Open-air Teaching, Children's Summer Camps and Semi-open-air Solutions

The decade from 1929 to 1939 saw the development of the so-called open-air school movement. The rise in the number of open-air schools across Europe and the spread of semi-open-air solutions to many schools demonstrate the popularity of the movement during the interwar period. The advances in education prior to 1914, the spread of ideas through publications and congresses on social hygiene, school hygiene, open-air teaching, combined

---

50 Kalafati, *Ta Skholika Ktiria tis Protovathmias Ekpaidefsis*, 217.
51 This view is held by Kalafati in her book *Ta Skholika Ktiria tis Protovathmias Ekpaidefsis*, 217.
52 These views were also carried by Miltos Kountouras and were recorded in his paper entitled "To Skholiko Ktirio," *Didaskalikon Vima* (November 23, 1930): 2–4; Giakoumatos, *Stoikheia gia ti Neoteri Elliniki Arkhitektoniki*, 80.

with the vigorous attitude of the open-air teaching advocates prompted local councils, municipalities, and the state to adopt novel proposals involving
both open-air teaching and New Education principles.[53]

6.1. The Spread of the Institution

Organizations, associations, committees, and international congresses on
open-air education set up between 1929 and 1939 contributed to the development and establishment of this novel institution. Case in point was the
French Association of Open-air Education (Ligue française pour l'éducation
en plein air), which aimed to regenerate the French race and help it survive
TB, alcoholism and other degenerative factors. Open-air education was one
method offered in various educational congresses—either of general or special interest—during this period (Paris 1922, Brussels 1931, Bielefeld 1936).
The international congresses on open-air education also facilitated the exchange of information and the spread of the institution. It was not coinci-
dental then that this movement developed in a period when new ideas on
education were spreading internationally.

The main characteristics of the open-air movement during the interwar
period included the pursuit of solutions that combined hygienic and educational principles and the involvement of pioneering educators who had
become fervently dedicated to spreading the principles of New Education
internationally. During the first international congress on open-air schools
organized by the *Ligue française pour l'éducation en plein air* and the International Child Welfare Congress, the delegate of the French Association of
Open-air Education stressed the need to prepare robust bodies, and vigorous and active individuals, in other words healthy future citizens both physically and morally.

Members of the congress stressed the need to set up a committee on
open-air schools in every city and replace all the conventional school build-

---

53 On the history of the open-air schools, see Anne-Marie Châtelet, Lerch Dominique and Luc Jean Noël,
    eds., *L'école de plein air. Une expérience pédagogique et architecturale dans l'Europe du XXe siècle* (Paris:
    Editions Recherches, 2003). Anne-Marie Châtelet, "A Breath of Fresh Air. Open Air Schools in Europe,"
    in *Designing Modern Childhoods. History Space and the Material Culture of Children*, eds. Marta Gutman
    and Ning de Coning-Smith (New Brunswick, NJ, and London: Rutgers University Press, 2008). Also,
    Cruikshank, M. "The Open-air School Movement in English Education," *Paedagogica Historica* 17, no. 1
    (January 1977): 62–74.

ings in cities with buildings based on an open-air or semi-open-air rationale. This proposition was justified in that it was considered necessary to
strengthen children's constitutions. Gaston Lemonier, who created the
League for Open Air Education in France in 1906,[54] suggested the introduction of open-air styles in all French schools, in order to apply the new pedagogical practices. These included restrictions on mental work, school trips,
personal and group observation, teamwork, physical education, training of
the senses, creation of playgrounds, open class promenades so that the students would explore their surroundings, visits to factories, museums and
ancient landmarks, as well as an overall family-like atmosphere. These pedagogical practices were converging with the New Education movement,
whose principles were often presented in the journal *Pour l'Ère Nouvelle*.

6.2 Open-air Solutions and New Education

Starting in the 1920s the open-air school attracted the interest of educators
who attempted to promote the principles of New Education and the Working School. The New Education movement aspired to become a "pedagogical isle," wherein students would develop into decent citizens, living away
from cities and culture, taking part in healthy outdoor activities dictated
by logic. A considerable number of practical open-air activities—physical
training, promenades, gardening, the commitment and the "obligation to
relax"—were exercises in self-discipline and an attempt to educationalize,
which had become very important for advocates of New Education. The
aim of education was to produce healthy individuals in body and mind,
driven by a strong sense of social responsibility and practical thinking. The
most important factors in this education were community life, isolation
in the countryside, agricultural and workshop activities and a manageable
programme of lessons and activities. Nature provided a suitable context
for the development of the new school as envisioned by the newly developed educational sciences: a school which promoted autonomy, action
and self-management in the child, as had been outlined in various international education congresses. These new practices were promoted in the

---

54 Vassiliki Theodorou and Despina Karakatsani, "École de plein air et éducation nouvelle et limites d'une
   tentative au début du XXe siècle en Grèce: influences," *Carrefours de l'Education* 23, no.1 (2007): 187–
   203.

atmosphere of internationalism and pacifism that characterized the International Bureau of Education (*Bureau International de l'education*) and the World Federation of Education Associations (WFEA), established in 1923. The former was established in 1929 to coordinate the institutions working towards intellectual cooperation, international solidarity and the revival of education. In collaboration with the LN and the International Labor Organization and inspired by the principles of international understanding promoted in the aftermath of World War I, the International Bureau of Education disseminated brochures, circulars and materials to teachers. Leading interwar personalities in educational sciences helped in this endeavor, educating teachers in many European countries and offering advice to governments on educational reform. Even nature-lovers were ardent supporters of the open-air education.

In the 1930s, the relationship of open-air schools and New Education developed and became stronger as open-air schools were considered to promote uniform education better than regular schools. This relationship was further strengthened by the creation of centers where staff were instructed on new teaching methods such as outdoor and indoor games, manual labor, theatre improvisation, nature observation, study of geographical and social surroundings, physical culture and modern views on children's psychology.

An important boost to these pedagogical and educational principles came from two leading personalities in the field, the president to the International League of New Education (Ligue internationale pour l'Éducation Nouvelle)[55] Adolphe Ferrière (1879–1960) and the Vice President of the French Group on New Education Georges Bertier (1877–1962). Jean Dupertuis, founder of the International Bureau on Open-air Schools in November 1920, also played an important role for the convergence of New Education principles and the open-air education.

According to Dupertuis, the open-air class was an energetic and sunbathed class, a "natural" school that combined the principles of medicine, pedagogy and puericulture. Considering this, one can recognize the impact of Ferrière who spoke of education in the countryside with special attention

---

55 It was established in 1921. Its principles were determined by Adolphe Ferrière, tireless proponent of the New Education principles. His work *L'École active*, published in 1922, served as a bible to contemporary educators.

to hygiene, controlled nutrition, continuous ventilation, and rest balanced with physical exercise. According to New Education proponents the acquisition of knowledge through the senses was an important objective as the direct observation of things and facts was considered to be the basis of this education.[56] Aside from that, other objectives included the close and democratic relationship between schools and parents, restrictions on the amount of memorization and the creation of a school that would be more popular and practical. The mental health of children was also highlighted in combination with elements of a special pedagogy (poor children's health was connected with immorality and led to degeneration) and a "functionalist architecture" (efficient and rational).

Open-air schools were a model of general educational reform in teaching methods and school space, initially in primary school and later in secondary education. The congresses on open-air schools in 1922, 1931 and 1936 examined the possibility of expanding the institution to include healthy children. The possibility of using these schools to promote mutual understanding between nations through exchange programmes was also discussed.

The rise of Nazism and the outbreak of World War II hindered these efforts. However, despite a general feeling of failure, the expectations of the organizers in the first congress had been fulfilled to a large extent. Many schools built in the 1920s and 1930s had open classrooms, open corridors, French windows and terraces. Architectural interventions to add semi-open air features such as the terrace or the open classroom had appeared in schools that had been built earlier and did not follow the open air rationale. The pedagogical methods of observation and the reduction of teaching hours also spread in education along with various hygiene practices and physical education. The open-air school set the example of smaller classrooms and a diverse curriculum.

6.3 The Spread of Hygiene and Social Welfare

Apart from New Education, the open-air schools also bear a strong connection to the hygiene movement. The supporters of the open air schools aimed

---

56 Daniel Hameline, "Adolphe Ferrière," *Prospects: the Quarterly Review of Comparative Education* (Paris, UNESCO: International Bureau of Education), vol.13, no. 1–2 (1993): 373–401.

to render children "health apostles" and hygiene reformers within the family. There was a tight relation between the open-air institution and eugenic pursuits, underlying the quest for a healthy childhood. The aim was to raise awareness of eugenics among young girls and boys, and help them to become good citizens.

In this context, the open-air school was considered the necessary step in preventive social medicine with the aim of targeting weak children and improving their health. The public reception of open-air schools was based to a great extent on the impact this educational and medical experiment had on regular schools. Many believed that the open-air school could be a useful tool in a defensive anti-TB campaign in that it could mobilize all the involved parties—both in the public and private spheres—as part of an appropriate social policy, while others thought of the open-air school as a locus where a collective spirit of solidarity could manifest itself or the principles of community socialism could be popularized.

However, some expressed reservations about the limits of this individual medico-educational intervention if it was not also accompanied by wider social measures. They also claimed that building schools in nature could not in itself cure the serious medical and practical family problems, or change socio-economic conditions. In other words, the open-air school could not be a panacea for complex social problems beyond the social and economic causes of illness and weakness. Although children spent time in the open air, followed a balanced diet and were inspected medically, their physical condition was not steadily improving. It was also found that diet, a hygienic regime and a special curriculum did not suffice for their continuous rehabilitation but rather for the development of their mental faculties. Critics purported that the full rehabilitation of students could only be achieved if the will of children to cure themselves was fully awakened. This would occur if children were put in self-administered student communities and were educated in issues of hygiene and physical care. Thus, in the context of community life, the pedagogical values of collective will, collaboration and solidarity would be combined with diet, hygiene lessons and practices.

Modern historians consider open-air education part of a larger effort to exert social control over people's bodies. Scholars have approached the open-air schools as "centers of institutionalized medical supervision and intervention,"[57] as spaces where ill children, considered to be dangerous, were isolated, thus making it possible to control and supervise their bodies.[58] According to Linda Bryder, open-air schools in England, apart from providing fresh air and a rich diet, also attempted to inculcate the Victorian values of self-help and self-discipline in working-class children. Removing children from school and sending them to the countryside was a kind of punishment for parents who were not able to follow the advice of visiting nurses. Experts in preventive medicine were interested in preventing both deviance and disease.[59] Contemporary studies look into the issue of danger,[60] the various means of managing it (medicalization, institutionalization, professionalization, marginalization)[61] and the resistance of children to these rhetorics and strategies.[62] However, some have questioned the previous interpretation, considering open-air education as evidence of medical progress, an architectural and pedagogical novelty[63] and analyze it as a privileged field of control, the inspection and surveillance of children's bodies and souls[64], on the basis of Foucauldian tools.[65] The medical and pedagogical influences on these vulnerable children, by means of medical treatment and moral regeneration, have also been studied in correlation with the rhetoric on national efficiency and racial robustness.

57 Peter Kelly, "Youth at Risk: Processes of Individualisation and Responsabilisation in the Risk Society," *Discourse: Studies in the Cultural Politics of Education* 22, no. 1 (2001): 23–5.

58 Sally Lubeck and Patricia Garrett, "The Social Construction of the "At-risk" Child," *British Journal of Sociology of Education* 11, no. 3 (1990): 327 and 329.

59 Linda Bryder, "'Wonderlands of Buttercup. Clover and Daisis': Tuberculosis and the Open-air School Movement in Britain, 1907–39," in *In the Name of the Child, Health and Welfare, 1880–1940*, ed. Roger Cooter (London: 1992), 72–95.

60 John Welshman, "Child Health, National Fitness, and Physical Education in Britain, 1900–1940," in *Cultures of Child Health in Britain and the Netherlands in the Twentieth Century*, ed. Marijke Gijswijt-Hofsta and Hilary Marlans (Amsterdam and New York: Rodopi, 2003), 63.

61 Jeroen Dekker, "The Fragile Relation between Normality and Marginality: Marginalization and Institutionalization in the History of Education," in "Beyond the Pale, Behind Bars: Marginalization and Institutionalization from the 18th to the 20th Century," *Paedagogica Historica* 26, no. 2 (1990):15–8.

62 Geert Thyssen, "The 'Trotter' Open-Air School, Milan (1922–1977): A City of Youth or Risky Business?" *Paedagogica Historica* 45, no. 1–2 (February–April 2009):157–70.

63 Jean-Noël Luc, "Open-Air Schools: Unearthing a History," in *Open-Air Schools: An Educational and Architectural Venture in Twentieth-Century Europe*, eds. Anne-Marie Châtelet, Dominique Lerch and Jean-Noël Luc (Paris: Éditions Recherches, 2003), 18.

64 It was noted that "fresh air could prevent criminality." Bryder, "Wonderlands of Butter Cup, Clover and Daisies," 83.

65 Thyssen, "The 'Trotter' Open-Air School, Milan (1922–1977)," 157–70.

6.4 The Establishment of the Open-air School in Greece:
The Second Attempt

In Greece, the issue establishing open-air schools for sickly children, which would use modern pedagogical practices, sparked a lively debate in various pedagogical and popular medicine journals during the 1920s. Pedagogues, doctors and feminists highlighted the importance of the open-air school in various international congresses, while pediatricians, like Lambadarios and Doxiadis, who were involved in school hygiene, participated in international congresses on open-air education and imported related views in the public discussion back in Greece.

These propositions seem to have become more specific in the late 1920s, when a second attempt was made to establish an open-air school in Athens. The open-air school may have been part of the 1929 educational reform when the Liberal government attempted to create institutions for various groups of students who were not able to attend regular school, i.e., working or sickly children. In the education reform bill, announced on April 2, 1929, the Minister of Education K. Gontikas stressed the need to set up schools for mentally and physically ill children. He emphasized that schools for sick children could prevent the spread of contagious diseases and the special curricula would not worsen the children's health. He contended that the establishment of one or two schools, initially on experimental basis, would not overburden the state budget. The climate of Greece was, according to the Minister, ideal for open-air teaching.[66]

Despite the commitment of the state, this attempt to establish an open-air school was once again due more to the collaboration between voluntary organizations and public services. It was the Greek Anti-TB Society, established in 1925 by G. Pamboukis, that provided the primary initiative. The society had spearheaded the anti-TB campaign, replacing the Pan-Hellenic Association Against TB, which had begun to dwindle following the death of its founder, V. Patrikios. Apart from publishing books and informative leaflets, the Greek Anti-TB Society had also founded an anti-TB clinic and a student soup kitchen in the center of Athens, with the aim of strengthening

---

66 Konstantinos Svolopoulos, ed., *Konstantinos Gontikas, 1870–1937. Thesmikes Allages kata ton Mesopolemo* (Athens: Etaireia Meletis Ellinikis Istorias, 2003), 186–87.

student health. It seems that the society suggested that a grove in the same area be allotted, aiming to set up an open-air, one-class school accommodating forty students under the aegis of the School Hygiene Department of the Ministry of Education.

As can be gleaned from the newspaper *Proia,* the inauguration of the school took place on June 10, 1929 with all the proper solemnities in the presence of the Ministers of Education and Health. The officials attended a gymnastics demonstration by students who had already started attending the open-air school. However, the school would only begin systematic operation the following year. Sickly students would attend the school on the suggestion of the school doctors in the capital. Students were taught all the lessons in the grove and occupied themselves with gymnastics and sports. A building constructed according to modern hygiene standards protected students from severe cold or heat and their desks were portable and very light. Students spent their days from morning until afternoon at school and their lunch was prepared by the Patriotic Foundation for the Protection of Children.[67]

On the basis of fragmentary information, we may assume that the school operated in the 1930s, possibly as late as 1940. As can be seen in pictures from the album of the National Council for the Protection of Motherhood and Childhoods in 1930, the school probably operated in the open air, staffed with two female teachers.[68] It seems that a wooden makeshift building was used for classes in case of adverse weather conditions. In 1938, the school was possibly under the supervision of the Greek Anti-TB Society. Yet, notwithstanding the success of this experiment, the government's plans to establish more schools for pre-tubercular children did not materialize.

However, the legislative and technical groundwork for the establishment of a modern open-air school had already been laid in the early 1930s. It is not certain whether the plans prepared in August 1931 by school architect Nikolaos Mitsakis for the Technical Service of the Ministry of Education materialized. It seems that the Ministry of Education planned to construct a modern building to accommodate the school in the same area where the

---

67 "Ta Khthesina Egkainia tou Protou Ypaithriou Skholeiou meta Pasis Episimotitos," *Proia* (June 11, 1929): 5.

68 Konstantinos Saroglou records, Hellenic Literary and Historical Archive. ELIA.

school operated temporarily.[69] These plans demonstrate the extreme care taken to secure the hygienic conditions of its operation. The plan envisioned seven classrooms in a simple building, with a sea water tank for baths, a sand tank, and a sun-porch on the roof. This plan clearly demonstrated the progress that had been made in open-air school architecture in Europe, which thrived in the interwar period, as well as the impact the European open-air school architecture had on Greek architects.

Although this open-air school building was never completed, government legislation on education continued, testifying to the willingness of the last Venizelos's government to create schools for special groups of students. In April 1932, during the Papandreou ministry, a legislative decree ordered the establishment of an open-air school. The school was named the "open-air primary school of the Greek anti-TB Society" and was to be accommodated in a building constructed by the Society in the Pedion of Areos area, close to Athens, and would operate under the supervision of the director of the School Hygiene.[70]

This open-air school was influenced by similar schools in Europe and America. School doctors chose both male and female students from the west region of Athens who were prone to illness to be admitted to the school. The pedagogical supervision of the school was to be undertaken by the Supreme Advisory Council while medical inspection was undertaken by the Greek Anti-TB Society in collaboration with the School Hygiene director. Its aim was to strengthen the constitution of sickly children, especially the ones that were suspected to have contracted TB, as an estimated 50% of the students were scrofulous, meaning that they carried the TB bacillus in dormant condition. Children would attend the school for a year, following the prescribed hygienic-dietary methods including exposure to the open air, sufficient and healthy food, suitable exercises and naps, ablutions, sun baths and respiratory exercises. The cost of lunches, the students' transportation and their summer vacations in the countryside was covered from school resources. Students would follow the curriculum of the primary school and be taught by one or two female teachers, seconded from other schools of

---

69 Archives of the Technical Service of the Ministry of Education, file 540, Ypaithrion Skholeion para ti Skholin Evelpidon, Genika Arkheia tou Kratous (GAK).

70 Diatagma, "Peri Idryseos Ypaithriou Dimotikou Skholeiou tis Ellinikis Antipthisikis Etaireias," Efimeris tis Kiverniseos, A', no.125 (April 22, 1932):830–31.

the same region. Female teachers with some knowledge of hygiene were preferred. The final programme was tailored to the children's needs and to medico-pedagogical teaching principles appropriate for children with fragile health, teaching them only the basics of each subject while avoiding overwork and not assigning homework. Four hours were allotted to lessons each day, skipping all the details and anything addressed to memory. The pedagogical principles of New Education included the idea that the spirit of love should inspire teachers and students should not perform memorization work. A school nurse would provide her services in the premises, appointed and paid by the Greek Anti-TB Society.

Questions regarding the cancellation of this school still remain unanswered. It is at least true that the portable makeshift construction did not allow the students' stay during adverse weather conditions and the socio-political changes further deterred the school's materialization. We cannot, however, doubt the interest Venizelos' government had in helping sickly and weak children, evident in other measures such as student soup kitchens, schools for children with special needs, and a prevantorium with a six-class primary school in Voula.

6.5 The Turn to Semi-Open Air Solutions

These open-air schools were abandoned in the late 1930s, at least by their advocates, possibly because of the influence of the international open-air school movement, which supported adopting solutions that were in the interest of more diverse groups of students. The high cost of their construction and maintenance and the large number of students in need of recuperation, led to the solution of semi-open-air classrooms. The Architectural Division of the Ministry of Education studied this system in cooperation with the School Hygiene Department.[71] This solution was considered to be ideal as it had the advantages of open-air teaching, yet with fewer expenses.

In the late 1930s, Lambadarios himself started to play with the idea of adopting the solution of semi-open-air classes, by converting normal classrooms into open ones. In a paper he delivered on June 9, 1938 in the Academy of Athens regarding the better orientation of school buildings, published as

---

71 Kalafati, *Ta Skholeia tis Protovathmias Ekpaidefsis*, pictures 99–101.

"Towards open-air education through the system of semi-open-air classes,"[72] he referred to the necessity of setting up a particular type of school. A plan for such a classroom was approved by the Technical Service of the Ministry of Education and served as the basis for more new buildings in Greece during the same period. The solution of semi-open-air schools, meaning the alteration of school buildings into semi-open-air classrooms with glass doors instead of windows, was an interesting practice that had been applied successfully earlier in England.[73]

A particular system of orientation and construction of buildings was suggested by the Technical Service of the Ministry of Education to leave open one of the sides of the classroom in case of good weather (semi-open-air class), and allow better natural lighting. At the same time, a corridor was also promoted. While in most countries the corridor attached to the classrooms faced north and the classrooms south, Lambadarios suggested the corridor face south and the classrooms north and that the corridor be totally open on its south side, closed with a simple parapet instead of a wall.[74] The corridors could be open terraces and serve as sunshades (brise-soleil) for the lower floors. This provided better and healthier light and ventilation to the classrooms; in good weather the doors could be opened, making the classroom semi-open, while the corridor-veranda facilitated open-air teaching.[75] In Greece, the Technical Service of the Ministry of Education applied this system to various newly-constructed buildings.[76]

6.6 Summer Camps and Child Welfare

The proliferation of children's summer camps can also be ascribed to the same concerns that led to the spread of open-air education. Along with the idea

---

72 Pragmateiai tis Akademias Athinon, Athens Grafeion Dimosievmaton Akadimias Athinon, ΙΓ΄ (ΙΓ and volume 7) vol. 7, no. 3, 1938 (June 9, 1938): 3–16.

73 Emmanouil Lambadarios, "I Ypaithriopoiisi tis Didaskalias dia tou Systimatos Imiypaithrion Skholeion," May 1938 (Lambadarios Archive (ELIA)).

74 Lambadarios, "I Ypaithriopoiisi tis Didaskalias" 3–16.

75 Giakoumatos, Stoikheia gia ti Neoteri Elliniki Arkhitektoniki, 79.

76 Particularly successful was the attempt of the architect of the Ministry of Education, N. Mitsakis to construct the school for highly challenged children in Kaisariani. A similar venture to change classrooms into semi-open-air ones was accomplished in a primary school in Moschato (Neo Faliro) in 1919 and a kindergarten in Agios Nikolaos in Pefkakia in Athens according to plans provided by Dimitrios Pikionis, a significant architect of the interwar period.

of a healthy childhood, Lambadarios highlighted eugenic ideas such as the robustness of the race. Health camps were themselves the outcome of efforts to strengthen the race, promoted, by means of various daily routines, the basic hygiene rules to be followed with military precision and extreme care. In this way, hygiene rules and practices were instilled in future generations. Lambadarios also laid emphasis on proper nutrition, considered indispensable for the protection of the body against TB. Gaining weight became a kind of obsession, while the routine of sunbathing became a daily ritual performed to build a healthier nation. In the span of twenty years, health camps developed from unofficial summer camps into real bureaucratic institutions. In them it was far easier for doctors to regulate children's lives in the name of health.[77]

The international congresses and the organizations that endorsed children's camps in the countryside dealt with strengthening vulnerable working class children's constitutions, especially those that they ran the risk of contracting TB. In a few cases, the main reason for establishing children's summer camps was not simply entertainment in the open air and trips but the restoration of children's health. Municipal governments, parents' unions, charities, associations and ministries would look for suitable areas in the countryside where summer camps could be built for city children during their holidays. Apart from strengthening the students' constitutions in the fresh air, children would be taught the principles of culture, politeness and discipline. After World War I, many camps or hospitals turned into colonies for sickly children.

During this period, efforts to systematize children's summer camps intensified in Greece. State officials and volunteers participated actively in societies that worked to institutionalize children's summer camps. Lambadarios and Doxiadis were the most active internationally; aware of the high numbers of sickly children in Athenian neighborhoods, they supported the social and pedagogical character of the children's summer camps. During the second international congress on open-air schools, which took place in Brussels in 1931, Lambadarios spoke of the importance of children's summer camps in the battle against TB, since he had realized how beneficial it was for children to spend time in hygienic conditions in the open air, follow

---

77 On the organization of children's summer camps in the interwar, see Margaret Tennant, "Children's Health Camps in New Zealand: the Making of a Movement, 1919–1940," *Social History of Medicine* 9, no. 1 (1996): 69–87.

a rich and balanced diet, and exercise to expand the thorax and breathe more easily. Participants in the congress also discussed issues pertaining to the children's summer camps, such as the instruction of the supervisors, the formation of a permanent council to oversee the camps and the close cooperation between various organizations of common good and social welfare and municipal governments, the Church and the State. They also looked into the issue of resources. The first international conference on children's summer camps also took place in 1931, where Doxiadis, as President to the Patriotic Foundation for the Protection of Child, participated and communicated to the rest of the delegates his experience from Greece. Participants in this conference discussed a plan to form an international permanent council to link different nations and collate the findings and experiences of various organizations involved in children's summer camps and "summer lodgings." Committees on "the hygiene of the child accommodated in summer camps in respect of choice, residence and diet, or its international transport" and a technical committee that would deal with the instruction of the technical staff were also formed.

In 1929, the state became interested in establishing children's summer camps on a larger scale. Lambadarios contended that, according to his own research in Greece, the estimated cost would be only half of what other countries spent. He also mentioned that the capital could create the necessary conditions for the running of open-air camps on a continuous and permanent basis and host a conference on children's summer camps because of the progress the capital had attained up until that time. According to the director of the School Hygiene Service, every city should have its own student summer camp run and financially supported by school resources.

In 1929, the School Hygiene Service prepared a bill for the establishment of student summer camps. The bill specified how the Ministries of Army, Navy and Hygiene would collaborate to provide tents, cooking utensils and other materials for the summer camps. This bill "on Summer Camps" emphasized the relationship between summer camps and the protection of health. It further stressed the therapeutic character of the student holidays in them. It goes without saying that this bill bore the indelible stamp of Lambadarios. The writers of the bill paid particular attention to the contribution of children's summer camps in fighting TB. Article no. 2 read specifically: "The aim of the students' summer camps is the rehabilitation and restoration of the health of scrofulous or sickly children by means of appropriate diet, sun and air baths, and exercise on the basis of the current findings of hygiene."[78] According to the same bill, the children's summer camps running under the jurisdiction of the School Hygiene Department of the Ministry of Education, were set up and operated by a special committee, paid for by the local fund of the students' summer camps, which comprised three to five members of both genders, appointed by the Minister of Education, with a three year tenure of office. The local school doctor and a high-ranking member of education also participated in the committee. According to article no. 4, the students' summer camps were set up in hygienic and, if possible, in sparsely populated places, in proportion with the available financial resources and current needs, following the proposition of the students' summer camp committee.

However, this bill was not passed for reasons that remain unclear. Following the failure to pass the law, Lambadarios was summoned to organize children's summer camps in various regions in Greece, relying on local authorities. As director of the Department of School Hygiene, he sent a circular stressing the moral and material support the Ministry would provide to local authorities if they were interested in establishing a summer camp for students in their area. The Patriotic Foundation for the Protection of Child participated dynamically in the cause and collaborated with various local organizations and authorities. These efforts finally came to fruition: in the 1930s, according to Lambadarios' testimony in the journal *Skholiki Ygieini* (School Hygiene), teachers, parents' associations and doctors took initiatives to set up children's summer camps in some regions in Greece with support from both local associations and large organizations such as the Patriotic Foundation for the Protection of Child and the Red Cross.

The construction of the first permanent summer camp for students began in Greece in 1930 on the coast of Glyfada, with donations from tobacco manufacturer Zirinis, after whom the camp was named. It seems that this was the first summer camp in the Balkans. According to one testimony, "The Zirineio Summer Palace for Children" had a capacity of fifty beds. During the same period, the Asklipeion in Voula faced problems due to lack of materials and was in danger of closing down without support from the state. The new two-storey building had four large classrooms and two isolation rooms

---

78 Lambadarios Archive, ELIA.

modeled after the Leysin sanatoriums in Switzerland which had been inspired by the doctor Rollier. According to the decree of November 2, 1929 an area in the woods in Voula was expropriated "for the Patriotic Foundation in order to set up a summer camp for tubercular children."

In 1930–31, the Ministry of Education allotted 1,000,000 drachmas to the Patriotic Foundation from the fund of educational taxes for the construction of another building in the summer camp of Voula with the aim of accommodating a summer camp for indigent and sickly students.[79] On March 23, 1930 the summer camps of the Patriotic Foundation in Voula were inaugurated.[80] It was not accidental that socioeconomic data on the children's families were entered in the card of each child kept in the summer camps of the Patriotic Foundation. Children were chosen according to the health level they had been classified into, but also according to socio-economic criteria (father's and mother's profession and type of permanent residence: number of rooms, dark or light rooms, and cleanliness).[81]

The staff of the summer camps took special care in providing the children's food; the quality, quantity, and preparation of the food were inspected thoroughly, and the goal was to increase the children's weight. At the same time, great attention was paid to the daily programme, which included exercise, baths, sunbathing, rest and games, group activities, cleaning of the camp and looking after the tents.[82]

7. NUTRITION AND THE ORGANIZATION OF SOUP KITCHENS DURING THE INTERWAR PERIOD

During the interwar period, nutrition evolved into a reliable indicator of the citizens' living standards and their health, and the country's social welfare infrastructure. Nutritional deficiencies during World War I hit hard large sections of the European population and highlighted the need for new state

---

79 Apostolos Doxiadis, "Ai Therinai Exokhai ton Paidion. Dia mia Kalliteran Genean," *Elefteron Vima* (August 7, 1930).

80 The journal *To Paidi* (The Child) provides information about the inauguration ceremony (May-June 1931): 41–2.

81 Lambadarios Archive, ELIA.

82 A list with the Twelve Commandments of the Children's Summer Camp of the Patriotic Foundation for the Protection of Child had been brought out. Each child taking part in the summer camp had to learn these twelve rules. "The summer camps give me health and make me a good and robust child. I always speak of it to my friends and acquaintances for the good it does me." "Paidiki Exokhi," Lambadarios Archive, ELIA.

policies to secure food surpluses and the importance of international collaboration in this field. The concerns raised regarding nutrition were linked to the reconstruction of health care systems in various European countries during the 1920s, the impact of the 1929 financial crisis had on the health of the working-class and, most significantly, the internationalization of the efforts to counteract health problems, now attempted by a group of experts working under the auspices of international health organizations.[83] Thus, there was a shift from the idea of nutrition being a necessary condition for the population's survival to the healthy nutrition as a factor conducive to the citizens' well-being and as a social right. International voluntary organizations set up in the aftermath of the establishment of the League of Nations, such as the Save the Children Fund, the Save the Children International Union, the American Relief Administration and the League of the Red Cross Societies, collaborated with one another and took action in order to fight children's famine in Central Europe between 1918 and 1921.[84] In the 1920s and 1930s, the international organizations played a key role in the establishment of nutritional habits and in the promotion of the respective policy and culture.[85] The League of the Red Cross Societies was the first health organization to employ experts on nutrition while the American Relief Administration made use of the advice offered by nutritionist R. Kellogg. Although supported by private funds and collections, these organizations had a great impact as they provided food to millions of children across post war Europe.[86] A more scientific approach and nutrition expertise was applied to various programmes they promoted which— among other things—aimed to bring social stability in Central Europe, already plagued by socialist insurrection.[87]

---

83 Iris Borowy and Wolf Gruner eds, *Facing Illness in Troubled Times* (Frankfurt am Mein and New York: Peter Lang, 2005). See the introduction, 3–13.

84 John F. Hutchinson, "Promoting Child Health in the 1920s: International Politics and the Limits of Humanitarianism," in *The Politics of the Healthy Life. An International Perspective*, ed. Esteban Rodriguez Ocaña, 131–50. Paul Weindling, "The Role of International Organizations in Setting Nutritional Standards in the 1920 and 1930s," in eds. Harmke Kamminga and Andrew Cunningham, *The Science and Culture of Nutrition, 1840–1940*, 319–21.

85 Harmke Kamminga, *The Science and Culture of Nutrition, 1840–1940*. John Burnett, Derek J. Oddy, *The Origins and Development of Food Policies in Europe* (London and New York: Leicester University Press, 1994). On the issue of child nutrition and its social parameters between 1890 and 1950, see Rima D. Apple, *Mothers and Medicine. A Social History of Infant Feeding, 1890–1950* (Wisconsin Publications in the History of Science and Medicine. Madison: University of Wisconsin Press, 1987).

86 For example, in July 1920, the American Relief Administration fed more than a million children in Central Europe.

87 Paul Weindling, "The Role of International Organizations in Setting Nutritional Standards in the 1920s and 1930s," in *The Science and Culture of Nutrition, 1840–1940*, 320–21.

7.1. New Scientific Data and Living Standards

Many of the health problems children faced in the 1930s were ascribed to lack of vitamin A and low in-take of milk, eggs, meat and fish and usually predicted a bleak future for them. The effect of their deficient diet was visible in the condition of their teeth. The conception of pre-tubercular children, as a condition and predisposition to illness, was correlated with deficient nutrition as well as with excessive labor, lack of hygiene and poor housing conditions. In fact, it was easier to measure malnutrition among schoolchildren rather than among other groups. Hygiene statistics recorded the cases of children suffering from adenopathy, as well as of weak and pre-tubercular children. Malnutrition was the result not only of ignorance but also of a number of socioeconomic conditions. In addition, the emergence of nutrition as a scientific subject, directly linked with the socio-political field, was connected to the means of approaching and combating starvation and poverty both at private and at state level. At the same time, research on physiology was giving rise to new scientific and instrumental ideas, such as the study of the ideal nutrition, and providing nutritional data on rural populations across Europe. Scientific models for nutrition emerged as nutritionists aimed to help people overcome their ignorance of the healthy food ingredients. Suggestions on proper nutrition became a vehicle for the spread of new cultural values, habits and attitudes among the population, especially among workers, farmers and children.

The discussion of nutrition in connection to the development of robust populations intensified during the interwar period. In some European countries, the discussion concerned whether family stipends should be distributed or soup kitchens for the destitute, workers, mothers and students be organized to help low income families facing the specter of malnutrition. At first, concerns centered on children's nutrition, particularly the issue of milk and its collection, distribution, and quality. Later on, people became more aware of the necessity of providing children with wholesome meals and balanced diet. They were also concerned with the energy content of children's meals. The proportion of the different ingredients in students' diets became the subject of in-depth analysis. The aim of the soup kitchens was to provide food to students who did not receive enough good quality food at home and as such could meet the requirements of proper physical development and the school. Food was given to students free of charge or for a small sum of money. School was to diffuse knowledge about the energy content of food and its importance for the proper physical development of children. Soup kitchens were undoubtedly a materialization of modern social welfare for students.

7.2. The Fight against Malnutrition

At the end of the 1920s, the frugal diet of the Greeks was cast into doubt. Articles by doctors featured regularly in educational journals evidence the serious concerns raised about nutrition. Soup kitchens were considered a measure of prime importance in Greece to counteract children's malnutrition which, according to the reports of school doctors, came near to starvation. The daily diet of students, some of whom walked long distances to school from neighboring villages, and spent the entire day at school was a hard stale piece of bread soaked in water with a piece of smoked herring or cheese. These dietary habits made students an easy target for malaria and tuberculosis.[88] A letter from a teacher in a mountainous village in the Peloponnese sent to the journal of the Greek Red Cross in 1930 aptly illustrated the dietary deprivations in Greece. The letter was just an example of the students' diet and was used to sensitize the authorities so as to increase the funds allotted to school hygiene. Yet, the diet of the students as described in this letter must have been very close to the average diet of rural children. Without strengthening the constitution of fragile children's bodies, every policy on the hygienic care of children seemed insufficient.

Starting in 1928, the Ministry of Education had been prompting educational authorities, especially school boards, to organize soup kitchens. In his attempt to spread the idea and give incentives for social welfare works, Lambadarios toured the provinces. His tour resulted in the establishment of School Welfare Committees with the participation of doctors and school principals. The role of teachers was also important for such initiatives.

---

88 "I examined the content of the basket or the cloth in which they kept their food and here is what I found! Their food was a piece of black hard bread which can be cut only with the hatchet. To eke out their meal they had a piece of herring or rather its scraps, or a bit of cheese and nothing more. I am sending you a piece of bread on purpose so as not to think that I am exaggerating. How are these children going to be fed, how will they grow up and how will they deal with the contagious diseases threatening them or with the Lernaean Hydra called malaria? Do not ask me! It's beyond my grasp! [...]" *I Skholiki Antilipsis kai idios peri ton Mathitikon Syssition en Elladi* (Perilipsis Omilias Genomenis kata to Progevma tis Rotarianis Evdomados tou Paidiou en Marasleio) (Athens, 1934), 5.

A report of the School Hygiene Service in 1931 stressed that "[the teacher] should be enlightened and be convinced that it is his duty to take the lead in establishing soup kitchens and consider it as important as teaching or even more important."[89] In just a few years, parents' societies, school inspectors, school doctors and committees set up especially for this aim, with the financial support of the Ministry and under the scientific supervision of Lambadarios, organized soup kitchens, most often in the school premises, intended mainly for needy primary school students, as the fight against TB required abundant and healthy food.

In the 1930s, meals were distributed to approximately 3,000 students on a daily basis at a price that ranged from 3 to 5 drachmas in soup kitchens in the refugee neighborhoods of Athens and Piraeus. A certain number of students received food free of charge. In the new schools, which had been built since 1923 according to hygienic standards, kitchens and dining halls were added.[90] The schoolchildren polyclinic also offered nutritional food in borderline cases of destitute children. The Patriotic Foundation of Welfare (PFW) also played an important role in the organization of soup kitchens for the destitute. Its contribution and the contribution of other philanthropic organizations, which had considerable experience in this field, were very important for the organization and funding of soup kitchens. Since 1925, when Doxiadis became president of the PFW, the number of children fed by the soup kitchens increased in both the capital and the provinces. In the aftermath of the 1929 crisis, doctors and state officials laid particular emphasis on malnutrition among Greeks as well. In their discourse the issue of malnutrition was linked not only with socio-economic parameters but also with the diseases it was likely to cause.

In May 1930, law no. 4376 gave the Patriotic Foundation the task of establishing soup kitchens.[91] In 1930, soup kitchens operated in three venues in Athens, offering 700 portions a day; yet, it is not specified which age range they were intended for and whether recipients had to pay or not. Later, the Department of Soup Kitchens of the Patriotic Foundation of Welfare prepared 2,500 portions a day, and another 12,500 portions on a daily basis for

---

89 Emmanouil Lambadarios, *Etisia Ekthesis tou Tmimatos Skholikis Ygieinis tou Ypourgeiou Paideias tou Etous 1930–1931*, Lambadarios Archive, ELIA.

90 See the architectural school designs of this period in the General State Archives, Archive of the Technical Service of the Ministry of Education, file 540.

91 Law no. 4376 amended law no. 4062 "Peri Patriotikou Idrymatos Prostasias tou Paidiou."

the soup kitchens run by the municipality of Athens. The same rationale of strengthening the constitution of poor students led to the distribution of raisin buns, starting in September 1931, to soldiers and students, following the raisin crisis, when raisin was promoted as a food that contained threpsini (raisin syrup).[92] The relation of TB and calorie deficiency raised concerns among columnists who discussed racial degeneration.[93] The head of the School Hygiene Service supervised the organization of soup kitchens, since it was he who designed the diet. Lambadarios had drawn up a table with a model diet[94] to be offered by student soup kitchens, detailing the calories required for students between the ages of 7 and 14, taking into account the necessary amount of leucoma (but also the combination of animal and vegetable leucoma at an expected rate of 60% and 40% respectively), fat and carbohydrates.[95] In Lambadarios's table, lunches for twelve-year old students should include at least 570 calories, with meat consumption daily. Hot lunches were preferred over a cold meal. This hot meal ideally would supply the student with half the calories required for their age.

Only the teacher's training college and a few more schools prepared the meals on the school grounds. Here, food was usually prepared by the lower staff, assisted by female students and members of the school board. Housekeeping courses were offered by quite a few schools to make female students more useful in meal preparation. In the 1930s, the newly-built schools had specially designated areas for a kitchen and a dining hall. In Athens, Piraeus and Thessaloniki, food was prepared by the Patriotic Foundation for the Protection of the Child, while in Thessaloniki it was prepared by the teachers' association "Merimna," which had been established in 1920 to aid destitute students.[96] The hygienic service of "Merimna" began in November

---

92 Anagkastikos Nomos (Emergency Law) no.5925, "Peri Kyroseos Anagkastikou Nomou peri Ypokhreotikis Paraskevis kai Katanaloseos Stafidopsomou," *Efimeris tis Kiverniseos*, A', no.372 (December 1, 1933): 2268–69.

93 Kostas Athanatos, *Patris* (November 14, 1928). "The most serious contemporary problem of the race! 80% of the Greek children are tubercular when finishing school! And 40% of them are blind due to trachoma. Our race could be wiped out in a century [...]."

94 This table was based on the calories and the fluctuation of price-index; it was the outcome of communication with the Patriotic Foundation for the Protection of the Child, which had undertaken the preparation and distribution of student meals in Athens during this period.

95 Lambadarios took special care so as to include meat, pulses, potatoes, pasta, bread, cheese, raisins, figs and fruit in the meals provided by the students' soup kitchens.

96 Special mention to its work was made in the first Pan-Hellenic Congress on the Protection of Childhood in 1930 by Ourania Boziana, president to the Association "Merimna," in her paper entitled "I Merimna Thessalonikis," *Praktika Synedriou Prostasias tis Mitrotitas kai ton Paidikon Ilikion*,389–92.

1925 and since then it kept a register of students that underwent medical examination, where their diseases were recorded. Tonic syrups and cod liver oil were also administered to children.

State funding for student soup kitchens gradually increased. The Greek state supported their organization, allotting to school boards funds ranging from 1,500,000 to 2,000,000 drachmas per year. At the same time, with the assistance of the state, school received support from local sources. In May 1932, under a new law (no. 5341/32) part of the money from tobacco taxes was allocated to student soup kitchens through the school boards. The cost of each student soup kitchen varied according to its organization and preparation, the menu and the energy value of foods. The price of food varied according to the source of funding. In 1930, the School Hygiene Service estimated that the average cost of each student meal amounted to 3 drachmas.

Circa 1930, 1/3 of the cost of the soup kitchens operating in most cities was covered by the Ministry, another 1/3 was covered by local philanthropic organizations, most often the Patriotic Foundation, and the remaining 1/3 by the students themselves, with the exemption of those certified to be destitute. Since 1934, the responsibility for the students' soup kitchens laid wholly with the Patriotic Foundation, which organized shared meals for students and destitute citizens. Yet, many problems arose due to the students and citizens mingling in the same place and having their meals at the same tables. For this reason, students began to take their meals separately after a while. The Department of Hygiene of the Patriotic Foundation took care to provide specially prepared food to sickly persons as well as to weak children who did not have the financial means to follow a special diet.[97] The development of soup kitchens was spectacular in the early 1930s. The number of students fed went from 525 in 1928 to 36,000 in 1933. Also, the number of cities that ran soup kitchens went from 13 to 28 during the same period. Student soup kitchens were set up in teacher training courses throughout the country beginning in 1931.

Although the development of nutritional science and international organizations[98] played a key role in the promotion of nutrition policy, we may assume that the soup kitchens were part and parcel of the social policy on

---

97 Department of School Hygiene, circular no. 102360/240/8.12.1937.
98 Harmke Kamminga and Andrew Cunningham, eds., *The Science and Culture of Nutrition (1840–1940)*.

children's health that the Venizelos government promoted. They were also part of the modernization trend that characterized the Liberals' policy on social issues. Finally, the promotion of student soup kitchens reflected the concerns raised about the health of the working-class, following the refugees' settlement and the financial crisis that led Greece to bankruptcy in May 1932. The organization and management of soup kitchens for students illustrates both the concern about nutrition and the interest in the development of robust bodies. Experts of international organizations in the 1930s believed that knowledge alone was not sufficient to improve the diet of the working class; instead financial measures were necessary, mainly an increase in wages and a decrease in the price of staple foods. Yet, since the latter was a very sensitive and complicated issue, experts emphasized changing cultural practices; training the working class in nutrition, especially mothers, seemed to be the key to this change.

8. EUGENIC PROPOSITIONS AND PUERICULTURE CONCERNS IN INTERWAR GREECE

Discussions about the necessity of eugenic steps began spreading in Greece since the beginning of the 1920s, as did scientific controversies over the use of hereditary theories and biological capital in planning policies on the improvement of the race. Doctors who held certain views on the value of hereditary theory and the means to confront the repercussions of dysgenics for the population took part in the debate, along with social scientists and jurists who were concerned with the moral, legal and practical aspects of eugenic measures.[99] The Ministry of Hygiene attempted to promote legislation on the control of the intending spouses in two phases, though unsuccessfully since the proposed laws never passed.

The earliest publication on eugenics dates back to 1917, when Michael Kairis's *Evgonia* (Eugenics) was first published.[100] However, Doctor I. Zallonis had already stressed the national dimensions of dysgenics in *Ypomnima pros tin Voulin peri Kolymaton Gamou apo Iatrikin Epoprsin* (Petition to

---

99   Sevasti Trubeta, *Physical Anthropology, Race and Eugenics in Greece (1880–1970s)* (Brill, Leiden, Boston, 2013).

100 The lecture "Eugenics" delivered by doctor Mikhalis Kairis in the Sinaia Academy on March 24, 1917 was published in installments in the Journal *Iatriki Proodos* 12, no. 22–24 (Athens, 1917): 261–5, 302–7, 336–9.

the Parliament about the Impediments to Marriage from the Medical Point of View). He had been an advocate since 1870 for the adoption of certain measures to prevent marriage between persons suffering from contagious diseases, in order to safeguard the robustness of the nation. The debate on the necessary eugenic measures to be taken featured in the daily press and in the journals *To Paidi* (The Child), *Ygeia* (Health) and *Paedologia* (Paedology) as well as in the *Praktika Synedriou tis Ellinikis Anthropologikis Etaireias* (Proceedings of the Greek Anthropological Society) in the 1920s and 1930s. However, despite the plethora of sources and the importance attached to eugenics in the interwar period, the history of Greek eugenics still remains an underresearched field. Interwar governments did not ultimately adopt negative eugenic measures such as sterilization or prenuptial health certification.

Debates started by scientific societies, feminist organizations and journals on the protection of children's health reflect the importance attached to the health of the population. By investing their energies into children's health, these parties were granted the chance either to directly affect the health of citizens or argue for the protection of their rights and the improvement of the nation in biological terms. More specifically, the formulation of the biological capital theory was associated with the decrease in infant mortality, eugenic education and the protection of children, including prenatal care and puericulture.[101] The Liberal government prioritized the issue of children's protection, associated with Venizelos's plan for urban modernization in correlation with the dictates for national integrity,[102] and the active role the state had assumed in the field of social welfare during this period. The state, as was often stressed by state officials,[103] should take certain measures to produce a healthy, new generation. These measures included mandatory medical check-ups of all the would-be couples, the medical examination of pregnant women and their well-being from the fifth month of pregnancy onwards, the financial support of mothers and the education of parents in biology.

People from various scientific, political, social and ideological backgrounds approached health problems from eugenics perspective. Leading

---

101 On eugenics and puericulture in the interwar period, see Vassiliki Theodorou and Despina Karakatsani, "Eugenics and Puericulture in Greece in Interwar Years: Medical Concerns about the Amelioration of the Biological Capital," in *Health, Hygiene and Eugenics in Southeastern Europe to 1945*, eds. Christian Promitzer, Sevasti Trubeta, Marius Turda (Budapest: Central European University Press, 2011), 299–323.

102 Giorgos Mavrogordatos and Khristos Khatziiosif, eds., *Venizelismos kai Astikos Eksykhronismos*.

103 Venizelos himself stressed this point in his electoral speech in Thessaloniki in 1928.

figures in the medical community that held posts in the governmental sector, voluntary and semi-voluntary organizations advanced eugenic theories. However, more often than not different and at times even contradictory arguments were employed with regard to the means of combating pre-, during and after-pregnancy related problems. The debate focused primarily on the social dimensions of the diseases, the degeneration of the nation, social hygiene, regulation of the size of the population through eugenics, the biological quality of the nation, birth control and the relationship between hygiene and eugenics.

In the 1930s, two issues caused a rift in the Greek intelligentsia that were both theoretical and practical: prenuptial health certification and sterilization. The issue of sterilization was whether it should be mandatory or not; its effectiveness as a means of preventing procreation in cases of established hereditary problems and diseases was also questioned. Lack of appropriate technological infrastructure and an organized health system were considered the main hurdles. In 1919, proposals for the adoption of negative eugenic measures were put forward in Parliament for the very first time. The occasion of the law on the establishment of anti-TB clinics urged the MP S. Papavasileiou to suggest that the tubercular be castrated and denied the ability to marry. Papavasileiou had come to propose these measures because of the rise in the number of tubercular patients during World War I. According to him, TB was a hereditary disease linked to syphilis. The views expressed about eugenic sterilization were presented in minute detail by gynecologist Moysis Moysidis in his book *Evgoniki Aposteirosis* (Eugenic Sterilization), published in 1934. This work traced trends in interwar eugenic thought and practices, with particular reference to sterilization and its types, the arguments for and against. Moyseidis presented the moral, social, religious, legal and scientific views, but also the views on and the objections to sterilization raised up until that time in Greece.[104] Moyseidis himself advocated voluntary sterilization and set down the eugenic criteria one should follow when choosing a spouse.[105] Stavros Tsourouktsoglou (1896–1966),[106] a renowned eugenicist active in Switzerland and Germany,[107] Kostis Kharitakis, direc-

---

104 Moissis Moyseidis published a relevant book entitled *O Malthoussianismos Allote kai Nyn* (Athens, 1932).

105 Moissis Moyseidis, "Ygieini tou Gamou," Vivliothiki Koinonikis Ygieinis, vol. 2 (Athens, 1933).

106 Tsourouktsoglou's views were aligned with those of other eugenicists and hygienists that were in favour of a scientific and legal approach to social diseases and the control of the population. See Trubeta, "Eugenic Birth Control and Prenuptial Health Certification in Interwar Greece," 282.

107 Trubeta, "Eugenic Birth Control and Prenuptial Health Certification in Interwar Greece," 271–98.

tor at the department of Social Hygiene, pediatrician and member of the Patriotic Foundation of Social Protection and Relief (PFSPR), and Professor Konstantinos Moutousis opposed obligatory sterilization, arguing on the basis of scientific and social grounds.

Prenuptial health certification attracted the attention of experts, as the number of articles in scientific journals and the daily press testifies to, was more widely approved of.[108] Its usefulness and necessity was recognized by most and was promoted as a milder way of dealing with genetic problems, the transmission of contagious diseases, and the birth of the mentally challenged. However, there were disagreements on whether prenuptial health certification should be obligatory or not, when it should be issued, the list of diseases that would deter prospective spouses from getting certification, the means of education and the financial resources for such a venture. Most persons involved in the discussion emphasized the difficulty in applying the measure, the insufficient infrastructure necessary for its implementation, and the difficulty in convincing the public.

It should be noted that in the end the attempts of the state did not come to fruition. In 1925, the minister of Hygiene K. Filandros filed a request to the Holy Synod, asking them to take a stand on the issue of people's good health as a prerequisite for marriage.[109] It seems that the Synod's reply was positive, but the matter was dropped a few months later because Pangalos's authoritarian regime dissolved the Ministry of Hygiene. In the early 1930s, prenuptial health certification was put back in the agenda as a series of health issues entered political discussion, following the Liberals' assumption of power and the appeal to the Health Committee of the LN. The number of the mentally ill and carriers of syphilis and TB and the spread of venereal diseases and marriages between the tubercular raised the concerns of doctors and politicians and made the adoption of hygienic measures imperative to counteract dysgenics.[110]

---

108 Nikolaos Drakoulidis was also an advocate of the eugenic prenatal examination and published extensively in the contemporary press and journals. Trubeta, "Eugenic Birth Control and Prenuptial Health Certification in Interwar Greece," 286.

109 Kostis Kharitakis, "Ta Zitimata tis Ygeias os Kolymata Gamou. I Evgonia, i Syzygiki Molynsis kai to Progamiaio Pistopoiitiko Ygeias," *Dimosia Ygieini*, no. 1 (January 10, 1931):13–6.

110 The issue was brought for discussion by Moissis Moyseidis in the first Pan-Hellenic Hygiene Congress that took place in Athens in April 1930. "I pro tou Gamou Iatriki Exetasis" (Eisigisis eis to A' Panellinion Synedrion tis Ygieinis), *Ergasia*, no. 1 (April 29, 1930): 19.

These concerns were reflected in the bill on venereal diseases as well as in the campaigns against TB and syphilis. The decision of the Ministry of Hygiene in December 1930 to align with the view of the then recently established Supreme Hygiene Council, which decided that would-be-couples had to sign a solemn statement prior to their marriage and that poor health bar people from marriage, was a decisive step towards the implementation of the law. Yet, a change to the Civil Code was required in order for the prenuptial marriage certification to take full effect. However, when the issue of certification was discussed before the Revisionary Committee of the Civil Code on March 12th 1931 the proposal of the jurists that diseases such as TB, syphilis, epilepsy and leprosy be included among the impediments to marriage was voted down.[111] Although the prenuptial health certification was not adopted, the views put forward then are most informative about the current biological theories such as genetic theory and its reliability, as well as about the practical problems the application of the prenuptial health certification would face such as insufficient health care infrastructure and medical training. The discussion on what the limits of state intervention in private life should be and possible infringements on personal freedom was also of great importance. Although the members of the Committee agreed on the value of eugenics as a modern means of reaching society, objections were raised on its compulsory nature.

While the adoption of the prenuptial health certification was discussed, doctors and social thinkers put forward interesting views. A few days before the matter was discussed before the Committee, Ioannis Koumaris, a professor of physical anthropology and president of the Greek Anthropological Society, a fervent proponent of prenuptial health certification, had connected the prenuptial health certification with financial measures in an article in the newspaper Estia (Εστία). He suggested fines be imposed on whomever provided false identification and taxes be lifted for would-be-couples if they proved they were healthy according to the health certification they submitted.[112] Koumaris asserted that everyone agreed on the necessity of the certification, but disagreed on the means of its application. He further stressed the importance of establishing consultation offices for pro-

111 Sevasti Trubeta, *Physical Anthropology*; Alexandra Saranti, "I Metarythmisi tou Astikou Kodika. Ta Kolymata tou Gamou," *O Agonas tis Gynaikas*, no. 15 (March 1931): 3–6.
112 Ioannis Koumaris, "Ena Ethnikon Zitima. Dia tin Evgonian," *Estia* no. 1 (March 1931): 1.

spective spouses. In 1933, Konstantinos Moutousis, professor of hygiene at the University of Athens, advocated for the compulsory character of pre-nuptial health certification in a lecture entitled "Hygiene and Eugenics in Contemporary Societies,"[113] in which he argued for the necessity of impos-ing the certification on those with negative genetic traits.

The National Council of Greek Women organized a series of lectures to educate mothers on child-rearing and to combat superstitions, prejudices and ignorance of child care, aiming to prevent disease and ultimately im-prove the health of the race. The National Council further suggested the government introduce a programme of preventative medicine and educa-tion including propaganda films, lectures on issues related to diseases and the means of preventing and fighting diseases, and set up consultation cen-ters. Those who believed that it was necessary to adopt strict eugenics and procreation measures in order to restrict and control births (even to impose sterilization) advocated the importance of state intervention and considered the educational campaigns insufficient.[114] There were also disagreements over propaganda as well. Some, among them Doxiadis and Drakoulidis, stressed the need to establish a wide network of consultation centers that would organize and disseminate educational propaganda. Drakoulidis also proposed the establishment of a eugenic society that would coordinate the centers. Presenting all the views on whether or not to implement eugenic laws is not an objective of this chapter; instead, we focus primarily on the discussion of infant mortality, the improvement of children's health, paedol-ogy and puericulture. The value of eugenics for improving the Greek race was not questioned. Most supported the adoption of mild eugenic measures by the state that would focus on educating citizens about their biological duties and preparing them for these duties. Advocates of mild eugenics laid emphasis on raising mothers' awareness of biology. Doctors, state function-aries and social thinkers who discussed sterilization and prenuptial health certification in the 1930s, all agreed that only education could increase peo-ple's awareness of biology, which was a necessary precondition for their co-operation with the state on private affairs of marriage and reproduction.

---

113 "Enarktirion Mathima eis to Panepistimio 9/11/1933," *Kliniki. Evdomadiaia Epistmimoniki kai Epangelmatiki Epitheorisis* no. 47 (November 25, 1933): 863–74.
114 Trubeta, "Eugenic Birth Control and Prenuptial Health Certification in Interwar Greece," 289.

The union of puericulture and eugenics was attempted mainly by three medical experts in the interwar period, Apostolos Doxiadis, Emmanouil Lambadarios and Kostis Kharitakis, who combined their medical backgrounds with the ability to make decisions from their high government positions in the public health sector. They all played a leading part in the establishment of social hygiene institutions for children. All three had been educated abroad, studied the organization of similar institutions in other European countries, played indispensable roles in the establishment of scientific societies for children's health and had attempted to import European eugenic theories into Greece.

Lambadarios argued that eugenic practices should include the establishment of puericulture centers for the better care of pregnant women and better preparation for child birth, and the instruction of the staff. He took as a model the Institute of Puericulture at the University of Paris (*L'Institut de Puériculture de l'Université de Paris*), a French-American institution for the theoretical and practical instruction of doctors, midwifes, and visiting nurses. He admired the French professor of pediatrics and president to the French Eugenic Society, Adolphe Pinard and adopted his views on the role puericulture should play in the improvement of the race. Moysis Moysidis, as a member of the Gynecological Society of Paris, the French Eugenic School and the International Institute of Anthropology in Paris and director of the journal *Ygeia* (Health), promoted the popularization of eugenics among mothers. He further identified the aims of puericulture with those of eugenics, using Pinard's own words: "Eugenics is puericulture before procreation ('puériculture antéconceptionnelle')."[115]

In the same context, Kharitakis diligently tried to organize the first state institutions for the protection of mothers since 1925. As director of the then recently established Social Hygiene Service, he attempted to initiate a new policy to reduce infant mortality and improve living standards for destitute families. In his book *Koinoniki Ygieini* (Social hygiene), he argued that eugenics constituted a branch of puericulture in conjunction with social hygiene. Considering puericulture to be the best means of preparing a robust young generation, he favored a puericulture policy that would include procreative puericulture, pregnancy and puericulture proper. The influence of

---

115 Adolphe Pinard, "De l'eugénique," *Bulletin Médical* no. 26 (1912): 1123–27.

neo-Lamarkian eugenics on Greek doctors, pediatricians and gynecologists who had studied in France are quite discernible. The neo-Lamarkian approach opposed its Darwinian counterpart, holding that both social and environmental effects (nature vs nurture) shaped hereditary characteristics. Social hygiene measures and education of parents, neo-Lamarkianists believed, were decisive in child birth and development. They emphasized the duty of the individual towards his or her society and race, and the need of the state to instruct families, especially women.

According to Kharitakis, mothers would be decisive for the improvement of the race. Mothers should be informed of their eugenic duties to society and the nation, mainly the value of breastfeeding and hygiene. Pediatricians tended to blame illiterate mothers who were ignorant of hygiene and proper nutrition for high rates of infant mortality. Having visited many infant medical centers in various European countries because of his office, Kharitakis suggested some urgent measures be taken by the state to improve the Greek race[116] including: the establishment of consultation stations for mothers, the spread of hygiene practices among young mothers and the education of visiting nurses. Kharitakis also stressed the great value of the prenuptial health certificate[117] to prospective parents, as they could be informed of the risks genetic diseases posed.[118]

The jurist, Elias Lagakos, in his article "The Prenuptial Health Certification. Legal and Sociological Views," published in 1930 in the journal *To Paidi* (The Child), argued that three steps of mild eugenics were feasible in the Greek case: the dissemination of propaganda material to would-be-couples; the establishment of centers staffed with experts who could give advice to prospective couples; and lectures delivered in universities, barracks, at the workplace and in schools. Through these steps, eugenics would become an "acculturation of the instinct of reproduction," rather than a strict enforcement of medical examinations on would-be-couples. During this period, Apostolos Doxiadis played the most important role in shaping

---

116 Kostis Kharitakis, "Koinoniki Ygieini," *Erevna*, Special Issue, no. 2 (April–May 1928), (Athens and Alexandreia: 1928): 15–6.

117 Kostis Kharitakis, "Ta Neotera Dedomena epi tis Koinonikis Ygieinis. Arkhai kai Kritiria Organoseos tis Dimosias Ygieinis," (Athens: Ethniko Typographeio, 1929).

118 See the series of articles by Kharitakis entitled "Koinoniki Ygieini," *Ellinis* 6, no. 11 (November 1927), 233–35; *Ellinis* 6, no. 12 (December 1927): 259–62; *Ellinis* 7, no. 1 (January 1928):10–2; *Ellinis* 7, no. 2 (February 1928):40–2. *Ellinis* 7, no. 3 (March 1928):63–5.

eugenic public views and promoting certain puericulture activities. In his interview to the newspaper *Patris* (Homeland) on November 14, 1928, he noted that "nothing is going to be accomplished unless we lay the foundations of a health policy starting from below, from childhood, which is the foundation of our society. For foundations are eroded, and our state and national edifice are nowhere rested. We will keep a watchful eye on the health of the Greek person, from his mother's womb to his conscription. This is most important and we should all pay attention to it. Accordingly, the Patriotic Welfare Foundation is transformed into the National Council of Childhood Protection [...]."

In his article "Paedology and Eugenics,"[119] in the journal *Paidologia* (Paedology) in 1921, Doxiadis wrote of the reasons for the hereditary predispositions for pathology among children. Following Sicard de Plauzoles, a French doctor widely known for his eugenic theories, Doxiadis maintained that parents' diseases, like syphilis, alcoholism, malaria and TB were responsible for the degeneration of youth. He also drew attention to both moral depravity and intermarriage with foreigners, which became all the more frequent after World War I. For the first time, Doxiadis stressed the need to raise awareness of biology and popularize the biological duty of the individual to the community. To eliminate pathological inclinations that led to the production of mentally challenged people, he proposed that a card be introduced with each citizen's genetic history, thus facilitating the production of healthy offspring.[120] The impact of French eugenicists is also discernible in the eugenic views put forward, especially by Doxiadis, on people as biological capital.[121] The influence of Sicard de Plauzoles's idea that the future of a nation's race rested on the quality of biological capital rather than on numbers of people is evident in Doxiadis's concerns about the degeneration of the Greek population.[122] Sicard de Plauzoles's proposals for the rights of people to protect children before and during pregnancy

119 Apostolos Doxiadis, "Paidologia kai Evgonia," *Paidologia* 2, no. 12 (April 1921): 14–22.

120 Apostolos Doxiadis, "Poian Taktikin Ofeilei na Akolouthisei I Koinonia kai I Politeia," *Elefteron Vima* (March 15, 1931): 3.

121 Apostolos Doxiadis, "Viologiki Politiki me Vasi tin Afxisi tou Plythismou tis Khoras," *Ellinika Grammata* 3, no. 3 (July 16, 1928): 95–8 and also by the same author "Koinoniki Viologia-Viologiki Politiki," *Ellinika Grammata* 3, no. 2 (July 1, 1928): 49–51 and "O Anaplythismos tis Elladas," *Elefteron Vima* (September 13, 1930): 1.

122 Apostolos Doxiadis, "Evgonia," *To Paidi*, no. 28 (November-December 1934): 5–15.

and during early childhood had been adopted in France by the Committee for the Protection of the Right to Healthy Life and the Central Committee of the French Association and had made it to Greece through the journal *Ygeia* (Health).[123]

Doxiadis also maintained that the sustainability of the nation was contingent on the biological capacity of the families comprising it. In the preambles of the Greek laws designed during this period, he stressed the relation of the population's fertility to the nation's survival and the need for the government to adopt a biological policy. Since children's health determined the biological quality of the race, it was the state's duty to secure the best childbirth conditions for mothers.[124] Doxiadis further claimed that in Greece the demographic questions were put in qualitative rather than quantitative terms. He noted that Greece did not face a problem of low birth, as had been the case in other European countries, because the refugees that surged into Greece after the Minor Asia Disaster infused new blood into the population, thus strengthening it. Yet, Doxiadis believed that this population consisted of persons mentally and physically burdened and biologically vulnerable who lived in adverse conditions, and as a result the biological quality of their children would not be of high value. Since TB, malaria and improper nutrition taxed refugees, infant mortality was high. According to his own research, infant mortality rates among the working class and agricultural workers came to 30%, while for the middle class it ranged from 10% to 12%. Therefore, although there was a surplus of births, a lot of people did not make it until the productive years of their life. Doxiadis estimated that in order to secure the viability of the Greek nation, each family had to give birth to four children on average and be able to sustain them in hygienic conditions until the age of five. If each family had only three children, there would be a decrease in population. He also purported that the Greek race had dangerously declined due to migrations, wars and revolutions; as a result, the inferior biological quality of lower class prevailed while the upper class dwindled because of the decrease in the number of children the latter group was having and the rise of mortality in South East Europe.[125] Thus, he

---

123 Apostolos Doxiadis, "Evgoniki kai Paidokomia," *Ygeia* no. 7 (July 1931): 153–54.
124 Apostolos Doxiadis, "Evgonia," *To Paidi* no. 28 (November-December 1934), 5–15.
125 Apostolos Doxiadis, "To Dimografikon Zitima," *Nea Politiki* no. 4 (April 1939): 416.

concluded that although Greece did not face the problem of childlessness, "we do not have the assets which could render our race very strong."[126]

Doxiadis believed that the state should intervene to improve the biological value of reproduction and a hygienic policy be drawn on a racial basis. In other words, he suggested a reconstruction of society based on race factors rather than class. Doxiadis thought that the biological value of families was indispensable for eugenic reconstruction, and the estimation of its value could be carried out by means of family statistics. He imagined this as a personal data file with information about the health of family members, genetic and contagious diseases, use of drugs and alcohol, the profession, residence and age of parents, number of births, and possibility of incest. With this information the impact these factors had on health could be estimated and families could be classified according to their biological value. According to this Tayloristic-like register, reproduction could be either subsidized by the state or hindered, depending on the individual.

Doxiadis further maintained that the risk of degeneration could be avoided, provided that the state financially supported poor families of superior biological value to encourage them to have many children, at least four. He argued that when states and governments want increased child birth, they must secure favorable birth conditions. Doxiadis imagined a society of physically eugenic and mentally healthy workers with many children who would have a strong sense of responsibility to the race, be aware of its value and control their sexual urges appropriately. Doxiadis suggested taxes be imposed on entertainment, the unmarried and the childless, which could thus help reform and reconstruct society.[127] Besides, it was a means to increase the meagre finances of the Patriotic Foundation for the Protection of the Child.

In order to popularize the issue of taxing the unmarried, Doxiadis spearheaded a large scale press campaign and gave a series of interviews to the press. In a letter to the Prime Minister (November 1930), he stressed that the protection of mothers and children should not be voluntary; instead,

---

126 *Elefteron Vima* (September, 13 1930) and March 1931. Apostolos Doxiadis, "To Dimografikon Provlima," *Ellinika Grammata* 3, no. 2 (July 1928): 49–51. Doxiadis referred to the issue of refugees and their future in Greece in an article hosted in *The Manchester Guardian* (May 11, 1923).

127 "I Epivoli Forologias eis tous Agamous. Ti Legei o Dagkeiologos k. Doxiadis," *I Pamprosfygiki* 805 (September 22, 1928): 1.

it should be mandatory through the new and necessary tax form he had proposed. The taxation of the unmarried should be regulated according to their family obligations, "on the basis of biology," as was the case in Germany and Italy. He further suggested that stipends for poor families come from a special fund paid for by those who did not have a family and thus did not help sustain society. In addition, the fund would inherit the property of the childless when they died, compulsorily.[128] Doxiadis also asserted that the childless and the unmarried should not inherit property, but instead their expected share of inheritance go to the Fund of Childhood Protection. The fund would enable a wide array of a large scale social work, like medical care, the provision of nutritious and healthy food to children, and the establishment of summer camps.

He maintained that it was a fair and efficient law for strengthening children and protecting mothers. The law had been previously applied by Mussolini in Italy in 1927 and had brought satisfactory results. In his view, it could facilitate the reform and reconstruction of the Greek society. In Italy, the decision to pass the law was made in December 1926 and was justified as a practice derived from the golden age of the Roman emperor Augustus, aiming to encourage marriage and redistribute national income among large families. France had passed similar legislation for unmarried couples in the 1920s. This law was meant to substantially help the Italian state, which was in deep debt. Priests and soldiers were exempted from payment in Italy while the ill, seniors and the destitute could ask for a special arrangement. As the law on the unmarried was tailored according to age and income, it burdened some population groups, especially men aged between 35 and 50. In addition, the tax tripled between 1927 and 1937. Initially, the income from taxes was channeled into social welfare, but in 1935 it was used to facilitate the African campaign and later to reduce the chronic state deficit.

Maria Sophia Quine argues that although the "penalizing" tax measures turned out to be inefficient they constituted the basic means of fascist population policy. The policy on curbing the "deliberate sterility" sometimes took the form of threatening to impose stricter measures and exclude people over 30 years of age, unmarried couples, or parents of children younger

---

128 In the newspaper *Elliniki* on September 20, 1928 the law on the taxation imposed on the unmarried is criticized. It is argued that young men should either get married or get taxed.

than four from relatively well-paid and secure job positions in the public sector. In addition, the law required that married couples with a small number of children be taxed for infertility, and the property of the deceased without an heir and of the unmarried be confiscated. Mussolini's advisers also suggested celibacy be penalized to force all citizens over 30 years of age to marry and bear children, and courts be able to annul marriages of those couples who had not had any children, after having been married for five years.[129] Even more extreme views were voiced, e.g. to make childlessness a crime against the state and the race punishable by imprisonment and other heavy sentences. In addition, similar to the French law put in effect in 1914, as part of 'a redistributive policy and justice' a series of tax privileges and tax exemptions were given to men who had many children in Italy in 1928. "Pronatalism gave a semblance of purpose to all policy initiatives under fascism. Fascism fought to redefine the exercise of citizenship and to make procreation appear as a patriotic duty."[130]

When Venizelos was asked about the fairness of this law noted:

[...] We are not, of course, able to determine the return of a tax which will be applied for the first time. However, we can approximate it on the basis of some evidence. We know, though, that the law on taxing the childless, which was applied in Italy in 1927, yielded returns of about fifty-six million lirettas, the equivalent of about two hundred and twenty-four million drachmas, during the first year of its application. By analogy with our population—one sixth of its Italian counterpart—we estimated that we might collect between thirty and thirty five million drachmas. But even if we get less, provided that the unmarried in Greece are not so many as in other countries—let's say about seventeen, even fifteen million drachmas for the first year—with this sum we will be able to do much work for childhood. In Italy taxes have been imposed on childless married couples since 1923.[131]

129 Maria Sophia Quine, *Population Politics in Twentieth-Century Europe*, 40–1.

130 Quine, *Population Politics in Twentieth-Century Europe*, 41.

131 It is underlined that there are many men that avoid marriage because they are either snobs or selfish, but hardly is there a woman that rejects marriage [...]. So, let the spinsters not worry." It also examines the case the law to include whoever is over thirty-five years of age and still single and whether the law should stop having effect at a certain age, as is the case in Italy–the sixtieth year of age–or the unmarried be taxed until their death. This tax policy included whoever of the unmarried paid taxes for income, starting at 1,000 drachmas and more.

In the 1930s, the discussion on eugenics in Greece did not result in negative eugenic measures. In contrast, emphasis was placed on educating citizens about the value of eugenics[132] and the establishment of social hygiene institutions for mothers and children alike to secure the robustness of the new generation. Hopes that the nation would regenerate were set on constant monitoring of the health of new generations through the school system by such means as the quantification of body measurements, health booklets and student health cards, but also examination of mothering conditions and hygienic infant raising, carried out by voluntary organizations and semi-state institutions such as the infants' ward and the ward for monitoring pregnant women of the Patriotic Foundation for the Protection of the Child. The mild eugenics and the linking of eugenics with puericulture and social hygiene can be attributed to the influence the French pediatricians who dominated the French Eugenics Society had on Greek doctors and to the objections raised by the Revision Committee of the Civil Code to the proposal of the Supreme Health Council to include serious diseases among impediments to marriage.

9. MENTAL HEALTH AND HYGIENE DURING THE INTERWAR PERIOD

In the early twentieth century, childhood attracted the interest of the mental health movement, which argued that childhood should be treated as a temporal and mental life stage that determined the course to and shape of adulthood along with various psychosocial changes. The debate over children's mental hygiene was organized around the principle that society could be improved and brought to perfection through the proper social integration of children, since happy and healthy children led to a healthy and productive adult population. The interest in children's mental hygiene was also linked to the development of pedagogical psychology, paedology and psychoanalysis. Sigmund Freud's *Three Essays on the Theory of Sexuality* published in 1905, analyzed the crucial role of childhood for adult life, and established the notional basis for child psychiatry. The Swiss and later American psychiatrist Adolph Meyer (1866–1950), president of the American Psychi-

---

132 See the article by hygienist and microbiologist Stavros Tsourouktsoglou "I Evgonia. Ta Tria Provlimata tis Evgonias," *Ygeia* no. 12 (1925): 246.

atric Association, emphasized the need to treat mental illness as a bio-psycho-social reaction and not as the result of biological origins. Promoting a psychobiological reading of mental problems and pointing out the connection between body and mind, he adopted a dynamic approach to mental illness, stressing developmental parameters and reasons.

The work of the pioneer American psychologist and pedagogue Stanley Hall (1844–1924), who had conducted research on children, and Clifford Beers's autobiography *A Mind That Found Itself* (1908) played an important role in the emergence of the mental hygiene movement. The child guidance movement was a major chapter in the field of mental hygiene, as it contributed to the emergence of psychiatric perception and care for childhood disorders.[133]

Mental health and intellectual hygiene attracted the interest of physicians and educators after World War I, especially during the interwar period, and led to special approaches to normality vs. abnormality as well as the imposition of social policy measures. In addition, since the early twentieth century, doctors and psychologists seem to have been convinced that deviant behavior was an indication of illness closely linked with the individual's mental health. They contended that timely medical intervention could not only decrease the severity of mental illness or even the illness itself. Throughout the 1920s, the child guidance movement targeted mainly the children of immigrant parents and children from the working class. During the 1930s, this movement started reaching mostly the native American middle-class and developed into a form of medical intervention that treated children with mild emotional and behavioral problems within the clinic.[134] The mental health movement, associated with the belief in the role of science in counteracting diseases and securing social progress, included diagnosis, scientific analysis of mental health problems and their treatment.[135] The men-

---

133 Margo Horn, *Before it's too Late: the Child Guidance Movement in the United States 1922–1945* (Philadelphia, Penn.: Temple University Press, 1989); Theresa Richardson, *The Century of the Child: The Mental Hygiene Movement and Social Policy in the United States and Canada* (Albany: State University of New York Press, 1989). See also Pâquet and Jérôme Boivin, "La Mesure Fait Loi. La Doctrine de l'Hygiène Mentale et les Tests Psychométriques au Québec Pendant l'Entre-deux-guerres," *The Canadian Historical Review* 88, no. 1 (March 2007): 149–79.

134 Kathleen Jones, *Taming the Troublesome Child: American Families. Child Guidance and the Limits of Psychiatric Authority* (Cambridge, MA: Harvard University Press, 1999).

135 William Sweetzer introduced the idea of "mental hygiene" in the USA in 1843. The American psychologist Isaac Ray was one of the thirteen founders of the American Psychiatric Association who defined "mental hygiene" as the art of maintaining the mind and curbing various influences that could damage

tal health movement was a scientific field aiming to solve social problems as well as a humanitarian movement with an interest in human rights and the alleviation of pain.

There were international congresses on intellectual hygiene in 1922, 1927 and 1930, which propped into various aspects of this field. During the same period, mental health clinics were set up to examine in detail the individual's mental ability and progress and determine them while offering special treatment. France had been a pioneer in the field of clinical mental hygiene; in 1925, the Medical School in Paris set up a clinic for persons with mental health problems that was attached to its psychiatric and pediatric clinics. In addition, in France mental protection, psychotechnics and clinical treatment of the illness were promoted, especially under the guidance of the psychiatrist Edouard Toulouse (1865–1947) who had studied the 'Emil Zola case' and explored the relationship between cognition and madness. Also, during the same period a special medico-pedagogical department operated in the Paediatric Clinic of the University of Vienna. Medico-teaching congresses began in German starting in 1922 to explore the same issue. They examined in particular the effect of psychology on character formation and the possibility of establishing a mental health institute. The German School, especially the Mental Health Society established in 1928, played an important role by promoting racial hygiene when mental problems were approached from the perspectives of eugenics and psychiatry. The development of paedology and the technical progress made in psychometrics enhanced the ability to measure individual mental and cognitive differences, combining this with the diagnosis and care of children with special educational needs. In the USSR the emphasis was laid upon psychohygiene, while Italy passed a law in 1925 that established clinics-asylums, special classes and institutions for "abnormal" children in every district. In 1926, the Belgian National Association for Mental Health established a similar clinic in Brussels, while teachers for mentally challenged children were trained at the Institute Jean-Jacques Rousseau in Geneva and the Zurich

---

its energy, quality and development. The management of physical strength in relation to exercise, nutrition, clothing, climate, reproduction laws, management of vices, response to contemporary feelings and views, mind discipline, all these were inscribed and impacted on mental hygiene. Dorothea Dix (1802–1887), a teacher who had devoted herself to helping people suffering from mental diseases and bringing to light their destitute living conditions was another important personality in the field of mental hygiene. The intellectual and mental hygiene movement was set up by Clifford Beers (1876–1943).

University medico-pedagogical seminar. For the measurement of children's intelligence, scales of mental development (psychometrics) and intelligence (IQ, grading intellectual ability) were used that led to a differentiated pedagogical and educational approach to children, according to their particular intellectual strengths.

Experimental psychology arose from the necessity to shape more suitable attitudes towards children and adapt teaching to students' individual needs. In connection with paedology experimental psychologists envisioned that the education of children would be more efficient, educational practices would reach the best possible degree, mortality rates would decline, care for children with special educational needs would improve and vocational education and choice of profession would allow each person to take the most suitable post for them.

Similarly, this attempt is evident in educational developments that took place in Greece. Nikolaos Exarkhopoulos (1874–1960), professor of pedagogy in the Faculty of Philosophy at the University of Athens wrote about the normality and deviance of school-age children in the 1920s, using three methods to do so: experimental anthropometry, psychometrics and systematic observation. Exarkhopoulos supported that physical and mental defects were genetically transmitted and underlined the necessity to take steps towards the improvement of birth conditions, recognizing the importance of eugenics. He stressed the therapeutic role of pedagogy in cases of genetic diseases but also the limits these diseases imposed on the child's mental development when these were incurable. He held that good moral qualities were likely to develop thanks to appropriate education, whereas intelligence was less likely to be cultivated by outside influence.[136]

Exarkhopoulos is considered the founder of scientific pedagogy in Greece; he set up the Experimental School at the University of Athens, where much psychological research was carried out. Affiliated with the Experimental School, the Laboratory of Experimental Pedagogy was established in 1923 and operated under the supervision of Exarkhopoulos and his partners. The laboratory was attached to the seat of pedagogy at the Faculty

---

136 Nikolaos Exarkhopoulos, "Psykhologia ton Atomikon Diaforon. I Diagnosis tou Vathmou tis Noimosinis epi ti Vasei Peiramatikon Erevnon. Nea Morfi tis Klimakos Binet-Simon," *Praktika tis Akadimias Athinon* (5th of November 1931): 356–74. In this article, Exarkhopoulos looked into the modification of this scale by him; at the same time, he pointed out its deficiencies.

of Philosophy at the University of Athens and served as a center of scientific paedological and pedagogical research.[137] Psychological experiments were carried out and applied to the educational process.[138] In addition, research was carried out for the diagnosis of the students' intellectual and mental condition and measurements of intelligence were taken through the Binet-Simon scale standardized in Greek. The laboratory aimed to cultivate and spread pedagogy in Greece; train students and public teachers in the use of scientific research methods and process of paedological problems; and carry out research on the physical, mental and moral condition of Greek children. An adapted version of the Binet-Terman scale that differed in the number and the type of tests was used while scales of the intellectual development of the Greek child[139] were applied in combination with foreign experimental methods adapted to local conditions. In addition, comparative studies were carried out to determine differences in physical development and intelligence between affluent and destitute Greek children; between boys and girls; and between children growing up in the countryside and their city counterparts. Studies were conducted on the relation between intelligence and school records, between the teachers' intelligence and judgment, and the students' performance in various subjects.

Other studies looked into the development of various mental skills and intellectual faculties, such as observation, attention, combinational, abstract, judgmental and reasoning skills, as well as performance in arts (drawing, plastics). Their end goal was to observe and diagnose individual peculiarities and idiosyncrasies using psychognostic tools (experimental method and systematic psychological observation), and appropriately instruct students on the right profession. Starting in 1923, the laboratory was equipped with special tools for these measurements. During this period, research was conducted on a sample 4,500 students from various schools, covering a wide age range. The sample included school age children, even toddlers from the municipal Foundling home and babies born either in the

---

137 *Epistimonikai Erevnai Genomenai en to Ergastirio Peiramatikis Paidagogikis tou Panepistimiou Athinon kata ta Prota 15 eti Leitourgias Aftou, 1923–1938* (Athens, 1938).

138 Nikolaos Exarkhopoulos, "Katanomi ton Ellinopaidon eis tous Diaforous Vathmous tis Noimosinis," *Praktika tis Akadimias Athinon* (14th of April 1932): 146–58.

139 Nikolaos Exarkhopoulos elaborated on the notion of intelligence in various articles, "I Ennoia tis Noimosinis," *Praktika tis Akadimias Athinon*, no. 6 (1931): 69 onwards. See also *Praktika tis Akadimias Athinon*, no. 5 (1930): 82 onwards and 107 onwards, and no. 5 (1930): 148 onwards.

municipal or the university hospitals and in private maternity clinics as well as university male and female students. The results led to the first comparative studies of Greek children with their counterparts from other countries, nations and races. Such studies resulted in diagrams depicting the curve of body development in relation to weight, height and thorax circumference.[140] Open-air institutions and the summer camps lent themselves to such measurements; within them, the role of regulated school attendance, a lighter school workload and educational activities in nature were quantitatively assessed by experts. During the same period, Sofia M. Gedeon, lecturer at the university laboratory of Experimental Pedagogy, taught the subject "Introduction to Pedometrie and Pedagogy."[141]

Another personality associated with psychological tests and measurements in Greece was George Sakellariou, founder of the psychological laboratory at the University of Thessaloniki. His scientific work extended to various experimental laboratories in Athens, where various psychological studies were carried out. He was the first to publish a textbook on child psychology in 1922, he standardized the Binet-Simon intelligence scale,[142] and he devised the Sakellariou-Terman scale, which he employed in much of his research.[143] After performing intelligence research on 540 people, he suggested special schools and classes be set up for gifted students and for students with a lower than the average I.Q. He further suggested group and individual tests be given to students to facilitate the students' admission to university and to determine their professional career. He insisted on the necessity to conduct research on the students' intellectual development and level of intelligence using psychometric procedures. He held that mentally challenged children and child delinquency should be dealt with through the existing special institutions. Intelligence measurements, framed within a discourse on "hereditary degeneracy," had been conducted by Sakellariou since 1926 during his professorship at the University of Thessaloniki. Sakellariou also conducted research on the emotional life of adolescents,

---

140 [521] Emmanouil Lambadarios, "I Somatiki Exelixis tou Ellinos Mathitou: Anthropologiki Afxisiologia," *Iatrika Khronika* no. 6 (December 1928): 354–56. Also by the same author, "I Somatiki Anaptyxis tou Paidiou," *Paidologia* no. 9 (December 1920):274–9 and *Paidologia* no. 5–8 (May-August 1921):145–57.

141 Sofia Gedeon, *Enarktirion Mathima tis Kathigitrias tis Paidometrias kai Paidagogikis Statistikis eis tous en to Panepistimio Athinon Metekpaidevomenous Dimodidaskalous* (Athens, 1930).

142 Georgios Sakellariou, *I Metrisis tis Efiias Atomikos kai Omadikos*, Self-edition (Athens, 1952).

143 Georgios Sakellariou, *I Metrisis tis Efiias met' Efarmogon eis tin Ekpaidefsin, ton Straton, ta Poinika Dikastiria kai tin Epaggelmatikin Katefthinsin* (Athens,1928).

employing a modified version of the Tendler method as well as research on the gifted in the area of Thessaloniki.

The Psychological Laboratory of the University of Athens operated since 1926 under the guidance of Theofilos Voreas. The next director of this laboratory was Geogios Sakellariou, a professor of psychology, who was the first to take the respective seat and set up a psychological laboratory in 1937.[144]

It seems that the interest in intelligence and mental health was combined with somatology, physical development, auxology, paedology and correlated directly with eugenic concerns. The idea of the direct relation between the child's physical and mental condition had gained ground. Various examinations of the bodies and minds of children led to a series of reforms in children's welfare. Venizelos's reforms, especially the one that took place in 1929, included regulations for special categories of children: girls, the sickly, the feeble-minded, non-native child speakers of Greek, the illiterate and working children. Already the 1913 bills included propositions for the establishment of special schools for children with learning difficulties. Article no. 11, Law 4397/16-8-1929, underlined that "[...] the Ministry reserves the right to arrange special teaching for the feeble-minded attending a primary school, or to set up a special class for them or even a special school, providing their number is sufficient."[145] In the early twentieth century, special institutions and schools were founded in Greece with the aim of protecting and educating the disabled (Home of the Blind, Lighthouse of the Blind, the Stoupatheio, National Institute for the Deaf, the Psychological Center of Northern Greece, the Educational Center for Spastic Children).[146] In 1923, the American philanthropic organization, Near East Relief,[147] which extended its services to assist and support orphaned children and cared for the health of rural people,[148] especially in Macedonia, set up the first school for the deaf, which was later moved to Syros and closed in

---

144 For the role Sakellariou and the psychological laboratories had played, see Panagiota Kazolea-Tavoulari, *I Istoria tis Psykhologias stin Ellada 1880–1987* (Athens: Ellinika Grammata 2002) 109–18.

145 Alexis Dimaras, *I Metarrythisi pou den Egine* (Athens: Ermis 1974), vol. 2, 172.

146 Dimitris Stasinos, *I Eidiki Ekpaidefsi stin Ellada* (Athens: Gutenberg, 1991) and Georgios E. Vasileiou, *Ta Ekpaidefsima Noitika Kathisterimena Paidia kai Efivoi* (Athens: Ellinika Grammata, 1998).

147 For more on this issue, see James Barton, *Story of Near East Relief, 1925–1930. An Interpretation* (New York: The Macmillan Company 1930); John Badeau and Georgianna Stevens eds., *Bread from Stones: Fifty Years of Technical Assistance* (New Jersey: Prentice-Hall Inc. 1956).

148 In 1929, this organization was renamed the Near East Foundation and continued to support the agricultural development and the establishment of public health stations in rural areas, where unfavourable health and hygiene conditions were very common.

1932. The same year "the National Home for the Deaf" commenced operation in Athens.[149] In 1936, Kharalambos and Eleni Spiliopoulou founded the National Institute for the Protection of the Deaf in Ampelokipi, Athens, following English and French specifications. Lambadarios, as director of the School Hygiene Service filed a report in 1931 underlining the lack of special schools for the mentally-challenged and the deaf and the lack of auxiliary schools or institutes for the blind, as was the case in other countries;[150] meager funding accounted for this lack. In 1933, in a public lecture organized by the Department of Child Protection of the National Council of Greek Women, Dimitris Moraitis, an advocate of Adler's theory and founder of the Society of Differential Psychology in Greece and professor of Psychology in Varvakeio and deputy director of Secondary Education, suggested a consultation pedagogical station be established. It materialized in 1934 by the Educational Department of the National Council of Greek Women. A few years later, in 1937, the first special school was established by the state.

---

149 Diatagma "Peri Idryses Ethnikou Oikou Kofalalon." *Efimeris tis Kiverniseos*, A΄, no.68 (March 15, 1932):454–56.

150 He referred to Bulgaria where an institute for the blind had already been set up.

PART III

Children's And Maternal Welfare During The Metaxas Regime (1936–1940)

CHAPTER VIII

SOCIAL POLICY AND THE IDEOLOGY
OF THE REGIME

The reform of social policy was instrumental in the success of Ioannis Metaxas's authoritarian regime that began in 1936, known as the 4th of August regime. Taking advantage of the political vacuum[1] and the fear of communism,[2] Ioannis Metaxas, ex-general and leader of an obscure party with royalist leanings, abolished democracy on the night of August the 4th. With the King's consent, he imposed a personalized authoritarian regime that lasted until his death in January 1941. During the four years of his regime, Metaxas criticized the interwar politicians on many occasions for the poor condition of the health care system, the slow pace at which refugees had been accommodated and politicians' indifference to childhood. To the rhetorical question "what is the position of Greece among the civilized states'?" regarding welfare, posed by Metaxas in one of his public speeches he responded: "[Greece] is almost last in the family of modern states, [its place being] even lower than [that of] other countries with less cultural claims."[3]

The association of "national regeneration" with a strong state appeared frequently in the public discourse of European authoritarian regimes after World War I. Following the model of Italian fascism, the dictator supported

---

1   It was created due to the difficulty of the two big parties to form a coalition government after the elections of January 1936; the death of the most important political interwar leaders was also a factor that contributed to this vacuum.
2   The communist appeal had risen during the 1930s, because of the economic crisis and the social problems. The possibility of the communist party toppling the bourgeois regime seemed exaggerated since the former had won only 5% during the elections in January 1936.
3   Anonymos "I Koinoniki Pronoia. Ta Pepragmena tou Ypourgeiou Kratikis Ygieinis kai Antilipseos kata to Proton apo tis 4is Avgoustou 1936 Etos," *Arkheia Ygieinis*, no. 6–7 (September-October 1937): 243.

a "New State" that differed from its liberal counterpart as it allotted more funds to citizens' welfare. According to Metaxas, the abandonment of the working class by Liberals was dangerous, because, among other reasons, it paved the way for the overthrow of the political system. According to the memorandum the dictator submitted to the King on the night of August 4, which abolished the main articles of the Constitution concerning political freedom, all social classes had been infiltrated by communist ideology, "fed by social discontent."[4] With this text, which was actually the instrument for the foundation of the dictatorship, Metaxas asked the King to abolish the Constitution and, in essence, to kill democracy.

The reform of social policy, connected as it was in the dictator's speeches with the nation's future, was important for the legitimization of the regime and Metaxas's elevation to the status of "the race's historical leader." Metaxas highlighted the inadequate social welfare services as one of the reasons why he abolished the parliament, claiming that the indifference of politicians and the clientele relationships with citizens accounted for this condition. Once more, in his discourse the quality of health and welfare services testified to the country's low cultural level and the future of the Greek race. The financial dimensions of health, that is the impact of citizens' health on the country's productivity, also pertained to the regime's propaganda. The reorganization of the welfare state and the preservation and strengthening of the nation's health were also recurrent themes in the regime's rhetoric.

The New State: Moral Reform and Cultural Mission

The dictatorship in interwar Greece was a period that can be better understood if seen in the context of the diverse authoritarian regimes in the interwar period. The way Metaxas's dictatorship was organized helps us identify the typical characteristics of totalitarian regimes, such as anti-parliamentarism, anti-communism and use of violence, censorship of the press, propaganda, the worship of the leader, centralization and intense policing. Despite its similarities to interwar fascist regimes, certain differences make the Greek dictatorship deviate from this well-known model. Metaxas's dictatorship was lacking in a strong massive party that could secure popularity and

---

4   See Ioannis Metaxas, *To Prosopiko tou Imerologio* (Athens: Govostis, 1960), vol. 7, 224–25.

impose fascist ideology. Metaxas's regime did not become a fully complete system as it lacked a solid theoretical foundation. The views formulated by the regime's advocates were the outcome of the development of the dictator's simplistic ideas influenced by foreign and Greek thinkers or simply derived from foreign theoreticians. The anti-parliamentarism belonged mostly to the 19th century tradition of "the Great Idea" rather than to the 20th century fascist ideology, as Metaxas did not welcome the plebeian elements of Nazism.[5] Besides, according to Metaxas, his regime bore more ideological affiliations with Salazar's regime in Portugal.[6] Most contemporary scholars agree that Metaxas's regime was not a fascist totalitarian state but rather a paternalistic dictatorship, a new popular right wing of the interwar period which never equaled fascism.[7]

The replacement of the government staff with people who supported Metaxas, the establishment of a police state, censorship and sweeping waves of prosecution against citizens for their political convictions evidenced the autocracy initiated by the "New State." Apart from the foreign affairs sector and the army leadership which were controlled by the King, all public sectors were controlled by Metaxas. The creation of the National Youth Organization (EON, Ethniki Organosis Neolaias) and the establishment of the third Greek civilization were key factors for the success of the moral reform attempted by the New State.[8]

The version of culture launched by the regime aspired to elevate the nation so as to win the respect of other nations.[9] To attain this goal, the Greek nation had to return to its roots and traditions, and break with liberal ideas.

---

5   For the character of the Metaxas's regime, see Khristos Khatziiosif, "Koinovoulio kai Diktatoria," in Khristos Khatziiosif ed., *Istoria tis Elladas tou 20ou Aiona*, vol. B2 (Athens: Vivliorama, 2004), 114–22; Constantinos Sarandis, "The Ideology and Character of the Metaxas Regime," in Robin Higham and Thanos Veremis eds., *Aspects of Greece 1936-1940: the Metaxas Dictatorship* (Athens: Hellenic Foundation for European and Foreign Policy-Vryonis Center, 1993), 152–63; Konstantinos Sarantis, "I Ideologia kai o Politikos Kharaktiras tou Kathestotos Metaxa," in Thanos Veremis (ed.), *O Metaxas kai i Epokhi tou* (Athens: Evrasia, 2009), 45–71; Vaggelis Aggelis, *"Giati Khairetai o Kosmos kai Khamogela Patera....."* *Mathimata Ethnikis Agogis kai Neolaiistiki Propaganda sta Khronia tis Metaxikis Diktatorias* (Athens: Vivliorama, 2006), 25–35.

6   See his discussion with British generals. Quoted in Sarantis, "I Ideologia kai o Politikos Kharaktiras tou Kathestotos Metaxa," 70.

7   Khatziiosif, "Koinovoulio kai Diktatoria," 119.

8   The third Greek civilization derived selective elements from its ancient and byzantine counterparts, which were considered important, yet incomplete.

9   Marius Turda refers to the cultural dimension of the national regeneration of the Metaxas regime, examining a wide array of European national regenerations in racial terms. Marius Turda, *Modernism and Eugenics* (New York: Palgrave Macmillan, 2010), 103.

As Greeks were thought to be the chosen people destined to civilize the world, the "New State" had to recreate Greek culture, aiming both to raise the standards of morality in Greek society and to spread this morality to other countries. Although this notion employed elements of modernity, it was built on the supposed continuity of the Greek race and on the culture of the "Great Idea." According to Metaxas, culture was the manifestation of "the vitality, the genius and the strength of the Greek race;" the edge it had over other races.[10] Spirituality and moral superiority were the main characteristics of this anti-materialist, anti-individualistic culture. The Third Greek civilization would resist progress and mechanization and thus opposed the European culture that led nations to disintegration. The legacy of Greeks' glorious past aroused feelings of pride and duty for Greeks. Because of its cultural superiority, the Greek race had the right to impose its cultural hegemony on neighboring countries. As the territorial expansion of Greece was no longer attainable, the Great Idea took on the meaning of the cultural spread attempted during the Greek antiquity rather than that of byzantine imperialism. The cultural dominance of Greece in the Eastern Mediterranean and the Balkans would give the Greeks a new mission to accomplish. To follow this mission, Greeks had to subdue their individual will to that of the nation. In this way, they could connect with their ancestors through thousands of years of history.[11]

1. The National Youth Organization (EON): the Cult of the Leader

With no mass movement, Metaxas attempted to legitimize his regime by undertaking vast welfare works for the protection of children. In line with other authoritarian states—Italy, Germany, Spain and Portugal—he tried to gain a strong footing among the young. Using modern means of propaganda, fascist youth organizations were an unprecedented undertaking to

---

10 In a series of articles entitled "Afterword," published in the newspaper *Kathimerini* in October 1935, Metaxas had analyzed his version of the Great Idea and the future of Hellenism. This version was inspired by the ideology of the late 19th century and was evidently influenced by Ion Dragoumis, a fervent advocate of the Great Idea. See Ioannis Metaxas, "Afterword" *Kathimerini*, January 23–6, 1935. In these articles, Metaxas formulated the main principles he would follow in case he assumed power.

11 "We have to believe in the continuity of the Greek race; we have evolved from the one and same race. To this testifies the contitunity of language." See Ioannis Metaxas, "Afterword" *Kathimerini*, January 25, 1935.

politicize childhood en masse. Established in November 1936, the National Youth Organization[12] was a systematic attempt to totally control the youth and the most advanced step towards the fascistisation of social life.[13] EON was high in the dictator's agenda as he expected that it would evolve into the fascist party he envisaged.[14]

According to its constitution, the EON aimed to promote the physical and mental condition of the youth through recreational activities and sports in their leisure time; offer vocational guidance; raise their national consciousness; inspire religious feelings; and foster solidarity and the spirit of cooperation. The regime's intention of indoctrinating youth can be detected behind these general statements. Children from various social classes were organized into two groups according to age and gender: the "diggers" from 7 to 13 years-old and the "phalangites" from 14 to 25 years old. Watching films, planting trees, celebrations,[15] Wednesday and Sunday meetings, and camp teamwork, were activities that allowed boys and girls to communicate without parental supervision and were the appealing aspect of Metaxas's massive effort to inculcate children. By targeting school-age children, the EON operated complementarily to school. Yet, their respective roles were distinctive: school aimed at the acquisition of knowledge, whereas EON aimed at molding children's character.

The importance the regime attached to physical exercise and hygiene is evident in the magazine *I Neolaia* (The Youth) which was published by the EON (1938–1941). Apart from the doctor's column, many popular articles were addressed to children and offered advice on diet, fighting popular superstitions with regard to health and the basics of hygiene. Articles and photos depicting gymnastic demonstrations, student soup kitchens, consulting for pregnancy care centers and convalescence facilities for children featured prominently in the magazine to highlight the regime's interest in improving the health of mothers and children.

Apart from instilling a moral sense in contemporary Greeks, the military preparation of the youth was also one of the main goals of the EON.

---

12 EON.

13 Robert Paxton, *I Anatomia tou Fasismou*, transl. Katerina Khalmoukou (Athens, Kedros: 2006), 192.

14 Giorgos Mavrogordatos, "Metaxy dyo Polemon," in *Istoria tou Neou Ellinismou, 1770–2000*, ed. Vasilis Panagiotopoulos, vol. 7 (Athens: Ellinika Grammata, 2003) 30.

15 The regime organised a wide array of celebrations among which were included national anniversaries and anniversaries for the commemoration of the establishment of the 4th of August regime.

The manuals given to children and adolescents were full of instructions on military drills. The uniforms, salutes and military hierarchy was meant to imbue children with military spirit. The youth's relationship with the army was also often highlighted in the leaflets distributed to the members of the organization. The break-out of the war made military training more urgent. Passive air-defense, marches, and instruction on the use of weapons were added to the organization's educational programme. In early 1940, the Ministry of Defense accepted the EON's request to provide spare officers to drill high school fifth and sixth graders.[16]

The connection to Greek antiquity is evident in all aspects of the organization in that it aspired to continue the educational institutions of ancient Sparta. Greek ancient symbols such as the double Minoan ax—symbolizing the eternity of the Greek race and its dual religious and royal power—ancient salutes, athletic and artistic events like torchlight processions, were means of resurrecting Ancient Greece, linking contemporary youth to the ancient models of physical beauty and strength and establishing the continuity of tradition. Athletic events were designed to popularize sports among youth, especially in Northern Greece, but with less focus on winning and merit. They were also meant to give children discipline, create strong and energetic bodies; and instigate enthusiasm for physical exercise among the masses, following the example set by their ancestors.[17]

A return to national traditions was expected to make the youth break away from the "rotten past" of recent times and the influence of liberalism and communism. The state's propaganda against communism was the main element of the youth's indoctrination. Organized in battalions, companies, platoons and squads, the young were instructed in political values, discipline and the personality cult of Metaxas, who was placed at the top of the hierarchy as the acclaimed leader of the organization. Uniforms and badges were indicatory of the rank, specialization and the adherence of the diggers and phalangites to the EON's principles.

The regime attempted to cultivate a new perception of childhood and family in conjunction with new political values. It was the first time that the politicization of youth had been attempted to such a great extent.

---

16 Aggelis, "Giati Khairetai o Kosmos kai Khamogela Patera ...," 225–7.
17 Sitsa Karaiskaki, "To Vathytero Pnevma tou Athlitismou," I Neolaia no. 33 (1939): 1074 in Eleni Makhaira, I Neolaia tis 4is Avgoustou. Fotografes. (Athens: IAEN, 1987), 134.

Although the regime's slogan was "Homeland, Religion and Family," Metaxas attempted to put limits on the power of the family and introduce a new perception of children's relationship to their parents and to the institutions of the New State. High rank members of the EON expressed fears that families might oppose the youth organization and hinder the devotion the dictator demanded from children. The family itself also took on a new meaning existing not for its own sake but for the nation's. This new perception invoked Spartan ideals and emphasized that the aim of the family was to strengthen the vital forces of the nation.[18]

Metaxas criticized parents for their possessive tendencies on numerous occasions.[19] Children did not belong only to their parents but also to the state and its leader. The dictator's address to the "diggers" is telling: "In a sense, you are my children, because your family brought you to this world; yet, you also belong to me because I brought you to the National Youth Organization, which we have laid our hopes and visions on; you are natives of the 4th of August New State and you have to imprint the goal of this State on your soul which is to raise national consciousness, purely Greek consciousness, so as to take pride in being Greek and set free in your soul all the forces that will help you enhance the greatness of your homeland[...]. On with New Greece!"[20] Children's upbringing was not to be left to parents alone. The EON could replace them as it was designed to be a new, large family that embraced all the Greeks. Parents had to limit their "selfish" power over their children and accept that the state was more responsible for raising them.[21] In order to alleviate parents' objections, the regime propagandized to local parents' associations and associations of large size families.

After 1938, the regime's attitude towards youth hardened. Youth organizations that operated before the dictatorship such as the Boy Scouts were incorporated into the EON, and students were now required to participate in it. Schools also became totally subordinate to the organization. In order to secure total control over teachers who refused to conform to his regime, Metaxas himself took over the leadership of the Ministry of

---

18 Propaganda leaflet, *Oikogeneia* (Athens: EON 1940).
19 Ioannis Metaxas, *Logoi kai Skepseis*, vol. 2 (Athens: 1938), 165.
20 *Oi Arithmoi Omiloun dia to Ergon tis 4is Avgoustou* (Athens: 1939), 45.
21 See Metaxas's speech to parents, *Ypothikai tou Arkhigou. Kathikonta ton Goneon pros ta Paidia ton. I Skhesis ton Goneon pros tin Neolaian* (Athens: EON , 1939).

Education.[22] In mid-1938 enrollment to the EON became mandatory; a campaign began to enroll all school and university students, even by force if necessary. Gradually, representatives of the EON infiltrated many institutions and public services, exerting control over citizens. Government provisions to organization's members increased, mainly social welfare and employment.[23] In this way, participation in the organization became a symbol of loyalty to Metaxas's regime, necessary for government jobs and other benefits.

2. Authoritarian and Modernizing Trends in Health and Social Welfare

In early January 1937, five months after the dictatorship began, in yet another programmatic speech, Ioannis Metaxas proclaimed a grandiose plan for immediately funding the government's social policy. Apart from regular allocations, an extra sum of 500,000,000 drachmas would be channeled annually into hospital care, the protection of mothers and children, the settlement of refugee and generally into health and welfare institutions. Accompanied by regulations designed to change the way health care was organized, the plan materialized the declarations the dictator had issued in June 1936, when he served as appointed prime minister of a provisional government. In his speech delivered in January 1937, he outlined the main directions and the philosophy of the social policy he intended to follow. The reform of social policy on health took on great importance for the success of the New State.

Indeed, among the key objectives of his programme, Metaxas emphasized "the development or rather the establishment of Social Welfare in our country so as to alleviate the most destitute and unhappiest classes."[24] Linked with the "future and the hopes of the nation, it was natural that childhood drew the full attention and the affection of the governor."[25] This is why the

---

22 According to circular no. 92606/137 issued in 1938 by the Ministry of Education, enrolment into EON was obligatory for all students. The same went for orphanage residents as well as for working youngsters registered in the clubs of working boys and girls.
23 Ioannis Metaxas Archive, EON, file 9, General State Archives.
24 Anonymos, "I Koinoniki Pronoia," 241–53.
25 "I paidiki ilikia einai to avrio kai i elpis tou Ethnous, gi'afto sygkentronei ameristi tin prosochi mas kai tin agape mas." Anonymos, "I Koinoniki Pronoia," 242.

protection of childhood was part and parcel of this social reform. Part of the money allotted to the programme would be covered from state revenue, as the government recognized its duty towards the working-class, while the remaining money would come from indirect taxes imposed on citizens.

Metaxas supported the view that the wars, the economic crisis and the arrival of refugees increased poverty and made nation's gradual degeneration visible as reflected in high mortality rates. Social scourges, like malaria, tuberculosis, venereal diseases and trachoma, accounted for them. The fight against these diseases was a priority for the government's health policy. Also the decline in infant mortality constituted yet another challenge for the government as infant mortality rates were high in Greece in comparison with other European countries. For example, the death of 134 infants for every thousand live births in the early 1930s, when that number was decreasing in other European countries, made Greece appear inferior.[26]

Metaxas considered the fields of health and welfare as key to the success of his regime. He severely criticized the preceding liberal governments in Greece so as to gain popularity by exploiting a field suitable for demagogy, a practice usually employed by interwar fascist regimes. Propaganda leaflets declared that "the state of the 4th of August, which emerged in a juncture of appalling danger for our country, a danger of total destruction, and swept all the hurdles standing in the way of the people is the state which responds to the deepest needs of the people [...]."[27] In this context, social policy on health became an effective channel for the regime's ideological legitimization. It was the vehicle for the success of the New State, which promised to reorganize Greek society on more ethical foundations as opposed to the earlier liberal regime. Thus, the work that would be accomplished in the fields of health and welfare justified the necessity of the establishment of his regime.

The publicity of social welfare by the regime was most useful as it allowed Metaxas to claim that he had introduced a novelty. The regime's economic and social policy was far less radical than its leader purported it to

---

26 For the indices of infant mortality in various European countries between 1880 and 1935, see Vasilios Valaoras, *To Dimografikon Provlima tis Ellados kai I Epidrasis ton Prosfygon*, thesis (Athens, 1939). See also Hilary Marland, "The Medicalization of Motherhood: Doctors and Infant Welfare in the Netherlands, 1901–1930" in *Women and Children First. International Maternal and Infant Welfare, 1870–1945*, eds. Valerie Fildes, Lara Marks, and Hilary Marland (London and New York: Routledge, 1992), 74–96. In 1931–1935, the index was 45 deaths in a thousand live births in the case of Netherlands, 45, 78 and 62 in the cases of Norway, France, and England and Wales respectively.

27 *Oi Arithmoi Omiloun dia to Ergon tis 4is Avgoustou*, 52.

be. Despite the criticism Metaxas leveled against liberalism 'as facilitator of the capitalist economy,' the financial measures he had adopted were not sufficient to change the social conditions of the working-class, as the regime's advocates propagated. Its policy was rather oriented towards establishing peace between employers and employees and the wealthy, securing their financial interests. The obligatory arbitration between employees and employers, the establishment of collective bargaining, the eight-hour working day, and the establishment of minimum wages were not as radical as they might seem at first glance since the trade unions were put under the control of the state and in essence were abolished. Rises in wages were lower than the workers had demanded and the right to strike was gradually abolished.[28] Metaxas maintained that the establishment of the Social Security Foundation (IKA, Idryma Koinonikon Asfaliseon) which began in December 1937, was one of his accomplishments. Its creation though had been the work of the liberal governments, especially that of Eleftherios Venizelos, with the contribution of the International Bureau of Work.[29]

Agricultural workers were meant to play a vital role in regenerating the nation as guardians of the time-honored values of the Greek nation.[30] Therefore, the regime's agricultural policies included the regulation of the farmers' debts, support to stabilize agricultural prices and the allocation of land to local sharecroppers and refugees. However, the dictator proceeded to abolish farmers' unions.[31] Despite the importance of agriculture for Greece's self-sufficiency, the regime's meager support of farmers was not consistent with its rhetoric. Metaxas's goal of alleviating farmers from their debts was undermined by his policy on the Agricultural Bank and the delays in mechanizing farming. The loans granted to farmers by the agricultural bank were not aimed at helping land reclamation works, which would have made the fields more productive.[32] Support to farmers was limited at

28 Khatziiosif, "Koinovoulio kai Diktatoria," 37–123 and more specifically 117–19.

29 Liakos, *Ergasia kai Politiki stin Ellada tou Mesopolemou*, 538.

30 Metaxas's empathy with the farmers can be seen in the context of the return to the roots and Greek traditions. The Greeks living in the countryside were considered "the pure representatives of our race," "unaffected by the influences the urban population were exposed to." Ioannis Metaxas, *Logoi kai Skepseis* vol. 2 (Athens:1940), 241–47 quoted in Konstantinos Sarantis, "I Ideologia kai o Politikos Kharaktiras tou Kathestotos Metaxa," in *O Metaxas kai I Epokhi*, ed. Thanos Veremis (Athens: Evrasia, 2009), 57.

31 Katerina Bregianni, "I Politiki ton Psevdaisthiseon: Kataskeves kai Mythoi tis Metaxikis Diktatorias," *Ta Istorika* 16, no. 30 (June 1999): 186.

32 Khristos Evelpidis, *To Agrotiko mas Provlima* (Athens: 1944).

the level of rhetoric in that it supported the public image of the leader as the "first farmer." In 1938, 83% of white-collar clerks and their families were below the poverty line.[33] The average income of farmers did not increase, nor was it enough to survive on. The average annual income of Greeks was $61, while in Belgium it was $309 and in France $389.[34] Considering this, it is understandable why the diet of Greeks during the interwar period was insufficient and why the rates of mortality due to diseases connected to poor diet were so high.

Metaxas's social and financial policy, especially during the first two years, was ambiguous and controversial. His rhetoric underlined society's duty to the destitute and the weak. Nevertheless, indirect taxation of the working-class was diametrically opposed to the regime's commitments to social justice. In order to fund its social policy, the regime imposed taxes on agricultural products, profits from shipping, tobacco consumption, lotteries, public entertainment and gambling, given that any rise in the taxation of the upper class would have been risky for the regime. As a solution, Metaxas sought to increase indirect taxes and better management of the state. Social injustice increased and public services were reorganized, but only people who were affiliated with the regime were appointed. In other words, centralization and authoritarianism were reinforced. Although the social policy adopted was presented as "national reform," it had some continuity with the pre-dictatorship regime. Some scholars underline the modernizing character of the social policies. However, many had been actually planned by previous governments, but had not materialized due to political changes.[35]

3. Social Policy on Health: Priorities and Limitations

As infant mortality and the spread of contagious diseases (tuberculosis, malaria, trachoma and venereal diseases) purportedly accounted for the high mortality rates, the emphasis of the regime's health policy was placed on campaigns that would curb these diseases systematically. Rationalization, state control, new institutions, and the reorganization of the scientific lead-

---

33 Kostas Vergopoulos, "I Elliniki Oikonomia apo to 1926 os to 1935," in *Istoria tou Ellinikou Ethnous*, vol. 15 (Athens: Ekdotiki Athinon, 1976), 340.

34 Georgios Trimis, *Ai Diekdikiseis ton Ergasomenon* (Athens: 1948), 15.

35 Khatziiosif, "Koinovoulio kai Diktatoria," 119. Panagiotis Vatikiotis, *Mia Politiki Viografia tou Ioanni Metaxa. Filolaiki Apolytarkhia stin Ellada, 1936–1941* (Athens: Evrasia, 2005), 309–12.

ership that coordinated these campaigns were the first steps taken by the government to implement this new health policy. The appointment of the banker Alexandros Koryzis to lead the Ministry of State Hygiene and Relief guaranteed the rationalization of health spending. The regime also attempted to change how hospitals operated by drawing up a series of laws. The regime thus secured the state's closer control of public life at large and public health in particular by appointing Metaxas's supporters in hospital administrations.

3.1 Changes in the Legal and Organizational Framework of Hygiene Institutions

The establishment of hospitals, sanatoriums, childcare centers and polyclinics in Athens and in a number of provincial towns, and the improvement of hospitals already in operation, can be placed in the context of these changes. State allotments for health care increased beginning in 1936.[36] The appointment of higher officials in the administration of health and welfare institutions aimed both at the reorganization of public health and the efficient financial management of health institutions.

One of the steps Koryzis took was to issue a law for the reorganization of health and hygiene institutions. The attempt to catalog all public and private health organizations and institutions across the country, their work, the members of their administrative boards, their movable and landed property, and their resources was also inscribed in the same context. Police colonels were assigned the task of supervising this venture. In addition, various professional unions were called to provide evidence of their support of the regime by donating some of their profits to the State Revenue Office, which would then go to funding welfare.

The government's work on health and welfare featured prominently in the regime's special propaganda publications with rich photographical material as well as in lectures and special magazine issues. Among these publications the ones on children's health and welfare repeatedly highlighted Metaxas's commitment to children by describing the works the regime ini-

---

36 See Koryzis Archive, Budget of the Ministry of State Hygiene, file 21, The Benaki Mouseum's Historical Archives.

.

tiated and by featuring hundreds of pictures of happy children's faces. Child welfare, health exhibitions and the capital's hygienic reorganization aimed at spreading new modern ways of hygienic living. In 1938, the Ministry of State Hygiene and Relief organized a health exhibition for the first time. The exhibition highlighted the achievements of health services and demonstrated the regime's general attitude towards health. The exhibition presented a model flat with modern amenities and a modern means of hygienic living for middle class families. The following year, the Ministry of State Hygiene and Relief organized in collaboration with the German Ministry of Propaganda the exhibition "Pleasure and Work" which put forward the organizational models Nazism applied to everyday life.

Not only did the regime publicize its achievements in welfare but it also wished to change the regulatory framework of the administration of welfare organizations. In early 1937, a committee for the creation of a unified organization of social welfare was established. As can be inferred by Koryzis's correspondence with Greek welfare experts, a new law "on the organization of public welfare" was to be passed. The draft law criticized the lack of state control over state-funded organizations. Yet, the draft law was disapproved.[37] The memos circulated between jurists, high-ranking state functionaries, institution directors and the president of the Pan-Hellenic Medical Association clearly indicate that there was no unanimity of opinion among them on a series of issues, such as the legal entity of the unified organization of social welfare, the duties of municipalities and voluntary organizations, their resources and even the meanings of the terms "social welfare" and "public relief." The employment status of the doctors and civil servants who would work together with this organization was another source of disagreement. The abandonment of the plan to create such a central state organization, clearly demonstrates that the line between state interventionism and private initiative in medical care was not clearly demarcated in the minds of policy makers.

Health care for the destitute was one of the most common subjects Metaxas's regime focused on since there was much room to criticize previous regimes and to gain public approval. A committee of experts had discussed the issue well before 1936 and as attempts were made to secure finan-

---

37 Alexandros Koryzis Archive, file 16.

cial resources for it. In October 1938, the government issued a decree that recognized the state's obligation to provide care to the needy, defined poverty and the means of proving it and provided free medical care to the destitute.[38] However, it was stressed that this could not be implemented until the government's programme for creating new health institutions had been completed. Due to limited resources it was impossible to provide free treatment to all destitute citizens. It would only be possible to provide for those who met the criteria of being Greek citizens, absolutely destitute,[39] ill and without social security. Poverty was categorized into regular and irregular. Both categories of destitute people could be offered health care either free or for a minimum fee. In order to establish citizens' finances a permanent committee of three members—the priest of the parish, a doctor and a local teacher—was formed in each parish.

3.2 Organizing the Campaigns Against Contagious Diseases

The regime attached great importance to the fight against diseases that were accountable for high mortality rates. The organization of the anti-tuberculosis, anti-malaria and anti-trakhoma campaigns took place between 1937 and 1938. It was the first time a venture of such an extent was undertaken in Greece. The organization of the fight against these three killers underlined the regime's resolve to start afresh, utilizing modern scientific knowledge and the state infrastructure. The main axes of the regime's welfare and health policies were the formation of special committees for the study of these contagious diseases, the nation-wide campaign against them and the establishment of new state services for the materialization of the proposals put forward by the committees.

As there were many children among the trakhoma and TB victims, these special committees discussed the means of counteracting disease. This discussion is of great interest for the purposes of our study as it offers profound insights into the correlation of power between the bureaucrats and scientists. It also reveals the simmering rivalries between doctors from different insti-

---

38 Diatagma "Peri tis Ennoias tis Aporias kai tou Tropou Apodeixeos Aftis pros ton Skopon Apolafseos Dorean i epi Ilattomeno Antitimo Iatrikis Voitheias," *Efimeris tis Kiverniseos*, A', no. 370, (October 13, 1938): 2449–52.
39 Those unable to meet the medical costs were defined as destitute.

tutions or specialties who had different priorities. The amount of funding required and the prioritization of needs were disputed as both bureaucrats and scientists claimed the largest share for themselves. The discussion also highlighted the need to establish a central agency to administrate responsibilities among the various state services, voluntary organizations and the state.

3.2.1 The Anti-malaria Campaign

Malariologist Grigorios Livadas, a graduate from Johns Hopkins University and director of the School of Hygiene, was in charge of the anti-malaria campaign committee. He suggested that a united coordination agency be created with administrative and scientific responsibilities based in the Ministry of State Hygiene and Relief.[40] High-ranking state functionaries and professors from the department of malariology at the School of Hygiene would act as counselors in the campaign.[41] In order to run the campaign with experts, malariologists and sanitary inspectors would be hired to strengthen the School of Hygiene.

The anti-malaria campaign committee knew that due to the scale of the malaria in Greece extensive field research would be required and a network of regional services and their reference back to the central service would need to be established. Each prefecture was to set up its own Hygienic Center as part of the anti-malaria campaign. The army and the school would cooperate with local health services to educate the public and drain swamplands.

In the spring of 1937, the Ministry of Education sent to schools material prepared by the School Hygiene Service. Circulars that drew attention to the national threat malaria posed to the Greek race urged primary and secondary school teachers to undertake not only instruction in the fight against malaria but also assisted by their students to carry out small scale water drainage of agricultural soils.[42]

---

40 "Praktika Epitropis Anthelonosiakou Agonos," *Arkheia Ygeinis*, no. 5 (May 1939): 197.

41 The contribution of Livadas who had apprenticed to the malariologists of the Rockefeller committee and studied on a Rockefeller scholarship in Baltimore must have played an important role in fostering a spirit of cooperation between the Ministry and the School of Hygiene. A few years back, the two sides had clashed; as a result, the attempt of the experts of the international organizations was abandoned.

42 See circular May 6, 1937 by the Minister of Education under the title: "O ek tis Elonosias Ethnikos Kindynos. To Ethnosotirion Salpisma tou k. Ypourgou tis Paideias pros tous Ekpaideftikous Leitourgous tis Mesis kai tis Dimotikis Ekpaidefseos," *Skholiki Ygieini*, no. 7 (May 1937): 3–4.

Given the scale of the disease and the high cost, the committee decided to first limit its efforts to certain areas of Greece rather than the entire country, following the example set by the Rockefeller Foundation.

3.2.2 The Anti-TB Campaign: Prevention or Treatment?

In September 1937, the Ministry of State Hygiene and Relief formed a committee for the organization of the anti-TB campaign. Ioannis Papakostas, a professor of social hygiene at the School of Hygiene in Athens who had studied TB, was responsible for submitting a report on the organization of the fight against TB. In this report he argued that targeting factors that contributed to the disease, like living conditions, personal hygiene, and sanitation, would be more efficient than fighting the disease itself.[43] Diet, he claimed, played the most important role and not housing, contrary to what had been claimed earlier. The poor diet of Greeks, the prevalence of infectious diseases—typhus, scarlet fever, measles, and malaria—and ignorance of hygiene due to poor education, were held accountable for the spread of TB. With an average mortality rate of 15.6 for every 10,000 people, Greece was among the countries with high tuberculosis rates. Yet, in the prefectures of Athens, Drama, Thessaloniki and Kavala, which had received a great number of refugees, the respective rates were between 23 and 28 per 10,000. These numbers were even higher, Papakostas claimed, for two reasons: many deaths went unregistered and medical statistics were still incomplete. Towns had triple or quadruple rates of deaths than rural areas; around 25% of deaths in towns were due to TB. The most affected age group was 20–24-year-olds, followed by 15–19-year-olds and 25–29-year-olds. TB was most prevalent among hotel and restaurant employees, typographers, shop-assistants, tailors and barbers.[44]

Despite the problem of high mortality, the anti-TB campaign was unsystematic and inefficient. Disease prevention was minimal and the few attempts that had begun after the 1929 reform were abandoned in the meantime for being too costly. According to Papakostas, the anti-TB campaign should include infirmaries for confinement and treatment of carriers, insti-

---

43 "Organosis Antiphymatikou Agonos," *Arkheia Ygeiinis*, no. 9 (December 1937): 333–84.

44 "Praktika Epitropis Antiphymatikou AgonosMetra Profylaxeos tis Mathitikis Ilikias apo tis Phymatioseos," *Arkheia Ygeiinis*, no. 1 (January 1939): 15.

tutions for meta-sanatorium care, prevantoria and anti-TB clinics. The number of beds required should increase from the available 3,385 to 8,500.

Papakostas laid great emphasis upon the protection of children because of the wide spread of the bacillus among them. He suggested 60–70 prevantoria of 1,500 beds be built for children who had curable types of TB. Children would spend 4–6 months in these prevantoria as if they lived in a boarding school under special conditions i.e., a special diet, ventilation, rest and open-air education.[45] Their stay at countryside institutions would strengthen and immunize their bodies. With the establishment of the prevantoria, Papakostas predicted that 90% of the cases would be cured and many resources would be saved.

Papakostas's proposal for the protection of childhood was received with reservations by the doctors who were involved in the anti-TB campaign. They argued that the proposed measure was of marginal importance in a country like Greece, which was unable to treat all of its sick people.[46] As N. Economopoulos, a TB specialist and doctor at the sanatorium Sotiria, argued the removal of all children that lived in a tubercular environment and their admission to prevantoria would be both costly and unsuccessful. The predicted number of children that might succumb to the disease was in the hundreds of thousands. Hospitalizing them would devastate the budget of the Ministry of State Hygiene and Relief. Despite the positive assurance of Papakostas that the cost of beds for prevantoria was lower than for sanatoria, most TB specialists favored building sanatoria.

Doctors who criticized Papakostas' proposal voiced reservations about how children should be selected for treatment, given that the carriers of the bacillus could also be children in healthy environments who were more difficult to detect. Despite their claims that the protection of children was of the utmost importance, doctors were divided in their support for "prevention or treatment," which actually meant targeting adults or children. Another group of doctors working in the sanatoria raised objections for financial reasons. They expressed fears that the funds allotted to prevantoria might be taken out of the sanatoria budgets. Hygienists at the School of Hy-

---

45 The latter would be based on the cooperation of doctors and female teachers who would also hold a diploma of a visiting nurse.

46 "Praktika tou Anotatou Ygeionomikou Symvouliou epi tis Organoseos tou Antiphymatikou Agonos en Elladi," *Arkheia Ygeiinis*, no. 4 (April 1939): 143–9.

giene also had different interests than doctors working in the sanatoria. The inter-professional rivalry between them prevented unanimity.

Invoking fears of state bankruptcy, the members of the committee for the organization of the anti-TB campaign expressed their reservations about the possibility of setting up a large number of prevantoria. Instead, the committee chose to increase the number of beds in hospitals-sanatoria to 9,000, since they considered these institutions the most suitable for accommodating a large number of tubercular patients. The majority of the committee's members favored treatment over prevention. In their final proposals the committee wanted to increase the number of children's summer camps and combine them with the prevantoria. Following the proposal of Kharitakis, director at the department of Social Hygiene, pediatrician and member of the Patriotic Foundation of Social Protection and Relief (PFSPR), a financially viable compromise was adopted: to use the children's summer camps for tubercular children during the nine months when the summer camps did not normally operate. In 1938, the summer camps in Penteli and Voula were used as prevantoria. The foundation stone for a children's TB sanatorium in Penteli was laid in October 1940 with a capacity of 200 children.

The committee also adopted the proposals of Dimitris Stefanou, who was in charge of the School Hygiene at the Ministry of Education. His proposals were to improve student and teacher health through more hygienic buildings, open-air teaching for 6–9 months, adjusting the school curricula to avoid mental exhaustion, and providing meals to students. He also wanted to subject all teachers periodically to TB-reaction checks and X-ray examination in polyclinics.[47]

The committee was concerned with the issue of diet and its relation to TB. Once more the poor Greek diet was condemned and a proposal was put forward to study foods that were "useful for feeding the common people" and to exempt them from taxation. A proposal that had been earlier formulated by N. Economopoulos, a TB specialist at the Sotiria sanatorium. The committee finally decided to reduce the prices of foods that "common people are in need of" such as milk and its byproducts, salted preserves, fats and oil, and to sell meat at different prices than entrails.[48] The committee

---

47 "Praktika Epitropis Antiphymatikou Agonos," 15.
48 "Praktika tou Anotatou Ygeionomikou Symvouliou epi tis Organoseos tou Antiphymatikou Agonos en Elladi," *Arkheia Ygeinis,* no. 3 (March 1939): 95.

also suggested that the destitute be entitled to all kinds of medical care, obstetrics and medicines either free of charge or for a reduced fee, and that the means of establishing poverty be determined. The committee also suggested TB-towns be set up under the aegis of the state and the fees of the TB-specialists serving at anti-TB clinics be decided on, following the model medical center that the Rockefeller Foundation had set up in Ampelokipoi. The committee also called for the rational use of funds in hospitals and sanatoria in various districts. Yet, the committee's proposal to teach the subject of TB subject as a compulsory course in medical school was not welcomed as pathologists raised objections. It seems that the separation of TB from medicine at large was still met with resistance.

3.2.3 The Fight Against Trachoma: The Establishment of Special Anti-trachoma Schools

Athanasios Economopoulos, the officer of the anti-trachoma service at the Ministry of State Hygiene and Relief who was in charge of the committee for the study of the anti-trachoma campaign, stressed that the scale of trachoma infection in Greece had reached such proportions that the country was "trachoma-ridden." The eight special clinics that had operated in the previous few years were not enough to counter the problem, particularly in Athens and Piraeus.[49] Economopoulos attributed the geographical spread of the disease to the migration of laborers and illiteracy. Trachoma was "the scourge of the weakest, poorest and most ignorant classes."[50] Based on studies that had been conducted in other countries, Economopoulos proposed a central institution be set up to look into the sources of infection, locate where trachoma was concentrated, educate the hygienists and teachers who would fight the disease, spread knowledge about trachoma through posters and films, and increase the budget of the anti-trachoma campaign.

Although the studies used by Economopoulos pointed out that the infection of children occurred mostly outside schools through the family of

---

49 "Praktika Epitropis Antitrakhomatikou Agonos," in Alexandros Koryzis Archive, The Benaki Mouseum's Historical Archives, file 26. It is mentioned that three anti-trachoma clinics had been set up in 1928, three more in 1930 in Athens and Piraeus while in 1936 two more were added. For the organization of the campaign 1,400,000 drachmae were allotted.

50 "Meleti epi ton Provlimaton tou Trakhomatos ypo Athanasiou Oikonomopoulou," in Alexandros Koryzis Archive, The Benaki Mouseum's Historical Archives, file 23, 24, 25 and 26.

infants and pre-school children, the committee stressed fighting trachoma in schools. Ten years after Lambadarios's *Diagramma Katapolemiseos tou Trakhomatos eis ta Skholeia* (Plan for the Fight against Trachoma at Schools) was published in 1927,[51] the establishment of student anti-trachoma clinics on school premises that would operate even during the summer holiday was seen by the members of the committee as a solution. In these clinics, school doctors or private doctors who were specially trained in trachoma treated students, while the latter's supervision was assigned to trained teachers who received a bonus for this service. The students were treated during morning classes, while in the afternoon locals would come to the schools to be treated. Special trachoma schools were built if the number of students was too high. Instead of setting up a central anti-trachoma institution, the committee built four anti-trachoma clinics (Athens, the Peloponnese, Thrace, Thessaloniki) where clinic staff and teachers were taught. The members of the committee for the study of trachoma suggested an orphanage be built for children suffering from trachoma similar to one in Cracow,[52] the assigned duties of the visiting nurse be increased, and makeshift clinics be set up to provide medical care to agricultural workers.

Anti-trachoma schools grew quickly in number. According to sources from the Ministry of Education, in 1938 there were thirty five anti-trachoma student clinics and thirty-six anti-trachoma schools in Attica, which were supported by the Ministry of State Hygiene and Relief and the Patriotic Foundation. 7,413 students attended these schools and more schools were scheduled to be built for the following year.[53] Three eye-specialist officers supervised the whole venture. The officers who were responsible for a district's schools examined all primary school students at the beginning of the school year and chose which students would undergo treatment. For each student they filled in a specially designated card with the type of trachoma, its development and the names of other family members in case they were also affected.[54] According to Theodoros Ioannidis, an eye-specialist in these schools, a well-supplied anti-trachoma station operated next to the classroom where the students were treated after class. A nurse and a doctor,

---

51   Emmanouil Lambadarios, *Diagramma Katapolemiseos tou Trakhomatos eis ta Skholeia.* (Athens: 1927).
52   In 1939 the Sikiaridio anti-trahoma orphanage was set up in Psykhikon, Athens.
53   *4th of August. O Apologismos mias Dietias, 1936–1938* (Athens:1938): 88.
54   Theodoros Ioannidis, "Skholeio dia Trakhomatika Paidia," *To Paidi,* no. 62 (January 1940):6.

trained for a three-month period in the treatment of trachoma in a certified ophthalmological clinic, staffed the anti-trachoma station.

In the late 1930s doctors were convinced that anti-trachoma schools were the most innovative step in the fight against the disease. Treatment was daily and compulsory for the students who had been diagnosed with trachoma. Doctors were certain that students who graduated from an anti-trachoma primary school would be cured, and that it was possible to help the students' sick families as well. Although treatment was carried out at the school premises, eye-specialists involved in this venture also tried to prevent students' families from contracting trachoma. In a study on both healthy students and students with trachoma in the Mesogia villages in Attica, Ioannnidis concluded that schools were not responsible for the infection, rather, it was the students' families as 85–90% of the students suffering from trachoma came from families who were already infected. Workers and farmers of Attica for whom the disease was considered a scourge as it rendered them unable for work attracted the interest of doctors. Most students in the first grade of primary school had already contracted the disease from a family member. In 1940 there were forty anti-trachoma schools operating in Attica alone: 16 in Athens, 10 in Piraeus and 14 in Mesogia. An average of 9.5% of students in the Mesogia villages were infected in 1940. Despite the state's continuous attempts since the 1920s to fight trachoma, the disease among students still persisted.

3.2.4 Zones of High Morbidity and Prenuptial Health Certification

As was mentioned in a previous chapter, in the 1920s and early 1930s the discussion between doctors, jurists and social thinkers about the imposition of the prenuptial health certification on prospective couples did not result in the adoption of legal measures. In 1937, the regime attempted to raise again the issue of negative eugenic measures with regard to trachoma and syphilis, which reveals the scale of worries caused by the spread of these diseases, especially among the peasantry and the young. Doctors protested that rural people did not understand the importance of cleanliness and never came to the clinics. Creating a register of people with trachoma and syphilis and forcing them to undergo treatment was a recurring concern of doctors for years-on-end. Emergency law no. 651/1937 attempted to bring a change in rural people's negative attitude towards the medical authority. In the law's preamble "on the fight against trachoma and hereditary syphilis," the legislator referred to provinces with infection rates as high as 60% where inhabitants did not visit the clinics. The new law dictated that state, municipal or village clinics had to be established for the fight against trachoma or syphilis; inhabitants from neighboring to the clinics areas would come there for treatment.[55] As a result, geographical zones which were considered dangerous for the spread of the diseases were demarcated and put under surveillance.

These clinics could be turned into vehicles of social control. Whoever did not wish to attend the clinic or children whose parents refused to take them to the clinic had to be entered into an inventory, provided they presented a medical certificate issued by the head of the clinic so as to verify that they had been treated by a private doctor. They also had to attend the clinic regularly to certify that they were continually being treated. If they refused to, the police took them to the clinic by force. People who refused to be treated had to pay a fine.

The law was the first attempt to penalize citizens' behavior on health issues. It was also an attempt to implement prenuptial health certification, which had garnered so much discussion among doctors, politicians and social thinkers in the previous decade. The importance of the prenuptial health certificate for the protection of mothers and children had been highlighted during the two Balkan congresses in 1936 and 1938. In 1934 and 1936 similar laws banning the marriage of those suffering from syphilis had been enacted in Yugoslavia and Turkey.

The emergency law meant that doctors in state or municipal anti-trachoma and anti-syphilis clinics in "dangerous areas" became regulators of birth control, since it was up to them who received marriage permits or not.[56] The ban reflected a spatial approach to the issue, in that areas with high rates of syphilis and trachoma sufferers were put under a special vigilance. According to the law, the Minister of State Hygiene and Relief re-

---

55 Anagkastikos Nomos no. 651, "Peri Katapolemiseos tou Trakhomatos kai Klironomikis Syphilidos," *Efimeris tis Kiverniseos*, A', no. 154. (April 27, 1937): 1005–6. See also the preamble "Peri Katapolemiseos tou Trakhomatos kai Klironomikis Syphilidos."

56 Trachoma was the second disease after leprosy that prevented people from receiving marriage licenses. In 1920, law no. 2450 "on the measures for the curtailment of leprosy," banned marriage between lepers or between a healthy person and a leper.

served the right to force would be-couples, whether they came from areas where trachoma and syphilis were endemic or were just supposed to marry in them, to produce a recent health certificate by the head of the clinic certifying that they did not suffer from any of these diseases. If the prospective couple failed to produce the health certificate, the marriage permit was not issued. Doctors who issued fake health certificates were penalized. Family registers that accumulated data on these two diseases were also to be set up in the clinics of these areas.

CHAPTER IX

THE POLITICAL USE OF MOTHERHOOD AND CHILDHOOD WELFARE

Mothers and children were at the center of the regime's national regeneration attempt since these two groups were thought to be linked not only with the nation's biological but also with its historical continuity. This is evident in the dictator's repeated claims that the New State was the protector of youth. If the policy on families in other European countries was linked with racial regeneration and territorial expansion, in the Greek case care for the protection of mothers and children alluded to the country's cultural traditions. In the regime's rhetoric, printed in thousands of various leaflets from the Ministry of the Press and Propaganda, improvement in the quality of human capital would protect Greece's historic culture. The attempts of the government to create a robust youth were inscribed in the long-standing tradition of the Great Idea, which dated back to the nineteenth century and generally based the superiority of the Greek race on its culture and the long-standing Greek history.[1]

Seen in the frame of cultural nationalism, the regime attempted to engage parents in its ambitious plans, attempting to instill in them responsibility for future generations as the nation's continuity was contingent on the good health of their children. In a simile of Greece's history, parents were likened to athletes in a relay race. Parents had to hand over the baton to a strong, younger generation that would continue the Greek race. It was stressed that if the necessary provisions were not made at the beginning of a child's life, the effects would be devastating, both for the children them-

---

1   Turda, *Modernism and Eugenics*, 103.

selves and for the future of the nation. Metaxas himself stated that "nations without a strong youth are powerless."[2]

The welfare works intended for mothers and children were presented in the regime's propaganda as a guarantee of the country's cultural superiority and as proof of Metaxas's affection for the youth. The "children's joy" was one of the many concerns of the "National Government." These upheavals, apart from enhancing the dictator's paternal image, were part of a national plan for the country's cultural elevation. The works targeted children and working-class families to improve the regime's image. Soup kitchens, nurseries and summer camps were innovative practices that took children away from the family, providing them a sense of belonging to a new group with new obligations. Apart from the EON's indoctrination of children, the welfare works helped internalize the regime's values in children and cemented their bond to Metaxas. "Born and bred of the new state," children grew up in better conditions and enjoyed good health and were therefore able to serve their country as future soldiers and citizens.

Although the relationship between welfare and the improvement of the "biological capital" was far from new, the regime's "nationalization" of welfare gave new meaning to the earlier practices adopted by liberal interwar ministers. The proliferation of welfare works for children was undoubtedly a source of good publicity for the regime as these works made it appear more child-centered and affectionate compared to previous governments.

As can be gleaned from the regime's leaflets, the emphasis on the young, at least during the first two years of the regime, can be explained by its modernizing, political and cultural priorities. It seems that Metaxas's absolute dominance after 1938 and the intensification of war preparation have made possible more biology-centered views on the relation between children and the race. As the war was approaching, references in the propaganda press to the cultural dimension of the welfare works became less frequent, while references to racial purity and the youth's duty to the motherland became more frequent. This tendency towards this racialized view of the child is evident in the changes in the way child welfare institutions were organized and in who staffed them. The publicity given to health care and welfare jus-

---

2   See Deftera Diaskepsis Perifereiakon Dioikiton kai Dioikitrion Ethinikis Organoseos Neolaias (May 19–26, 1940), *Praktika* vol. 1 (Athens: EON, no. 72, 1940): 246.

tified Metaxas's demand for children and adolescents to make sacrifices for the nation. As the likelihood of war increased, so did the need for children to be prepared to sacrifice themselves. Parents had to accept this sacrifice, to understand that "children do not belong to them but first and foremost to the state." One of the regime's theoreticians noted that "the children of the Greeks belong to Greece [...]. Parents take pride in their children only when the latter are able to respond to the needs of the society, the nation, the homeland."[3]

1. "CHILDHOOD IS THE FOUNDATION OF THE NATION'S FUTURE": WELFARE FOR STUDENTS

The policy on the protection of mothers and children can be distinguished into two parts: protection for mothers and infants, and protection for school age children. In the latter case, the regime tried to make children robust through sports, school meals, summer camps, children's sanatoria, and trachoma schools. It seems that these works, especially those for sick children, absorbed the majority of funds allotted for social welfare.

1.1 The "Policy of Joy": The Regeneration of the Youth

According to the publications of the Subministry of Press and Tourism, sports were the best means of recreation and the most important factor in promoting the health of the young. The New State initiated the "policy of joy." The New State, realizing that "edification was necessary for the Greek people so as to abandon their fatalistic attitude to life" put emphasis on recreation, particularly exercise and games.[4] Setting up recreation grounds in many neighborhoods evidenced the paternal care of the government. Sports were supposed to be the link between modern youth and the values of ancient Greece. Metaxas stressed that robust bodies played a crucial role in the preservation of the ancient Greek traditions. As descendants of the ancient Greeks, modern Greeks should follow the example of the ancient Spartan

---

3   Panagiotis D. Iliadis, "I Paidiki Egklimatikotis kai ai Prospatheiai tou Neou Kratous," *To Neon Kratos* 4, no. 29 (January 31, 1940): 305.

4   Neoellin, "I KHARA apotelei simera tin Vasin tis Ethnikis Diapaidagogiseos ton Neon," *To Paidi*, no. 70 (September 1940): 1–3.

model to improve their physique. Schools and the EON emphasized physical exercise and sports. Physical education was upgraded to be a major subject in school curriculum, school gyms were established and funding provided for sports equipment, and the School of Physical Education was also upgraded in that graduates could become sport instructors in the EON.

Physical exercise was meant to build strong constitutions that the state needed for the coming war and the necessary increase in the country's productivity. Physical exercise and pleasure were linked with the regeneration of the youth. The following passage from a volume on the regime's fourth anniversary reveals how the state imagined physical exercise would create a new man:

> The state says: me, the state, I will make you strong with all the means Science recognizes: physical exercise, trips, games, discipline and habitation to work analogous to your age. But you'll exercise in a pleasant way, since pleasure makes a man love working. A sulky man tends to be lazy and he is unable to work profitably and productively while the state is in need of citizens working willingly and intensively with no exception whatsoever.[5]

If physical exercise was an important issue for other countries, in Greece, because of national traditions, it was presented as a pressing need. As descendants of the ancient Greeks, the young had to exercise to become robust and strong not for the purpose of conquering other countries, but to pay tribute to their noble Greek origin. The "genuinely Greek spirit of sports" was one of the principles of the EON "according to our Olympics tradition."[6] In its attempt to create Greek culture, the government could not overlook the development of physical education and the organization of athletic contests. "Greece as the mother of the Olympic Games and as the birthplace of the balanced development of the mind and the body"[7] had to do both. The appointment of physical education teachers, the establishment of municipal and school gyms, the support of all kinds of athletic unions and the organization of school athletic events, all evidence the care the government took for its students and their physical exercise.

---

5   *Oi Arithmoi Omiloun dia to Ergon tis 4is Avgoustou*, n.p.

6   September 13, 1937, n.p.

7   In the propaganda album *Oi Arithmoi Omiloun dia to Ergon tis 4is Avgoustou* many pictures of young people who exercise can be seen; captions of these pictures stressed the connection of the ancient Greek spirit with the care provided by Metaxas's government.

1.2 School Hygiene: Continuities and Discontinuities

Apart from certain measures in the fight against malnutrition and trachoma, important changes in the supervision of student health were not recorded during the first three years of the regime. However, in June 1939,
two laws were enacted that were presented as "a landmark in hygiene and
education."[8] The reorganization of the School Hygiene Service and student
meals were publicized by the regime as part of the new direction the medical supervision of children took during Metaxas's personal leadership of the
Ministry of Education.

As was the case with other social policy institutions, the reorganization
of the School Hygiene meant closer control, a more centralized structure
and the appointment of members loyal to the regime in key posts. The preamble of the emergency law "on the organization of the School Hygiene Service" highlighted the regime's attempt to bring changes.[9] It criticized the
way the service had operated for twenty five years with all of its insufficiencies and irregularities. Its poor functioning made school doctors unable to
perform their main task, lowering student morbidity. The preamble further
stated that parents were not only illiterate but also very poor and it further
contributed to the poor condition of student health.

Establishing Student Welfare Centers and hiring suitable staff to treat
students were publicized as the most important novelties of the law.[10] The
law stipulated the appointment of 117 school doctors in order to have one
school doctor for every 10,000 students, although it was known that twice
that number would be needed to reach the ideal ratio. These school doctors
were hired following a public contract and four months of training. Their
wages were satisfactory, but they would not have the right to work privately
on the side, as had been the case up until then. The director of the School
Hygiene Service would have increased disciplinary responsibilities. The law
also called for only eight female school doctors who would serve in towns

8   Anonymos, "Ta Pepragmena apo tis 4is Avgoustou kai Entefthen. Diefthynsis Skholikis Ygieinis," and
    "I Nomothesia peri Skholiatrikis Ypiresias. Aitiologiki Ekthesis epi tou Skhediou Anagkastikou Nomou
    'Peri Organoseos tis Skholiatrikis Ypiresias'," Skholiki Ygieini, no. 31 (September 1939): 13.

9   Anagkastikos Nomos no. 1805 "Peri Anadiorganoseos tis Skholiatrikis Ypiresias," Efimeris tis Kiverniseos,
    A', no. 252 (June 20, 1939), 1639–46.

10 Anonymos, "Ta pepragmena apo tis 4is Avgoustou kai Entefthen. Diefthynsis Skholikis Ygieinis," and
    "I Nomothesia peri Skholiatrikis Ypiresias. Aitiologiki Ekthesis epi tou Skhediou Anagkastikou Nomou
    'Peri Organoseos tis Skholiatrikis Ypiresias'," Skholiki Ygieini, no. 31 (September 1939): 13–41.

where there were female secondary schools. Female school doctors could not be promoted to medical officers.

It was expected that the establishment of student welfare centers in the capitals of the counties would serve not only the detection of the sick but most importantly their treatment. Student Centers in Athens and Thessaloniki, would be staffed with a full range of experts: a director, school doctor, dentist, otolaryngologist, eye specialist, X-ray specialist, specialist in therapeutic gymnastics, psychiatrist and two more doctors, one responsible for career counselling and the other for the organization of hygiene propaganda. Ancillary staff included four school nurses, graduates from the School of Visiting Nurses. The rest of the student clinics would operate under the supervision of school doctors in cooperation with the polyclinics that would be established by the Ministry of State Hygiene and Relief in the capitals of the counties.[11]

The board of School Hygiene was another novelty.[12] Its job as a coordinating body was that it submitted proposals to the ministry, drew up regulations for student welfare centers and supervised the school hygiene services. The board was made up of Metaxas's advisors, the professor of Paedology and School Hygiene at the University of Athens, the director of School Hygiene, the director of Social Hygiene at the Ministry of State Hygiene and Relief, the general inspector of the School Hygiene Service. Emmanouil Lambadarios, Dimitrios Stefanou, Kostis Kharitakis and Khristos Georgakopoulos sat on the first board. During its first session in July 1939, the members of the board expressed their satisfaction with the serious attempt the national government had made in protecting student health by providing the School Hygiene Service with staff and funding.

In order to fund the school hygiene institutions, students had to make a compulsory annual contribution.[13] Only poor students could be exempted on the suggestion of the respective school board, but this could not be more than 20% of the students in each class. In the student welfare centers, school doctors were required to provide medical care to EON members, providing they had a certificate of penury. On his speech to the newly appointed school

11 "Peri Organoseos tis Skoliatrikis Ypiresias," 19–33.
12 Anonymos, "Symvoulion Skholikis Ygieinis," Skholiki Ygieini, no. 31 (September 1939): 10–13.
13 Primary and secondary school students had to pay each year 10 and 30 drachmas respectively in order to get registered.

doctors in March 1940, Metaxas prompted them to employ the 1,000,000 child members of EON as assistants, since in the ranks of EON the "pioneers" (skapaneis) were trained in first-aid and hygiene.

Metaxas's views on the protection of children's health in a totalitarian regime can be extracted in this speech, as he elaborated on how he expected the Student Welfare Centers to contribute to the regeneration of the Greek race. He estimated that their effects would become visible after fifteen to twenty years. He presented children as the part of society that had suffered the most due to poor living conditions, wars and all the causes that had led the race to degeneration over the last thirty years. The fight against child malnutrition, TB, malaria and trakhoma would pay off in the future through better war preparation. It would also raise the country's productivity. It is clear that Metaxas perceived the reorganization of the School Hygiene Service as an investment in the future of the Greek race and the productive value of the population "so as to make our people stronger, men and women with better build, better mental health and therefore women and men with better results and higher performance."[14] The political benefit derived from similar ventures was obvious since it was expected that they would undermine communist discourse. Thus, permanent school hygiene institutions were expected to form "an irresistible weapon against all the subversive powers, a means to consolidate the psychic and emotional unity of the nation's various classes."[15]

1.3 School Meals and 'National Regeneration'

As was the case with other European countries, by reorganizing the school meals scheme, the regime attempted to solve the problem of malnutrition of schoolchildren and other physical defects they suffered from (like glandular fever, weakness and pre-tubercular conditions which were recorded in health cards by school doctors).[16] Research conducted in the 1930s pointed out that 30 to 40% of agrarian and working-class people suffered from malnutrition. Their diet was indicative of the gap between Greece and other western European countries, especially regarding the consumption of meat,

---

14 Anonymos, "I Titaneios Prospatheia pros Anatasin tis Phylis," *To Paidi*, no. 64 (March 1940): 4.

15 "Ta Pepragmena apo tis 4is Avgoustou 1938 kai Entefthen," *Skholiki Ygieini*, 13.

16 Harry Hendrich, *Child Welfare 1872–1989* (London: Routledge, 1994), 108–10.

eggs and dairy products. As already mentioned, the committee responsible for the anti-TB campaign, had proposed lowering the prices of basic necessities to avoid starvation. The regime seems to have reached the conclusion that in order to deal with nutritional deficiencies, it was preferable to control the prices of primary necessities and organize school meals and soup kitchens instead of paying family and maternity stipends. The government expected that the political benefits would be greater in the first instance.[17]

In the dictator's public speeches, the building of a robust young generation was linked with the growth in loyalty to the regime and the intensification of Greece's war preparation after 1939. Emergency law no. 1787/1939 put school meals into effect. As mentioned in the preamble to the law, "if in other countries emphasis is laid on other issues, here we must launch a real crusade taking into account the malnutrition of the Greek people."[18] The proliferation of school meals granted the regime the chance to prove its affection for children,[19] striking a blow to the rival ideologies of communism and liberalism. School meals are a characteristic example of the way the regime understood social benefits for its citizens. Since the meals were intended for the working-class, publicizing them was expected to enhance the paternalistic image Metaxas promoted and shape the kind of citizenship the regime was keen on. As propaganda leaflets often highlighted, the regime's advocates expected that children who were in regular contact with state-run institutions, would feel gratitude and express their respect towards the society and the state. In this way, "[they would promote] not only their health seriously in danger of malnutrition but also raise their consciousness as citizens, [showing them] that the state today is a benevolent power and the Greek society [is] a mother figure for all its children."[20] The regime disdained previous attempts at providing food for youth presenting

---

17 The organization of meals for the vulnerable sections of the population was one of the most common steps European governments had adopted in the 1920s. However, there were dissent voices against this policy. Delegates of parties and women's organizations took part in the discussion about the suitability of the means of assistance to families afflicted by the crisis. For this discussion in England in the 1930s, see Jane Lewis, *The Politics of Motherhood. Child and Maternal Welfare in England, 1900–1939* (London: Croom Helm, 1980), 171–90.

18 Nikolaos Spentzas, Aitiologiki Ekthesis tou Anagkastikou Nomou "Peri Organoseos ton Mathitikon Syssition," *Skholiki Ygieini*, no. 31 (September 1939), 41–3.

19 The involvement of the dictator's wife who embraced the whole venture stressed the dictator's personal interest in maintaining the health of lower class children.

20 "I Nomothesia peri Mathitikon Syssition. Aitiologiki Ekthesis epi tou Skhediou Anagkastikou Nomou 'Peri Organoseos ton Mathitikon Syssition'," *Skholiki Ygieini*, no. 31 (September 1939): 41–55.

them as acts of charity towards the poor rather than as a duty that the "National Government" performed. Given the inability of many families to provide their children with a balanced diet, the help of state services was presented by the regime as a national need. According to emergency law no. 1787/1939, parents had to fulfil their responsibilities. The family was obliged to register their children for free school meals, which was publicized as a family duty not only for the benefit of their children but also for the nation's benefit since the provision of sufficient food would guarantee that children would later serve their country efficiently. School meals were linked with national regeneration and evoked respect for the motherland. Children who were not fed well could build neither a strong body nor a strong mind. They would remain sickly with little vitality, "inferior and unsuccessful," a burden to themselves and their country.[21] Thus, school meals were meant to evoke feelings of dignity in children, raise their national consciousness, and inspire a feeling of obligation towards the regime.

School meals were the basis of the school welfare since other measures (i.e., student clinics, open-air schools, summer camps, prevantoria, etc.) would not bear fruit unless each student was provided with a sufficient quantity of food. According to the regulations for school meals published in 1938, school meals were the most efficient step towards "the preventive care of sickly and malnourished poor children."[22] Their systematic distribution was dictated by hygienic, social and pedagogical needs. School meals aimed at the provision of food "either for free or for a small fee" to those students who were not sufficiently fed at home to meet the needs of their developing bodies and school requirements. As a circular of the Ministry of Education addressed to school officers stressed, educational authorities should not remain indifferent "to the empty stomach of their students." It is impossible for "starving or malnourished students" to attend classes. They cannot excel as "the development of brain cells requires food."[23]

The benefits from school meals were not only related to student performance, but also to the cultivation of dietary habits on the common table. It was expected that informed students would instruct their parents on de-

---

21 "Ti Zita to Kratos apo emas (tin Koinoniki Ergatida)," Ioannis Metaxas Archive, file 022, Genika Arkheia tou Kratous (General State Archive).

22 *Kanonismos Mathitikon Syssition* (Athens: 1938).

23 Circular no. 240 Pros tas Ekpaideftikas kai Skholiatrikas Arkhas "Peri Organoseos kai Leitourgias Mathitikon Syssition." Ioannis Metaxas Archive, file 022, Genika Arkheia tou Kratous (GAK). .

veloping good eating habits, as it was believed that "malnourishment was mostly caused by illiteracy rather than poverty."[24] In this way, students, especially female students, would learn about the nutritional value of foods and domestic economy, and subsequently contribute towards improving the nutrition of the working-class. However, the cultural benefits of the provision of school meals were related to the instruction of good manners, namely eating in a decent and civilized way. School nurses and female volunteers tried to impose standards of cleanliness of face and hands. As was the case with summer camps, school meals aimed at the improvement in the behavior of children. The initial selection of children eligible for school meals was carried out by the Board of School Meals and by school doctors and nurses who were well aware of students' financial status and living conditions. The selection was based either on the physical condition of the child or on the family's economic and social circumstances. The Board preferred students whose parents were "established as poor," undernourished, lived far from school (and thus could not return home for lunch), lacked motherly care, or "their fathers are either prodigal or drunkards."[25] Hygienic evidence was examined by the school doctor on the basis of weight and height measurements, and diseases (rickets, anemia, glandular fever, TB, anorexia). Inappropriate decorum on behalf of the students could result in discontinuing the service. Students who committed moral wrongs also would not receive school meals.

The board was responsible for supplying the necessary kitchenware and equipment for cooking, while students had to bring their personal cutlery. A specially designated hall was used as a dining hall and if there was no such hall, the corridor of the building or a shed in the yard was used. A female cook and a cleaning lady were hired for the preparation of food and some female EON members worked as volunteers. During the first year of state-provided school meals, the Ministry of State Hygiene and Relief rose the funds allotted to the Patriotic Foundation of Social Protection and Relief by 300% to increase the number it benefited, improve their organization and acquire permanent premises for the preparation of meals and storage rooms in Athens, Piraeus and Thessaloniki. Gradually, the meals became more organized

---

24 *Kanonismos Mathitikon Syssition*, 4.
25 *Kanonismos Mathitikon Syssition*, 6.

and their provision was centrally controlled by the government. School meals were organized at central, county, district and school level. In July 1939, the Central Committee of Student Meals was set up led by the Archbishop of Athens. Other members were bankers. The committee supervised the distribution of school meals across the country, secured resources for them, and publicized about them. Taking into account the reports of the county committees, the Committee of Student Meals recommended the Ministry take measures for their effective distribution. County and district committees and school boards were responsible for the coordination of school meals at local level and reported back to the central committee. In these intermediate committees, the place reserved for high-ranking EON members was very important. The committees explored the necessity of school meals and decided on the location of school dining halls. They also tried to secure local resources, approved the menu, funded the building of kitchens and buying of kitchenware, and organized the bids for food supplies.

Milk was offered with breakfast and lunch was a clean hot meal with sufficient calories. The menu was planned by the committee with suggestions from the school doctor and was adjusted to the resources of each district. It included mainly beans, pasta, vegetables, rice, cod, and meat once a week. If financial resources permitted it, either a sweet or fruit was offered, most of the times donated by civilians. In order to save resources, two or more schools could share the same kitchen.

There was a gradual increase in the number of students registered for school meals, reaching its climax just before the breakout of World War II. In 1939, this number reached almost 100,000, roughly 20% of the student population. Most students attended schools in Athens and Piraeus. Yet, as can be gleaned from the reports of the school officers, it was impossible to provide hot meals for all students on a daily basis because kitchens could not be built in every school. Most of the expenses were covered by the county committee of school meals and less by local resources and student fees.

Although destitute primary school students might have secured their food to a certain extent, working children from the provinces who swarmed in Athens in order to find a job faced starvation since there was hardly any soup kitchens for them. Barefoot, filthy and hungry children wandering around in urban or working towns, begging for bread or snatching food from the plates of inattentive customers would have been a common sight.

1.4 "Childtowns of Health" and Summer Camps

The expansion of summer camps was the regime's second method to strengthen the constitution of weak children with pre-tubercular symptoms or the children who were from poor families unable to afford summer vacations. According to the articles written by the pediatricians working for the Patriotic Foundation of Social Protection and Relief, children had to be removed from their family in order to be saved. Poor parents were not suitable to raise their children properly as they lacked both the means and the knowledge.[26] Sun, light, pleasure, good food and a change in environment would ideally contribute to "the child's regeneration," away from their unhygienic hovels. In these pediatricians' articles, it is evident that an attempt was made to disparage the working-class house which did not meet the hygienic standards for the proper development of robust children. As one member of the summer camp staff put it, strengthened by a three-week stay in a summer camp, children were able "when back in the bosom of [their] family to face efficiently the adventure of the unhygienic environment, bad diet, and unsatisfactory living conditions."[27] The main aim of the summer camps was to deal with the pre-tubercular and tubercular conditions of childhood. The expansion of summer camps followed the proposals that had been put forward by the committee of the anti-TB campaign for the protection of childhood.

During this period, two therapeutic childtowns or children's villages, one in the seaside area of Voula and the other on the mountainous area of Penteli, were set up. The institution of "children's health villages" was a novelty in the field of strengthening and treating children. It was the outcome of collaboration between pediatricians, architects, state functionaries responsible for health issues and summer camp staff members.[28] It was a place es-

---

26 The paediatrician Panagiotis Mitropoulos, director of the mothers' and children's department of the PFSPR, pointed out in 1939 that "the squalor of the lower classes of society, the lack of means to feed their children sufficiently, the inability of the families to send their weak children or those who live in dark, unhygienic houses or in cellars to summer camps and the morbidity entailed by these unfavourable conditions [...] as well as the development of children into weak lads or men, made the establishment and operation of Summer Camps imperative." Panagiotis Mitropoulous, "Skopos kai Organosis ton Paidikon Exokhon," *To Paidi*, no. 59 (October 1939): 8–9.

27 Emmanouil Vrontakis, "Irkhisen I Leitourgia ton Paidikon Exokhon tou Patriotikou Idrymatos eis Olin tin Ellada," *To Paidi*, no. 67 (June 1940): 24.

28 For their architectural conception, see Panos Dzelepy, *Villages d' Enfants* (Paris: ed. Albert Morange, L'Architecture Vivante en Grece, 1966).

pecially designed for the children's recreation and treatment. It included health centers, aeriums, summer camps, prevantoria and a school. Both summer camps and health childtowns ran with the support of the PFPC, however, it was necessary to mobilize local authorities, school staff and the private sector for their operation.

The facilities, which had been operating in Voula since 1923, were complemented with the construction of two more wings for the treatment of children that suffered from bone TB.[29] In the summer of 1939, the complex including open and covered pavilions, dining rooms, kitchens, baths, dormitories, an amphitheater, the Bakala and Pesmatzoglou wings, the wing for impaired children and the Zirineion Summer Palace for Children was completed, forming "a cheerful childtown."[30] Approximately 5,000 children were accommodated in the summer camps and 400 children were treated in the convalescence wards. The number of members and employees reflects the sheer magnitude of the endeavor. In 1937, eighty-one people were employed, including educators, administrative and working staff. In 1938, the regime also sent young workers below the age of eighteen to the summer camps.

Following the proposal of the committee of the anti-TB campaign, convalescence wards or prevantoria for students operated in the premises of the summer camps during the school year when summer camps did not operate. Children that were sent to the summer camps included destitute children from seven to twelve years old, weak, sickly and anemic children suffering from closed TB (non-contagious), children recovering from serious diseases of the respiratory system or from childhood diseases (measles, whooping cough, scarlet fever or other infections) and children who were generally in good condition but had been "in direct contact with a person suffering from open TB." During their stay, children underwent rigorous hygienic and dietary treatment, which meant contact with nature, good and abundant food and medicine. A small hospital where children suffering from minor diseases were admitted and a primary school also operated in the summer camp. Children stayed in the convalescence wards until they recovered their stamina. Apart from the energy

---

29 Drawing on the architectural archive of the Benaki Museum and features in technical journals, it can be inferred that during this period "the Pesmatzoglou wing," donated by the banker on his child's death, and a series of buildings known as the "Piraeus buildings" because they were targeted at weak children from Piraeus, were built; all of them were drawn by the architect Kitsikis.

30 Thalia Flora-Karavia, "Liges Ores stis Paidikes Exokhes tis Voulas," *To Paidi*, no. 71 (October 1940): 16–8.

and weight gained (three to six kilos), moral change was also mentioned among the recorded benefits. Members of the summer camp staff claimed that children grew more disciplined and willing to work.

In 1938 a new therapeutic childtown was set up in Penteli, a mountainous countryside area on the outskirts of Athens. Here the regime established a series of modern institutions for the treatment and rest of sick children, mainly those who had TB, since many children were discharged from the Convalescent Home in Voula (Asklipiion Paidon) either uncured or having gained a little benefit from their long and expensive treatment. Soon, mountainous summer camps were set up in Penteli—as also called Penteli infirmaries—and the plans were drawn for an asylum of incurables, specially designed for children with a hundred beds, a children's sanatorium with 150 beds and a sanatorium for the treatment of children suffering from bone TB with 200 beds.

The building of the mountain summer camps, designed by the architect Panos Tzelepis and promoted as a novelty in interwar architecture journals, was inaugurated in 1939. It was an attempt to meet the contemporary standards of a therapeutical childtown in a hygienic environment.[31] The foundation stone of the Children's Sanatorium for closed TB, expected to serve 600 children annually, was laid down on October 17, 1940 with great pomp and circumstance.[32] The building, estimated to cost 20,000,000 drachmas, was described as simple, like the Greek family, where "children of the Greek people could be hospitalized under circumstances analogous to the potential and simplicity of the Greek family."[33] Metaxas delivered a speech on the occasion, stressing in it the importance of these works for the restoration of the race and the benefit of the poor classes.

In 1937, the regime announced the establishment of new summer camps in nineteen towns and the operation of mountain summer camps in Hortiatis, an area not far from Salonika. The facilities in most of the camps were quite simple. Permanent facilities included kitchens, WC, and tents for the children to sleep. Gradually summer camps spread. In 1940, the regime's policy makers expected that summer camps would be founded in new ar-

---

31 For the plans, see Khatzipanagiotou Archive, Archives of Modern Greek Architecture Benaki Museum, file 46.

32 Anonymos, "To Sanatorion Paidon tou Patriotikou Idrymatos eis tin Pentelin," *To Paidi*, no. 71 (October 1940): 27. Male and female members of the phalange took part in the inauguration ceremony.

33 Anonymos, "To Sanatorion Paidon," 27.

eas (Metsovo, Hortiatis, Drama, Thassos, N. Makri-Alexandroupolis etc.) to provide 1,700 extra spots for 6,800 children to vacation. They also estimated that the new camps would add 5,500 spots for 22,000 working-class children. By 1940, 30,000,000 drachmas had been spent on building the old and new summer camps.

In 1938 student exchanges began between Greece and other Balkan countries, following the decision of the First Balkan Congress in April 1936 in Athens. The Congress had entrusted the International Union of Child Protection with organizing the exchanges. This practice was meant to foster peace in the Balkans. In 1938 a mission of thirty children from Yugoslavia spent their vacations in the summer camps of Voula and a group of children from Greece spent their holidays in the summer camps of Yugoslavia.

Apart from strengthening the constitution of sickly children, the summer camps were designed to inculcate values and attitudes in children that served the regime. Training children in discipline and obedience to their superiors, national and social education, and cultivation of respect for the country's leader, were appreciated as benefits equally important to increasing children's weight. The militarization of everyday life, instruction in discipline and the presence of the regime's ideological goals in the summer camps generally are evident in the articles the members of the summer camps published in the journals *The Child* and *The Youth*. Similarly to the regime's political discourse, the articles made references to miasma, discipline and elevation of the race. Also, many common elements can be traced back to the summer camps and the EON military camps. Emmanouil Vrontakis, who was responsible for the summer camps in Chania, underlined that order, discipline and self-government turned the summer childtown into a military camp. "The little campers" were trained in a system of government. The division into communities and groups under the surveillance of leaders, deputy-leaders and assistants created "a perfect, decentralized system and in this way it is possible to impose an exemplary order on each group with the children as disciplined as soldiers." In this open air military camp "there are no social classes."[34] All members are equal and disciplined. Unified, "free from every corruptive taint, little children are lined up every night in front of the altar to thank the almighty God and

---

34 Vrontakis, "Irkhisen i Leitourgia ton Paidikon Exokhon," 25.

experience some patriotic elation when they attend silently the lowering of the flag." Summer camp members always stressed the social role of the summer camps. There "the child is within a self-ruled and disciplined community wherein the feelings of religion, family, solidarity and sacrifice are cultivated so as to form the most important pillars whereon Society will be supported in the future."[35]

2. Care for Sickly Children

2.1. Schoolchildren Polyclinics and Special Clinics

For the protection of sickly children the regime built pediatric wards in provincial general hospitals and set up two children's hospitals, one in Athens and the other in Thessaloniki. In Thessaloniki, the Children's Hospital was set up in 1937 with 100 beds, with five million drachmas spent for its construction. In Athens, thanks to the donation of Aglaia Kyriakou and a state grant of 1.5 million drachmas, a new wing with a hundred beds for destitute children was added to the children's hospital "Saint Sofia," which had been in operation since 1900. The new wing was built according to modern architectural trends. The two pediatric hospitals, "Saint Sofia" and "Aglaia Kyriakou" worked jointly and constituted the Children's Hospital which admitted children from across the country.

The two hospitals were managed by professors of pediatrics at the University of Athens because the hospitals would also be used to train medical students in pediatrics. In the 1930s, pediatricians gained higher prestige, a fact reflected in the establishment of the Greek Paediatric Association in 1931. Renowned pediatricians, professors at the University of Athens, and members of the Patriotic Foundation of Social Protection and Relief, such as Apostolos Doxiadis, Georgios Makkas, Konstaninos Khoremis, Emmanouil Lambadarios, Konstantinos Saroglou and others, played a leading role in its establishment. In addition, a building was constructed for the training of nurses who specialized in the hospitalization and treatment of children under the directorship of an American expert.

---

35 Amalia Gkioka, "Pos Eida tin Apostolin ton Paidikon Exokhon tou Patriotikou Idrymatos," *To Paidi*, no. 59 (October 1939): 28–9.

Considerable funds were allotted for the fight against incurable diseases, especially TB among children. The regime publicized children's sanatoria, prevantoria, anti-trachoma clinics and homes for incurable children as modern institutions for children's health, although only a number of these were completed and in operation before the war. Polyclinics and special clinics for children, aimed at the treatment of children with emphasis on dental and ophthalmological care. These clinics followed the initiatives of previous governments. Three new anti-trachoma children's clinics and two new stomatology centers in Athens, Piraeus and Thessaloniki were established. In addition, the Patriotic Foundation was given funding by the government to build two new polyclinics for primary school students in Athens and Piraeus,[36] and in Thessaloniki a similar polyclinic was to be funded by the association "The Child's Care."

During the same period, two children's medical centers opened: the Paedological Center in Athens and the Model County Hygienic Center in Ampelokipi, which collaborated with the Ministries of Education and State Hygiene to provide medical services to students in Athens. The Paedological center included ophthalmological, dental and otolaryngological departments and a department of soup kitchens.[37] Visiting nurses accompanied doctors to schools where they referred students to the paedological center for checks as needed, gave vaccinations, filled out students' personal health cards, measured the weight of children taking their meals in soup kitchens, examined the children in open-air schools every week, taught hygienic rules to students, and examined students' homes that were of doubtful cleanliness to pinpoint the origin of the infectious diseases detected in schools.

The Model County Hygienic Center in Ampelokipi, established in 1935 with funding from the Rockefeller Foundation and organized according to its scientific standards, was one of the very few institutions that survived the health reform plan on health in the Venizelos government. Innovative

---

36 It seems that in 1938, the architectural plans of Panos Tzelepis for the construction of a students' polyclinic in Athens, in Vathis square, were approved by the directorship of the Technical Services of the Ministry of Hygiene. Yet, it seems that the polyclinic did not open before the war. For the architectural plans of the Polyclinic, see Student Polyclinic of Athens, plans of Panos Tzelepis, Archives of Modern Greek Architecture Benaki Museum, files 445 and 446. In 1939, the plans for the construction of the schoolchildren's polyclinic in Piraeus were under way.

37 Anonymos, "Paidologikon Kentron Athinon, Examinaia Ekthesis Pepragmenon," *Skholiki Ygieini*, no. 7 (May 1937): 37–9.

programs for observing the health of local residents were implemented at the center, where a school hygiene department also operated in collaboration with the Ministry of Education.[38] The protection of students from infectious diseases and the cultivation of hygienic values in children were all part of this department's work. School nurses there played a similar role to their counterparts in the Paedology Center. They filled in personal health cards according to the template provided by the Ministry of Education and categorized students into three groups according to the condition of their health: "fully satisfying," "almost satisfying" and "non-satisfying at all."[39] The names of children found to suffer from various diseases (trachoma, heart diseases, lung conditions or pediculosis) were entered into a different list and their parents were summoned to the center to be given medical advice. According to the Center's minutes, in 1936, approximately 50% of the parents came.

Destitute students suffering from contagious diseases were referred to the outpatient department, the anti-TB department, or the anti-syphilis department in the center. In addition, investigations were carried out that included "social screening," i.e., home visits by the nurses, to decide on which children were eligible for a stay in the summer camps of Voula. Nurses notified the Patriotic Foundation about the results of their investigation. Drawing on the Center's statistics derived from the personal health cards, it was found out that in 1936 28% of the students suffered from kyphosis, 10% from scoliosis, 2% from trachoma and 8% from conjunctivitis. The percentages that correlate to nutritional and developmental problems are worth noting: 62% of the students suffered from tonsillitis, 40% from cervical adenopathy, 32% from malnutrition, and another 48% had vision problems generally.[40]

2.2. The Special School

The policy begun by the Liberals in the early 1930s concerning students with special needs continued during the totalitarian period with the construction of anti-trachoma schools and semi-open air classrooms, while the open-air school run by the Anti-TB Society continued operating.

38 Dimitrios A. Messinezis, *I Protypos Ygeionomiki Organosis Ambelokipon tou Dimou Athinaion kai tis Ygeionomikis Skholis. To Programma kai ta Pepragmena mias Topikis Ygeionomikis Ypiresias, Octobre 1935–Decembre1936* (Athens: 1937).
39 Messinezis, *I Protypos Ygeionomiki Organosis Ambelokipon,* see the appendix.
40 Messinezis, *I Protypos Ygeionomiki Organosis Ambelokipon,* 34.

The most important step was the foundation of the first "School for anomalous and mentally impaired children" in Kaisariani in 1937,[41] later renamed the "Model Special School of Athens" by law no. 1049/1940.[42] The school operated until 1940 and gave physical, moral and mental care to "anomalous" and impaired children who could not keep up with the pace of regular schools due to their mental conditions.[43] According to the law, students aged 8 to 15 who were capable of being educated, but unable to follow regular education, attended the special school. The "feeble-minded," "deaf-mute," and blind children, those suffering from contagious diseases and street urchins were not to be admitted. During the early stages of its operation only local students from the suburb of Kaisariani attended the school.

The architect of the school took Lambadarios's recommendations for semi-open air classes into consideration. In addition to five classrooms, the building had a crafts workshop, infirmary, bath, gym, playground, yard, garden and chicken shed. A boarding house and special rooms for vocational training were planned for the future.[44]

Although doctors and educators had said that it was necessary to establish schools for children with special needs, efforts were unsuccessful. Lambadarios estimated that the number of "feeble-minded" students aged 6–14 who could not be educated was between 7,000 and 8,000. His proposals to set up a special school did not materialize until 1936 because of financial constraints and shortage of suitable staff, despite the fact that a law passed in 1929 mandated a school be set up for the "feeble-minded."[45]

Known for her progressive ideas both in pedagogy and politics, educator Rosa Imvrioti seems to have played a leading role in establishing the school. Her background made her the most suitable person for such a venture. During her graduate studies in Paris and Berlin, she witnessed European developments in reformative and special education and she had followed the

---

41 See Anagkastikos Nomos no. 453 "Peri Idryseos Skholeiou Anomalon kai Kathysterimenon Paidon etc.," *Efimeris tis Kiverniseos*, A´, no. 28 (January 30, 1937): 175–6.

42 Antonia Kharissi, *I Rosa Imvrioti sto Protypo Eidiko Skholeio Athinon (1937–1940)* (Athens: Epikentro, 2013), 230–3.

43 The terms used in this section to describe the children with special needs are derived from the greek legislation of the 1930s.

44 Rosa Imvrioti, "I Ergasia tou Protypou Eidikou Skholeiou Athinon (1937–1938)," *Skholiki Ygieini*, no. 18–19 (September-November 1938): 18.

45 Emmanouil Lambadarios, "Symvoli eis tin Psykholmetrian tou Anomalou Ellinos Mathitou kai Arkhai Organoseos tou Protou Skholeiou Anomalon Paidon par' Imin," *Skholiki Ygieini*, no. 7 (May 1937): 5–16.

principles of Edward Spranger.[46] Influenced by the Swiss educator Heinrich Hanselman and his work *Heilpaedagogik*, Imvrioti adopted a much more medical approach to her pedagogy, stressing the cooperation of the doctor with the educator. In her articles, she attempted to shed light on the difficulties that arose in the treatment and the instruction of children with special needs. She also highlighted the shortages in this field of education in Greece. Affiliated with the Left from very early on, Imvrioti stressed the social and cultural dimensions of special schools.

Although she was opposed to Metaxas's ideologically, he selected Imvrioti to direct the school and choose the teachers she thought were the most suitable according to their expertise in didactic and psycho-pedagogical issues. Apart from her, Lambadarios's role in the special school was also significant. He was appointed member of the supervisory board of directors and deputy president, which was responsible for the evaluation and selection of the students.[47] Metaxas's decision to establish a special school in response to Imvrioti's and Lambadarios's publications on the need to set up such a school might be better understood, given that members of his family suffered from mental diseases.

Lambadarios and Imvrioti undertook the organization of the school and the selection of students. Questionnaires were distributed to local teachers of Kaisariani in order to determine the ability of the students who were evaluated as mentally-challenged. The students underwent a medical, psychological and pedagogical examination, on the basis of psychometric and cognitive tests designed by Imvrioti and Lambadarios.[48]

In its first year of operation, 130 students were referred to the Special School, but after examination only 68 were admitted. According to their mental age, students were characterized "moderately and mildly" impaired.[49] Students, both male and female as co-education had been introduced to the

---

46 According to Spranger, the teacher is "an educator by birth." He/she allows the student enough space and grants them many opportunities for self-action and participation. Spranger Edward, "I Synkhronos Germaniki Paidagogiki," (trans. K. Vourveris) *Deltion Omospondias Leitourgon Mesis Ekpaidefseos*, no. 71 (May 1932).

47 Besides Lambadarios who served as president to the committee, Khristos Georgakolpoulos, doctor and director of the Paedological Center in Athens, Nikolaos Kharalampoulos, school officer of the Primary School of the First Educational District in Athens, and Rosa Imvrioti herself, served as members to the committee.

48 Lambadarios, *Skholiki Ygieini*, 11–4.

49 Rosa Imvrioti, "Ekthesis peri tis Leitourgias tou Eidikou Skholeiou Athinon. Apo 1ois Maiou Mekhri 20is Iouniou," *Skholiki Ygieini*, no. 8 (June 1937): 22–38.

school, came from working-class backgrounds and faced many personal problems: neuropathy, psychopathology, hysteria, emotional problems, social ineptitude and speech problems. The number of difficult, nervous and undisciplined children was quite high.

Special medical cards were made for each student upon admission that listed their individual conditions and in which teachers confirmed if the student was unable to adjust to the conditions of mainstream schooling and therefore in need of special care. Three more information cards described the student's intellectual state after they had been admitted to the school: a "health card," designed by Lambadarios, an "information card" and an "individuality card" both designed by Imvrioti. The health card and the information card were completed by the visiting nurses of the paedology center. The third card was filled in by the psychiatrist who examined the child's parents first in order to establish whether or not there were any hereditary factors at work. He then examined the child from a psycho-pedagogical view using the Binet-Simon-Terman scale. The Rossolino profile was used to measure powers of cognition: attention, memory and observation. The individuality card was completed with a fourth card, the "medical card" that included information about the child's condition upon their release from school. This card was completed by both the psychiatrist[50] and the school personnel.

Teachers at the school used special methods aimed at improving the children morally and socially. School work played a central role as it helped students become more observant, cultivate their physical and mental capacities, develop their creativity, strengthen their will and increase their sociability. It was the first time that the principles of the Arbeitschule and the New Education methods[51] were implemented in special education. Material such as sand and clay were used in teaching. Classes were short and physical education, crafts, gardening and animal breeding were essential subjects. Theatre, puppet shows and shadow plays, music and games were interspersed in the curriculum. School festivals were also a normal part of school life.

The school was divided into three levels: lower, middle and upper; each one corresponding to two grades in regular school. Apart from these lev-

---

50 Rosa Imvrioti, *Anomala kai Kathysterimena Paidia. Protos Khronos tou Protypou Eidikou Skholeiou Athinon.* (Athens: Elliniki Ekdotiki Etaireia, 1939): 147.
51 For this method, see Ioannis Khristias, *Theoria kai Methodologia tis Didaskalias* (Athens: Grigoris, 2009): 196.

els, there was a preparatory level during which games and singing strengthened the mental and physical powers of the students, unearthed talents and prepared them for school life. Children learned to behave freely in a class that bore little resemblance to a typical school. Then, students were directed to the lowest level (corresponding with the first and second grades of primary school) where the particular needs of the children determined the material taught.

In the first year of their studies at the lower level, crafts and drawing were the most important subjects, while in the second year teachers emphasized object lessons. Teaching was reinforced with trips to nature and the neighborhood where children observed their surroundings. The intermediate level stressed team work; playing was replaced by structured activities, writing and reading. In this way, students were prepared for the upper level, which corresponded to the fifth and sixth grades of primary school. At the upper level, professional education was the most important, while the therapeutic element receded yet was not totally neglected. The aim was for children to be able to earn a living and integrate into society.

Imvrioti considered children's professional education as a tool of social integration and intended to set up a boarding facility within the special school. The therapeutic mission of the school was as important and necessary as education. Doctors regularly examined students and sometimes children were referred to the Paedological Center of Athens and to public hospitals for treatment. Provisions were made for sunbathing, aquatic therapy and the administration of cod-liver oil. Milk and meals were provided by the Patriotic Foundation, which also took care of the children's clothing. The staff responsible for the pedagogical and psychotherapeutic work at the special school focused their attention on dealing with the anti-social tendencies some of the children displayed. According to Imvrioti, the educator's aim was to remove all the sources of irritation for the children, control their instincts and their temper, help them integrate into society, fight their anti-social tendencies, and generally make them useful to both themselves and society. Staff sessions were often held to analyze and comment on daily issues in the school. Staff were encouraged to discuss pedagogical issues, to experiment with new teaching methods, and to pursue further training in therapeutic treatment through special classes. On the initiative of the headmistress gatherings and lectures for parents were held to fight alcoholism, drug addiction and in general to raise the hygienic standards of family life for the benefit of the children.

The medical and pedagogical involvement in the special school produced satisfactory results in the children's health. Their behavior improved, their socialization was reinforced and the learning results were so positive that after having attended the special school for a year some students were able to return to a regular school.[52] However, due to World War II the ultimate goal of spreading this new pedagogical institution was not attained.

3. The Policy on Motherhood and Infancy

3.1 The Reorganization of the Patriotic Foundation, Statism and Racial Orientations

During Metaxas's dictatorship, the Patriotic Foundation became the regime's instrument for protecting mothers and children. Gradually, it undertook larger and more numerous welfare projects, however, its main function was systemizing propaganda for working-class families. Its work brought more new mothers and children closer to the regime who benefited from its welfare policies. At the same time, this placed mothers and children under the control of services that closely monitored their health and behavior. Mothers and children were the target group of the communication policy that promoted the Metaxas's personality cult and stressed their obligation to the regime for the aid it had given them. Government funding for the welfare of mothers and children grew in step with increasing despotism and infiltration of the board of directors of the Patriotic Foundation by the regime's followers, which by the outbreak of the war had turned into another tool of the authoritarian state for implementing its racial policies. The regime dissolved the General Society for the Protection of Childhood and Adolescence (Geniki Etairia gia tin Prostasia tis Paidikis kai Efivikis Ilikias), turned volunteers into obedient servants of the regime and replaced members of the board of the Patriotic Foundation that voiced dissent against the regime with high-ranking EON members. In this way, the New State left its mark on an institution known for its modernizing practices in the pro-

---

52 Ivrioti, *Anomala kai Kathysterimena Paidia*, 149.

tection of mothers and children, practices that had been promoted by the League of Nations in the early 1920s.

According to its amended constitution in January 1936, the Patriotic Foundation once more shifted gears. Apart from children's welfare, it now also aimed at satisfying other social needs like aiding the destitute and victims of natural disasters. However, during Metaxas's dictatorship, most of the Foundation's funds were channeled into projects for children: building new summer camp lodges, new medical centers, and expanding the institutions that had been in place since the previous liberal government. Increased funding and closer state control were the main characteristics of the regime's policy on child protection. The generous increase in the Foundation's funding from 1936 until 1940, which fluctuated from 30% to 50%, as compared with funding during the pro-dictatorship period, points to the importance the regime attached to social work for children.[53] In 1940, the budget of the Ministry of State Hygiene and Welfare reached 240,000,000 drachmas, second only to war funding. State involvement in the administration of the Foundation was increasing although private funding continued, yet to a lesser extent. During this period, the state also determined the role of the volunteers. They were expected to play at the Foundation's consultation centers the role of "soldiers [...]obedient to the state for the general benefit." Therefore, in its new form "the Patriotic Foundation is directed towards and managed by the state."[54]

In October 1939, the General Society for the Protection of Childhood and Adolescence, founded in 1925, was dissolved and replaced by the Press and Propaganda Department, later renamed the Popular Enlightenment Bureau. The Bureau published the journal The Child, which previously had been published by the General Society. The change in the journal's layout and content, the decrease in the number of scientific articles, the increase in popular articles written for mothers in a very authoritative tone, and most of all the influence of Metaxas's cult of personality and the regime's racial policy, turned this scientific journal into a magazine that served the best interests of the regime. The increase in articles that highlighted the importance

---

53 Ekthesis ton Pepragmenon tou Patriotikou Idrymatos Koinonikis Pronoias kai Antilipseos. Chrisis 1934–1935 and 1935–1936 (Athens: 1938).
54 Anonymos, "I Eklaikefsis tis Paidokomikis. Ai Dialexeis tou Tmimatos 'Laikis Diafotiseos' tou Patriotikou Idrymatos," To Paidi, no. 66 (March 1940): 15.

of the Patriotic Foundation for advancing the regime's racial policies and the publication of Metaxas's speeches and the Press and Propaganda Department's lectures cast no doubt as to its new orientation.[55]

The publication of the emergency law no. 1950/1939 "on the organization of the Patriotic Foundation of Social Protection and Relief" was yet another step towards increasing state control over the Patriotic Foundation.[56] Since the first months of Metaxas's dictatorship, the state's oversight of semi-state welfare institutions was a critical issue for the regime. To this end, a committee was set up to establish a unified social welfare agency. The members of the committee considered that state control of the Foundation was lax as most responsibilities lay with its administrative board, which was partly composed of volunteers, rather than with the Minister of State Hygiene and Welfare.[57] Because of the amount of funding it oversaw, the Patriotic Foundation was in need of stricter control by the ministry. The new law created a labyrinthine organization influenced by the Opera Nationale Maternitaed Infanzia,[58] which was set up by Mussolini in 1925.[59]

The General Board and the Committee of Directors were established in 1939 to manage the Patriotic Foundation, with members appointed by the Minister of State Hygiene and Welfare. The General Board comprised scientists such as professors of obstetrics and pediatrics, high-ranking state functionaries as well as twelve distinguished civilians. The Committee of Directors was the preparatory organ which submitted proposals to the General Board for approval and proposed staff appointments. There were two advisory committees, one for issues regarding mothers and the other for all other issues. The Central Service in Athens, which comprised four divisions—the general division, the division for the protection of mothers and children, the

55 The reference to the social welfare as a factor conducive to racial regeneration and the contribution of EON to child care apart from highlighting the dictator's personal interest in "the titanic effort put into the elevation of the race" signifies also the dominance of control mechanisms within the Patriotic Foundation.

56 Anagkastikos Nomos no. 1950, "Peri Organoseos tou Patriotikou Idrymatos Koinonikis Pronoias kai Antilipseos," *Efimeris tis Kiverniseos*, A', no. 371(September 7, 1939): 2473–5.

57 "Paratiriseis peri Organoseos tis Dimosias Pronoias kai Antilipseos." Alexandros Koryzis Archive, The Benaki Museum's Historical Archives, subfile 16, February 15, 1937.

58 Michela Minesso (ed.), *Stato e infanzia nell'Italia contemporanea. Origini, sviluppo e fine dell'Onmi, 1925–1975* (Bologna: il Mulino, 2007) and Michela Minesso, *Madri figli welfare. Istituzioni e politiche dall'Italia liberale ai giorni nostri* (Bologna: il Mulino).

59 Sileno Fabri, "To Ethnikon Idryma Prostasias Mitrotitos kai Paidikis Ilikias," (transl. Kharil. Prokopidis), *To Paidi*, no. 54 (May 1939): 24–7 and Quine, *Italy's Social Revolution*, 144–47.

division of welfare services and the division of financial services—and the district branches implemented the decisions of the General Board. High-ranking officials, prefects, mayors, bank managers, high school principals and merchants, some of whom were the local supervisors of the National Youth Organization, were appointed as members of the local branches. It is interesting that Metaxas's wife, Lela Metaxa, served as a member of the board of directors beginning in 1938.

The inauguration of these two overseeing bodies took place in the presence of the minister Ilias Krimbas and signified a transition to a new era of social policy. Apart from trying to improve its reputation among the working-class, the Foundation was expected to materialize the regime's racial policies. According to the Krimbas, the Foundation's mission was not so much to offer aid to the destitute, as a voluntary society would do, but rather to achieve "the regeneration of the race; it is this very race that our Leader has many aims for."[60]

The new General Board, which was set up in October 1939, was in addition to the high-ranking state functionaries made up of Konstantinos Logothetopoulos, a professor of obstetrics and gynecology; Konstantinos Khoremis, a professor of paediatrics at the University of Athens; members of the EON such as its director Alekos Kanellopoulos, industrialists and wives of members of the government.

4. The Medicalization of Birth

The health and welfare of mothers and infants were the main topics of the public debate during the interwar period in Western Europe among political parties, women's organizations, the medical community and experts on social security.[61] The public debate revolved around birth control, the cost of health, the policy on benefits, the desirable size of the family and the place of women in their families and therefore their emancipation. In addition, this discussion led to the organization of health services and the regulation of the education of doctors, midwives, nurses and social workers.

---

60 "Pos Skeptetai o Neos Ypourgos mas k. Ilias Krimbas," *To Paidi*, no. 59 (September 1939): 1.
61 Jane Lewis, *The Politics of Motherhood. Child and Maternal Welfare in England, 1900–1939* (London: Croom Helm 1980); Gisela Bock and Pat Thane, eds., *Maternity and Gender Policies. Women and the Rise of the European Welfare State 1880s–1950s* (London and New York: Routledge, 1994).

The medicalization of child birth reformed power relations between doctors specializing in different fields, the relationships between doctors and midwives, and between mothers and doctors. Medicalization of child birth became also a contested space between feminist organizations and governments. The medicalization of birth took on different meanings for each of the groups involved. Gynecologists and obstetricians attempted to increase their clientele and become more prestigious than pathologists. This is why, they tended to deal with birth as if it were a medical problem. Although obstetricians wanted mothers to give birth in hospitals, without generous state funding needed to improve hospitals, a decline in mortality rates among mothers, attributed to hospital infections and puerperal, was far from possible.

Women's organizations and working-class women were not against delivering a child in hospital as long as it meant better conditions for child birth. They claimed stipends, social insurance benefits, and assistance at home, usually in the presence of a midwife during birth. Dire housing conditions, physical exhaustion and the lack of hygiene threatened women's lives. Women who participated in the discourse over declining infant and mother mortality highlighted their financial difficulties which were otherwise ignored by state officials and doctors who tended to deal with the issue in medical or bureaucratic terms. Despite the different approaches taken in various countries, the increasing medicalization of birth, the instruction of mothers in their maternal duties and the relationship between demographic policy and birth policy were the common characteristics of this period.

In Greece Metaxas's regime focused on how to combat high infant mortality and on the importance of instructing women in their maternal duties. As other authoritarian regimes had previously done, the regime paid homage to "women at home" and glorified "motherhood" and the family.[62] Two Balkan congresses in 1936 and 1938, popular journals for mothers and medical journals serve as rich sources for understanding the views of doctors, child experts, and high-ranking state officials who affected the policies on the protection of mothers. Yet, women themselves remained silent since women's organizations were dissolved by Metaxas and the organizations' publications were banned. In the following sections, we examine the

---

62 Anna Cova and António Costa Pinto, "Women under Salazar's Dictatorship," *Portuguese Journal of Social Science* 1, no. 2 (2002): 129–46.

attempts in the observation of mother and infant health, as well as the debate on the means of fighting infant mortality.

4.1 Consultation Centers for Mothers and Infants in Cities

In order to insure safe births and raise healthy infants, a plethora of already existing infrastructure invested in the medical supervision of mothers. The consultation centers for mothers and infants at the Patriotic Foundation were maintained and funding increased to start new consultation centers, especially in the working-class neighborhoods of Athens and Piraeus. Doctors attached great importance to the examination of prospective mothers in the consultation stations since it was found that half of the infant deaths occurred during the first two months. The infants' deaths were attributed to poor conditions during pregnancy and constituted a considerable part of the overall rates of infant mortality.

In 1933, thanks to the donation of Elena Venizelou, the prime minister's wife, the maternity home "Marika Iliadi," a modern building in the center of Athens, was constructed.[63] There was a school of midwives in the maternity home and a consultation center in its outpatient department that offered advice and examined expectant mothers free of charge. This maternity home was a representative example of the modernization attempts in the supervision of mothers. The erection of a new maternity home with an estimated number of 300 beds, "Alexandra Maternity Home," was under way in the same area in the late 1930s.

The 1936 annual report of the Patriotic Foundation mentioned that although the number of women who visited the consultation centers had increased, a high number of births still posed a risk for mothers and babies due to the limited number of beds in the maternity clinics or "due to lack of scientific means at births occurring at home."[64] Gynecologists and pediatricians suggested two maternity vans be bought in 1937, which would have an obstetrician, a midwife graduated from the School of Nurses and a

---

63   The donation was made in the memory of her friend Marika Iliadi.
64   According to statistics which are far from representative, since they refer to expectant mothers who were registered at the consultation stations in the capital and therefore to a small percentage of women, it seems that around 1938 at least half of births occurred at home. It is not known if they occurred in a scientific way, i.e., with the help of a graduate or an empirical midwife. *Ekthesis Pepragmenon tou Patriotikou Idrymatos Kratikis Pronoias kai Antilipseos*, 12.

female assistant to secure safe births in the homes of women who lived in remote Athenian neighborhoods and were unable to reach the maternity home in time.[65]

Two new departments were set up for the medical observation of infants along with two new departments for pre-school children in working-class neighborhoods of Athens. Health centers also aided mothers and infants, which were a new institution created in large cities, i.e., Athens, Piraeus, Thessaloniki, Ioannina, Herakleion and Kavala. They included a consultation center for laboring mothers and infants, children's clinics, a day-care center, nurseries, a radiology department, and microbiology clinics.[66]

There was a consultation center for expectant mothers and an observation center for infants in the Model County Hygiene Center in Ampelokipi, which operated as a branch of the outpatients' department of the "Marika Iliadi" maternity home and was staffed with its obstetricians. Nikolaos Louros, the manager of the maternity home, required women in the area of Ampelokipi who came to the maternity home to give birth be registered at the consultation center, at least by the seventh month of pregnancy. According to the center's report, this measure provided expectant mothers with a great incentive for their registration. Half of the expectant local mothers and 45% of the infants were under observation in 1936, rates high even by American standards.[67] The mortality rate of the infants under observation was below 5%, considerably lower than the national average infant mortality in Greece.

The maternity and family health cards, which might have been designed by social workers who had experience with the American system, reflected a scientific approach to recording data. These cards reveal a lot about how those in charge of the Model County Hygiene Center understood the relation between social conditions and social diseases. Data such as the number of rooms in the family's house and their hygienic condition, the husband's occupation and financial status, and diseases such as TB, venereal diseases

---

65 According to the information provided by paediatricians, the construction of makeshift maternity clinics was Nikolaos Louros's idea and were built thanks to the funds offered by Papastratos Brothers, see Georgios Tsoukalas, Ioannis Tsoukalas, "Diakomides Neognon apo tous Mythologikous Khronous Mekhri Simera," in Istoria tis Ellinikis Paidiatrikis, ed. Dimitrios Karaberopoulos (Athens: Elliniki Paidiatriki Etaireia, 2009): 27.

66 Anonymos, "I Koinoniki Pronoia," 243.

67 Messinezis, I Protypos Ygeionomiki Organosis Ambelokipon, 38.

and mental disorders were entered in these cards. As for infants, data like development rhythms, nutrition and condition of their teeth, were recorded in diagrams and indices.

4.2 The Role of the Visiting Nurse in the Eradication of Traditional Child-rearing Practices

Doctors were deeply concerned with how to approach mothers and convince them to let go of superstitions surrounding birth and traditional ways of raising infants. They reached the conclusion that mothers' ignorance and poor education impeded this effort. As can be gleaned from the Ampelokipi case, it was much easier to approach lower middle-class mothers in urban centers, especially those who had turned to a maternity home to give birth. The problem was much more acute in the provinces where tradition kept women tied to superstitions and the advice of the older relatives, especially mothers-in-law.

As had been the case in other countries during the same period, aid to mothers came mostly in the form of advice and less in material means, like milk, swaddling-clothes or money.[68] The consultation stations, in other words, operated mainly as "bureaux de consultation" rather than as "gouttes de lait." Individual instruction, especially supervision at home with discretion, was preferable to financial aid. The scientific community was convinced that the decline in infant mortality depended on the mothers' instruction in hygiene and instilling in them a sense of responsibility for their role: to work within the confines of the home or, for farmers, not to work excessively; to improve the hygiene of the home; to take baths; to dress babies suitably; to care for babies with affection; and to breastfeed them. Mothers were instructed in their maternal role by means of special leaflets, and individual advice at the consultation centers. Material aid, when it did come, was limited to swaddling clothes, milk and in exceptional cases money.

During this period the role of the visiting nurse was strengthened. Apart from the work they did at consultation stations as doctors' assistants, it was expected that they acculturate the working class mother, by encouraging better hygiene habits in them and their families. Through the visiting mid-

---

68 Hilary Marland, "The Medicalization of Motherhood: Doctors and Infant Welfare in the Netherlands, 1901–1930," in *Women and Children First. International Maternal and Infant Welfare, 1870–1945*, eds. Valerie Fildes, Lara Marks and Hilary Marland (London and New York: Routledge, 2013):74–96.

wife, the consultation center observed not only the expectant mother but also the entire family.

Nurses served "as the eye of the Foundation so as to clearly perceive what happened in the infant's environment."[69] Their main goal was to record information and change the women's habits. They paid great attention to the housing and hygiene conditions of families, especially of farming families. Nurses' investigations had to be conducted with great discretion and politeness. The visiting nurse would gather valuable information on families that was necessary for proper hygienic and financial aid.

Monitoring families was the first step of the cultural changes the regime attempted. The example of the Model Health Center, which was established by the Patriotic Foundation in Keratea, Attica in 1938, is quite characteristic of the cultural mission the visiting nurse had to accomplish. The center included a consultation station for expectant mothers, an infants' station, a children's clinic and an anti-trakhoma clinic.[70] Three months before the center commenced operation, the Foundation had sent a visiting nurse and a graduate midwife to visit all the village houses and observe how farmers lived. The visiting nurses described the difficulties they encountered in convincing farming women to change their habits: sleep with the window open, bathe their babies, avoid swaddling, breastfeed regularly and turn to the graduate midwife for help and advice instead of the practical midwife. The center launched a campaign to eradicate dietary habits—the frugal diet of the Greeks deeply rooted in the mentality of the peasantry—and convince men not to exhaust their wives with their selfish behavior.[71]

Apart from changing the material conditions of the families they visited, the visiting nurses had to change mothers' attitudes, as they saw that mothers were often tough and indifferent towards their children. The financial aid was ineffectual if the mother did not display the necessary affection.[72] The compliance of working class mothers with the advice of the vis-

---

69 Margarita Khrysaki, "Ai Peristerai tou Politismou. I Episkeptria Adelfi apo Arkhaiotaton Khronon mekhri Simeron," *To Paidi*, no. 66 (May 1940): 20–3.

70 Anonymos, "To Protypo Kentro Ygeias stin Keratea. I Ypaithros Ekpolitizetai," *To Paidi*, no. 51 (February 1939): 29.

71 The habit of men to return from the fields riding an animal while women were loaded with wood, children, etc. was condemned.

72 "One of the most important issues is the necessary affection that it should be forced when it is nonexistent in families and mothers." See Ioannis Aravantinos, "I Symvoli tou Patriotikou Idrymatos eis tin Exygiansin tis Neas Genias," *To Paidi*, no. 67 (June 1940): 3–5.

iting nurse was crucial to the provision of aid. The infants' stations supplied milk, swaddling clothes and other items according to the opinion of the visiting nurses. If the mother did not cooperate, did not attend the consultation center or did not comply with the doctors' advice, the consultation center reserved the right to strike the names of the undisciplined mother and her infant off the register. On the other hand, the willingness of the mothers to come to the center and the regularity of their visits were taken as evidence by the doctors and the nurses of the center for its successful work.

The regime's advocates interpreted mothers' cooperation with the Patriotic Foundation's consultation centers as evidence for people's trust for the state and its services and as a contribution to the regeneration of the race. The statements of the regime showed the national importance of the consultation centers. In 1940 the general director of the Patriotic Foundation, Ioannis Aravantinos, stated that mothers had to entrust their children to experts not only for their physical development, but for their education, which only the state was able to provide since illiterate mothers could not. Aravantinos launched an appeal to mothers to register at the branches of the Patriotic Foundation where they would learn to take care of their babies "not only because as mothers they were obliged to but because of their sacred duty to bring up the future healthy Greeks."[73]

Despite the rhetoric on mothers and infancy used by the regime, the funding given to benefit them was rather low and its welfare policy on motherhood and childhood was not particularly innovative. Although infant centers and consultation centers were set up, especially in the poor neighborhoods of Athens, the pace of development was not much different from that of previous years. Compared to what the Liberals had accomplished in the wider area of Athens, the increase in the number of consultation centers was not that impressive. It was certainly lower than propagandists presented it.[74] Children's diseases and infectious diseases were still on the rise, especially in refugee quarters and in poor urban neighborhoods where no hygiene measures had been taken.[75]

---

73 Aravantinos, "I Symvoli tou Patriotikou Idrymatos," 4.

74 In 1932 in Athens there were in operation four consultation stations for expectant mothers and fourteen stations for the protection of infants in various working class quarters; in 1942 there were five stations for mothers and twenty-four infant stations.

75 In Attica in October and November 1938, 187 children of infant, preschool and early school age came down with diphtheria; during the early summer months, 580 children came down with measles and

5. DEMOGRAPHICAL TRENDS AND PRIORITIES: THE GREEK PARADIGM

If we compare the policy on childbirth implemented by Metaxas's regime with that of other contemporary fascist regimes, we see certain similarities and differences. Totalitarian interwar regimes enforced particular bio-politics regarding births and families. Social welfare on women as prospective and potential mothers took on a more racial and national character. Marriage stipends—thanks to the taxation of the unmarried—and the financial support for those that met the racial criteria set by the government, penalization for abortions, support for large families, the establishment of welfare organizations for mothers and children, and the decisive role which scientific communities played in the adoption of eugenic measures were characteristics that many contemporary European governments who were interested in increasing their population and its biological quality shared.[76] Italy and Germany serve as illustrative examples of the importance bio-politics on childbirth had for materializing imperialist aims and of the way in which fascist ideology combined with demographic, racial and gender policies.[77]

During Metaxas's regime, the decline in infant mortality became a social issue of prime importance. It was associated on the one hand with the development of social policy programmes for childbirth and on the other hand with the education of mothers and the training of nurses, midwifes and social workers. However, in contrast with the policy on families adopted by other authoritarian regimes during this period and despite the

---

nearly as many from chicken pox, whooping cough and parotitis while in September and October typhus counted ten victims in neighbourhoods where flies proliferated. See "Ekthesis peri tis Ygeionomikis Katastaseos tis Perifereias tou Ygeionomikou Kentrou Attikovoiotias kata to 1937 ypo tou T. Triantafyllou" *Arkheia Ygeiinis*, no. 6 (June 1938): 171–91.

76 Maria Sophia Quine, *Population Politics in the Twentieth Century: Fascist Dictatorships and Liberal Democracies* (London: Routledge, 1996).

77 For Nazi Germany, see Gisela Bock, "Antinatalism, Maternity and Paternity in National Socialist Racism," in *Maternity and Gender Policies. Women and the Rise of the European Welfare State 1880s-1950s*, eds. Gisela Bock and Pat Thane (London and New York: Routledge, 2008): 233–55. For fascist Italy, see Chiara Saraceno, "Redefining Maternity and Paternity: Gender, Pronatalism and Social Policies in Fascist Italy," in *Maternity and Gender Politicies*, 196–212; Ipsen Carl, *Dictating Demography: The Problem of Population in Fascist Italy*. (Cambridge: Cambridge University Press, 1996). See also Maria Sophia Quine, *Italy's Social Revolution. Charity and Welfare from Liberalism to Fascism*, especially the chapter entitled "Racial Regeneration through Welfare. The National Organization for the Protection of Motherhood and Infancy under Fascism," (New York: Palgrave, 2002), 129–72. For Spain, see Mary Nash, "Pronatalism and Motherhood in Franco's Spain," in *Maternity and Gender Policies*, 160–77.

emphasis laid on family values by the regime, Greece was lacking in measures aimed at increasing its population: loans were not given to newlyweds nor there were taxes for the unmarried and the childless, although Doxiadis had suggested a similar measure in 1929. Similarities were limited to the level of discourse. Stipends and social security benefits for mothers were not proposed. Women secured the right to maternity leave but not to maternity stipends. The country's financial difficulties did not allow for maternity stipends even when the law on the establishment of the Social Security Foundation took effect.

These choices might have been due to the lack of "hysteria" about the decline in births and population in interwar Greece that was present in Italy and Germany. Financial incentives to strengthen racially valuable marriages or large families were not given, nor were measures taken to promote birth control. We assume that the development of demographic sizes accounts for the lack of similar measures. And this is why the demographics of Greece inspired optimism, in contrast with the pessimistic Western European delegates at the International Congress on Demographic Studies in Rome in 1931 who predicted that if fertility and mortality rates remained the same, the population of developed countries would drop. In the 1920s and 1930s Greek doctors and social thinkers who had taken part in the debate about eugenics had been concerned more with the quality of the population rather than its size. It was then that they voiced their worries about the consequences of overpopulation for the quality of the biological capital, especially after the arrival of the refugees and their concentration in towns.[78] In the early 1930s, the discussion turned to the biological value of the offspring and fertility rates across the social spectrum. Some proposals were put forward for the distribution of birth control according to the biological value of individuals and the social class of their parents. However, as suggested above, these proposals were wishful thinking since other proposals prevailed, prioritizing education and the preparation of society for the introduction of negative eugenic measures.

In Greece the first demographic studies that examined the issue of population under a more strictly technocratic perspective using indices and mea-

---

78 For the related discussion, see Sevasti Trubeta, *Physical Anthropology, Race and Eugenics in Greece (1880–1970s)* (Chicago: Brill, Balkan Studies Library, 2011): 207–23.

surements, i.e., the studies of Konstantinos Karanikas and Vasilios Valaoras, were published in the late 1930s.[79] In their publications Karanikas and Valaoras attempted to compare demographic changes in Greece and other countries to construct a developmental paradigm.[80] They were mainly interested in estimating the total change in population in conjunction with the European concerns about depopulation. They more or less reached the following conclusions: regarding fertility and mortality, demographic trends were not alarming with the exception of the period 1923–1925 due to the effects of the Asia Minor Disaster, and that Greece was demographically similar to other Balkan or Mediterranean countries.

The authors found that in the last decade the population of Greece had increased. As can be seen from the 1928 census, due to the settlement of refugees, the population increased from 5,017,000 to 6,204,000 residents. Between 1930 and 1935, marriages fluctuated from 44,000 to 47,000 a year and births between 199,000 and 208,000, with the exception of the two low years 1932 and 1933. Births followed an upward trend, while the mortality rate decreased. For example, in 1934, there were 31,2 births for every 10,000 residents, which was very close to that of Bulgaria (30) and Romania (32), while the respective index for Italy was 23.[81]

According to Valaoras, Greece was a particular case demographically speaking. The surplus of births after 1926 reached 50%, while mortality rates dropped to 15.9%. Such sudden change in demographic indices was observed only in Greece. He underlined that it was not a numerical influx but a different demographic trend. Valaoras suggested that the increased fertility in Greece was due to the refugee influx since the refugee population had much higher birth rates compared to native Greeks. Thus, it was the refugees that contributed to this "increasing vitality." In contrast with other

---

79 Vasilios Valaoras (1902–1996) had studied medicine at the medical school of Athens and was further trained in hygiene in Paris and London. He cooperated with Balfour in the anti-malaria campaign. At his instigation, he studied at the School of Hygiene in Athens. He also studied on a Rockefeller scholarship public hygiene and biostatistics at John Hopkins University. In 1939, he was elected reader in hygiene at the University of Athens. Later, in 1962 he became professor in the same seat and established the Center of Biometric Demographic Studies.

80 Scientific studies that looked into the development of demographic sizes in connection with the policy on births were first published during the dictatorship; their publication is indicative of the interest in similar issues developed in Greece. See Vasilios P. Valaoras, *To Dimografiko Provlima tis Ellados kai I Epidrasi ton Prosfygon* (Athens: 1939); Konstantinos Karanikas, *La Crise de la Population en Europe et les Données Démographiques de la Grèce* (Athens: éditions Flamma, 1937).

81 Valaoras, *To Dimografiko Provlima tis Ellados*, 123.

scholars, like Doxiadis, who in the 1920s had stressed the negative impact refugees had on the quality of the biological capital due to the hardships they had experienced, Valaoras clearly underlined the positive contribution of refugees to Greece.[82] He concluded that their influence was crucial for the "biological vitality of the race." His analysis of the demographics in the areas where refugees had settled confirmed that in these areas the fertility indices were higher. Thanks to the refugees' higher fertility, Greece climbed in the ranking of European countries with regard to fertility from the fourteenth to the fourth place between 1932 and 1936. "Youthful blood" streamed into the Greek population.[83] The surplus of births gave a feeling of safety. Compared to Sweden, the surplus of births in Greece was five times higher. Compared to Bulgaria and Yugoslavia it was almost the same.[84] The moral backwardness and the high number of large farming families had protected Greece, Karanikas claimed, from the problems other Western and Scandinavian European countries encountered. Karanikas expressed fears that that if the western European model, which argued the nuclear family, women's emancipation, abortions and smaller families, would be adopted in Greece would lead to the decline in births.

Karanikas and Valaoras concluded that in demographic terms Greece was South-Eastern European in its high birth and mortality rates. The latter was attributed to the high infant mortality. This is the reason why Metaxas's regime turned its attention not to increasing childbirth, as there was no such need, but lowering infant mortality. This is confirmed by doctors and state officials who considered infant mortality to be the main problem of the Greek population. Births were enough and could balance out mortality, but many infants died during their first year of life. This explains the concern about the biological quality of the race, referred to by Doxiadis. In 1934, the ratio of infant to general mortality was 23.3%, while in 1933 it was 21%, and only 20.5% in 1932. Approximately 25% of deaths were of infants below the age of one. Moreover, 12–15% of the live infants at birth died during the first year of their life. For instance, in 1932, 185,523 infants were

---

82   Valaoras, *To Dimografiko Provlima tis Ellados*, 56. Doxiadis's attitude was ambivalent. In 1939, in a lecture he delivered in the Parnassos Association, he supported that refugees were an element of fine biological quality despite his earlier reservations. See Anonymos, "Ai Dialexeis tou Tmimatos Propagandas tou Patriotikou Idrymatos," *To Paidi*, no. 54 (May 1939): 31.

83   Valaoras, *To Dimografiko Provlima tis Ellados*, 58.

84   Karanikas, *La Crise de la Population en Europe*, 20.

born, but 23,875 babies died during the first year, which was 12.9 % while the respective percentage for England was 6.5%, for Norway 4.6%, Bulgaria 15% and Yugoslavia 16.7%. Infant mortality dropped from 170 deaths per 1,000 live births in 1900 to 115 in the 1930s, but it still remained high in comparison with Western European countries where it had been under 100 since 1920.[85] In 1931–1935, the index for the Netherlands was 45 deaths per 1,000 live births, 45 for Norway, 78 for France, and 62 for England and Wales. Balkan countries were similar to Greece. In 1928, life expectancy was 49 years in Greece. In this respect, Greece was similar to its neighboring Balkan countries.

The authors estimated that a drop in births in Greece should be balanced by a decrease in mortality rates, especially among children and infants with mortality caused by starvation, dire hygiene conditions and the low crop yields.[86] Thus, whereas other countries emphasized increasing childbirth, Greece emphasized improving living conditions, securing better conditions for safe births in the countryside and the provision of facilities for the observation of children's health.

6. THE BALKAN CONGRESSES: FINDINGS AND PROSPECTS

As the demographic problems in Greece were similar to those in other Balkan countries, it was not accidental that the two Balkan congresses organized in 1936 and 1938 focused on the living conditions in the countryside and on the preparation of qualified medico-social staff who would help women, especially women farmers, improve hygiene and housing conditions to have safe childbirth. As the economies of these countries were mostly agricultural—the percentage of people engaged in agriculture ranged from 70 to 80%—the interest of their governments rested in a healthy agrarian population. Thus, governments of Balkan countries had started since the 1920s to examine how they could secure better reproduction conditions for the agricultural family in an effort to modernize agricultural infrastructure as

---

85   Hilary Marland, "The Medicalization of Motherhood: Doctors and Infant Welfare in the Netherlands, 1901–1930," in *Women and Children First. International Maternal and Infant Welfare, 1870–1945,* eds. Valerie Fildes, Lara Marks, and Hilary Marland (London and New York: Routledge, 1992), 74–96.

86   For Karanikas, the yield of land in connection with living conditions and the educational level of the agrarian family were very important for the development of demographic sizes. See Karanikas, *La Crise de la Population en Europe,* 47.

the yield of land and the density of the agricultural areas depended on the health of the agricultural family.

These congresses took place to inform social welfare experts in the Balkans about how their neighbors had dealt with similar problems and to find common solutions between them. The delegates of the congresses also wanted to benefit from the experience of delegates from international organizations. Participants included doctors, nurses, ministers and high-ranking officers of the Ministry of Health and Welfare, and delegates from international labor organizations, welfare and child protection organizations, women's associations, voluntary organizations, scientific associations and solidarity funds. The participation of the child protection associations that were affiliated with the International Union was instrumental.[87] M.J.C. van Notten, vice president of the Union Internationale de Secours aux Enfants, made reference in his inaugural speech to the inspiration for international children's aid organization, Englantyne Jebb. The idea of cooperation between the welfare organizations of the Balkan countries was supported by the diplomatic collaboration that had begun during the same period and resulted in the Balkan Pact in 1934.[88]

The first Balkan congress took place in Athens in 1936. Yet, the decision to hold it had been made four years earlier by members of the International Union for the Protection of Children. In the early 1930s, the Union promoted the idea of international cooperation between its members. Since 1928, the Union had increased its efforts outside Europe and in 1931 it organized the first international congress on African children.[89] The adop-

---

87 The international associations for the protection of childhood represented in these congresses were the Union International de Secours aux enfants, the Save the Children Fund, the Ligue des Sociétés des Croix Rouge, and the international youth associations: Alliance Internationale des Unions Chretiennes de Jeunes Filles (YWCA), Alliance International des Unions Chretiennes de Jeunes Gens (YMCA), and the international feminist organizations: Alliance international pour le Suffrage et Action Civique et Politique des Femmes and Conseil International des Femmes.

88 The convention signed on February 9, 1934 between Greece, Yugoslavia, Turkey and Romania aimed to reconcile their differences and establish peace in the wider vicinity. It also provided for the promotion of cultural exchanges between these countries.

89 For the action of the International Union between 1920 and 1940, see Anonymos, "Ta Eikosakhrona kai i Drasis tis Diethnous Enoseos pros Perithalpsin tou Paidiou," *To Paidi*, no. 62 (January 1940): 13. For the cooperation between local and international unions on child protection in the Balkans, see Kristina Popova, "Combatting Infant Mortality in Bulgaria. Welfare Activities, National Propaganda and the Establishment of Pediatrics 1900–1940," in *Health, Hygiene and Eugenics in Southeastern Europe to 1945*, eds. Christian Promitzer, S. Trubeta and M. Turda (Budapest: Central European University Press, 2011), 143–63.

tion of common approaches to social work took on a particular character in Balkan countries. Old national antagonisms and the economic crisis of 1930, which further strengthened the introversion, were major hurdles in overcoming national boundaries.[90] The members of the Greek branch of the International Union advocated international intellectual cooperation between agents, individuals and institutions from different countries and stressed the benefits drawn exchanging experiences. Greece, Bulgaria, and Yugoslavia played a particularly active role in the first Balkan congress, while Turkey, Romania and Albania were underrepresented. High-ranking officers from France, Great Britain, Germany, Belgium, Hungary and Latvia attended the congress. The organization of the congress by Greece was a chance for the government to publicize the work of public services and voluntary organizations for child protection. Delegates could visit the institutions and evaluate the progress they had achieved. In his inaugural speech, in a period of political unrest a few months after the imposition of the authoritarian regime, the Greek Minister of State Hygiene and Relief asked the congress to make a practical plan for the protection of children in the Balkan countries, but without moving away from the fundamental values of religion, family and tradition.

6.1 The Acculturation of Mothers in Rural Space

The problem of high infant and child mortality in the countryside was high in the agenda of both congresses. Most pediatricians and high-ranking officials who took part in them distinguished between urban and rural children and stressed the negative impact of state indifference towards the latter. In the first congress, the higher infant mortality in the countryside—twice that of towns—was attributed to the lack of safe labor and to ignorance of hygiene.[91] In contrast to the progress achieved in urban areas where there were centers for the protection of mothers and children, the countryside lagged behind in the medicalization of birth. The strain on mothers in the countryside and the primitive conditions they lived in, the absence of mid-

---

90 Konstantinos Saroglou, "Anagki Diethnous Synergasias dia tin Prostasian tis Mitrotitos kai tou Paidiou," *To Paidi*, no. 37–38 (May-August 1936): 58–70.
91 Union Internationale de Secours Aux Enfants, *Congrès Balkaniques de la Protection de l'Enfance*, Premier Congrès (Athens: April 5–9, 1936).

wifes and prenatal consultation stations combined with the general moral backwardness accounted for the high numbers of premature births.[92]

In his paper, pediatrician Konstantinos Saroglou, drawing mainly on empirical knowledge, argued that the infections of umbilical cord and tetanus of the infants caused by the fact that births occurred in places where animals lived, led to high infant mortality in the Greek countryside.[93] Many houses were just one room hovels, with no floor, where people and animals lived together. There were no consultation centers for expectant mothers in the countryside and despite the efforts for the establishment of midwifery schools, most midwifes were empirical, dirty and superstitious. Saroglou attributed the lack of nursing knowledge to mothers' illiteracy, superstitions and her low social status in the countryside. Due to the lack of transportation and the long distances between villages, it was impossible for doctors to observe infants as was the case in urban centers. Farmers' ignorance and the rough way they treated their children accounted for the high child mortality and exhausting child labor, which in turn resulted in high numbers of men not being able to join the army. Children fell victim to superstition, isolation and backwardness.

Most delegates at the first Balkan congress, mainly pediatricians and obstetricians, highlighted the need to "acculturate" the agricultural family so that they would cooperate with doctors. For instance, Solon Veras examined the possibility of appointing nurses to instruct expectant mothers in hygiene and Konstantinos Saroglou proposed offsetting up makeshift consultation centers in the capital of each prefecture. Visiting nurses would go about the villages once a week to see whether doctors' instructions were being followed. Because establishing small maternity units led to financial problems, Saroglou suggested that storage rooms with sterilized material for births be built, which would be taken to the houses by the nurses since empirical midwifes lacking in sterilization skills ignored the risks involved. He also suggested that nurses visit new mothers in the first week following

92 Aristotelis Koutsoumaris, ex director of the Criminal Investigation Department of Athens, supported that the impressions formed about the condition of social welfare for children in the first Balkan congress did not correspond to reality since the sick, poor and delinquent child was not the subject of state welfare, see Aristotelis Koutsoumaris, "I Koinoniki Pronoia gia tin Prostasia tou Paidiou ston Topo mas," *To Paidi*, no. 41 (January-February 1937): 5–17.

93 Konstantinos Saroglou, "I Prostasia tou Paidiou stin Ypaithro Khora," *To Paidi*, no. 39–40 (September-December 1936): 5–17.

delivery with an assistant to clean and care for the farmer's house. Doxiadis also put forward the idea of extending social insurance benefits to farmers and the idea of educating female teachers in hygiene, as was the case in other Balkan countries. He further proposed the number of midwives, nurses and polyclinics be increased. In addition, some pediatricians argued that the family structure of Balkan countries, women's inferiority and the interference of relatives in raising infants accounted for the high infant mortality.[94] They also stressed that removing close relatives was important to instruct mothers that it was their exclusive responsibility to raise their children. Congress delegates also attributed the backwardness of the farmers to the fact that Balkan governments were negligent in adopting supportive measures. In their conclusions, delegates emphasized the necessity of passing legislation on the protection of children. They also argued for the general, social and hygiene instruction of the lower classes. They also suggested that children born out of wedlock be taken care of by families rather than at institutions. Besides, they proposed building more soup kitchens, summer camps and nurseries and that school hygiene be reinforced, especially in rural areas. They were unanimous in improving the health of rural children and the financial condition of mothers working in the fields.

The second Balkan congress took place in Belgrade in October 1938 in an anxious atmosphere as the war neared. Delegates from various western countries presented the progress accomplished in children's welfare, and referenced its political consequences. The Italian representative, Marquise Medici del Vacello, referred emphatically to the role of the Italian fascist party and especially of women in organizing aid for children in rural areas.[95]

Although it was suggested that zones of safety be established for children during wartime, the emphasis once more was laid on protecting children in the countryside. This time, however, more complete propositions were put forward to organize aid for rural families. The protection of rural children was linked to the poor economic condition of the countryside due to the effects the economic crisis had on agriculture. The representative of the International Bureau of Work, George Thelin, referred to the work ac-

---

94 For the views on the backwardness of the agricultural society in the Balkans, see *Congrès Balkaniques, Premier Congrès*, 57–67.

95 *Deuxième Congrès Balkanique de la Protection de l'Enfance, Compte Rendu, Belgrade*, October 1–7, 1938, Union Internaltionale de Secours Aux Enfants (Genève: 1939), 56–61.

complished by a permanent committee for the protection of the working child in rural areas while the representative of the International Union for the Protection of Children, Jan Harm Tuntler, stressed that planning protection in the countryside should take many factors into account such as the economic, social and hygiene conditions of the area, the geographical conditions that affected crop yield and consequently nutrition, means of transport and distances.

Resorting to solutions adopted by other western countries for the protection of countryside children, Tuntler looked into how these could be applied in the Balkan countries. At a demographic level, he suggested that the precise causes of infant mortality in each area be explored different agencies collaborate with one another. Tuntler contended that the village health center should be the site of primary action.[96] He further argued that medical work should be combined with social work, especially regarding nutrition, food conservation, housing, clothing, nurseries, public baths, drinkable water, summer camps for children, games and sports. The protection of children was not disassociated from the village's economic and social welfare at large. Therefore, the protection of children in the countryside was contingent on the farmers' health, education and material welfare.[97]

Bulgarian and Yugoslav delegates at the second Balkan congress referred to the everyday life conditions of the farming woman and to infant mortality. Doctors and the state officials spoke of the cultural characteristics of the agricultural societies, the role of gender and the work of women in the fields. For the very first time they spoke of the husband's role in the family. The medical conseiller (medical consultant) of the Central Institute of Hygiene in Belgrade, Dr V. Yvkovitch, argued that infant mortality was higher in plains than in mountainous areas because poor farming mothers whose families had small holdings were forced to work in the fields of the rich landowners far from their villages, leaving their children alone, in contrast with the mountainous areas where mothers used to take their children with them.[98] The Bulgarian pediatrician G. Tabakoff referred to the unequal

---

96 He distinguished between primary health centers addressed to mothers and infants, staffed with visiting nurses, midwifes and assistant-midwives who would undertake instruction, and secondary health centers which would include polyclinics for the treatment of students and the training of nurses and doctors, *Deuxième Congrès Balkanique de la Protection de l'Enfance*, 58.

97 *Deuxième Congrès Balkanique de la Protection de l'Enfance*, 76–82.

98 *Deuxième Congrès Balkanique de la Protection de l'Enfance*, 93.

division of work between the farming couple, the husband's despotic behavior and women's exhaustion due to many births.[99] Therefore, the improvement of the child's place required the improvement of the woman's position and the instruction of men in their paternal duties.[100] Tabakoff suggested a committee be set up in each village to educate mothers in child-rearing and protecting their children from alcoholic fathers. The experience of female teachers in Bulgaria who had undertaken the instruction of mothers brought to light the hardships women went through, venereal diseases and alcoholism among men.

Everyone agreed that the instruction of mothers in hygiene would play an instrumental role in the modernization of the family. Feminist delegates to the congress stressed that mothers and fathers had equal rights and commitments, a view that required the preparation of men for the paternal role. Most delegates supported that it was necessary for each country to pass a law for the protection of children to pool resources derived from special taxation: i.e., from taxing inheritance or the childless. These taxes would go to a special fund, the National Fund for the Protection of the Child, which would be managed autonomously. The proposal for the establishment in each country of a central organization for the protection of the child with local provincial branches, following the model of the Italian Foundation for Motherhood, gained ground. A lengthy discussion was held about the make-shift consultation centers, the portable hygiene exhibitions and the maternity clinics in the countryside. These maternity clinics were considered insufficient if not run by permanent staff who would conduct systematic work over a long time period to build up steady relationships with mothers. On the contrary, the proposal for the establishment of a medical center to meet the needs of the rural population in general was most welcome. This medical center would be the central organ of the local committee for the protection of the child and would be staffed with a visiting nurse who specialized in many fields and a doctor further trained for this work.

The delegates reached the conclusion that women in the Balkans were very fertile, but lacked good advice during pregnancy, labor and the first

---

99   According to the research of Bulgarian agronomists, women were already exhausted by the first births while men worked for 96 days per year maximum.

100 It was suggested lectures for prospective fathers be delivered to the army and awards be handed out; the same went for mothers.

months of the infant's life. As a result, mothers' mortality rate was high and they had many diseases due to the unhygienic birth conditions. The discussion about the medicalization of birth centered on the training of suitable medico-social staff. Although the mode of training varied from country to country, the distinction between qualified staff and empirical midwifes, especially in the provinces, was generally accepted.[101] The visiting nurses were expected to be well educated and have the ability to establish trust with mothers, while midwifes could be young village girls who after intensive practical training in obstetrics, infant nutrition and child protection generally could be hired by the community to offer their services to female farmers during pregnancy and the first months after birth.[102] According to Kharitakis,[103] midwifes of peasantry origin with poor education had more chances to be accepted by the farmer's family in contrast with qualified midwifes who were considered suitable for the urban environment. As far as the doctors' education was concerned, the congress suggested that Balkan medical schools increase students' practical training in pediatric and maternity clinics, and that local community doctors attend compulsory lessons at the school of health and do their practicum at a model center for six weeks.

In the discourse of doctors and high ranking state officials of the regime who were responsible for drawing up social policy, the backward ideas and primitive living and hygiene conditions of farmers, were decried, as was the subordinate place of female farmers. The education of rural mothers in hygiene was considered crucial for the improvement of the biological capital of rural children. Under the pressure of traditional patriarchal structures, it was difficult for doctors and visiting nurses to approach mothers, and accept the influence of science. Despite the grand promises, the regime did not adopt effective measures for farmers to overcome chronic weaknesses, feudal vestiges and technical backwardness. The regime attempted to improve the condition of women with no expenses whatsoever; only advice was provided to husbands so as to change their attitude towards their wives. As a

---

101 The School of Visiting Nurses of the Greek Red Cross which operated since 1924 offered two options for the study of midwifery; the first after two years of study accredited primary school graduates with practical midwife while the second after three years of study led to the degree of the skilled midwife offered to high school (gymnasium) graduates.

102 *Deuxième Congrès Balkanique de la Protection de l'Enfance*, 143.

103 Kostis Kharitakis, "To Provlima tis Maias idia eis tas Agrotikas Periokhas. Dynatai I Maia na Ekteli kai Ergon Adelfis Episkeptrias?" *Arkheia Ygieinis* 3, no. 6 (June 1939): 248–51.

result women's exhaustion, which was destructive for the regime's demographic aims, could be avoided. In spite of its propaganda and criticism levelled at Greek farmers, the regime did not have an effective social policy for rural mothers.

CONCLUSION

The questions raised at the end of the nineteenth century by doctors, social thinkers and state officials in relation to the Greek state's indifference to the medical supervision of children were inscribed in a wider discussion on hygiene and improvement of the body, which were prevalent across many European societies in the last quarter of the century. The progress achieved in microbiology and its contribution to the fight against certain epidemics, the attempts to sanitize cities, the enhancement of doctors' position, as well as the emergence of a wider hygiene movement shaped the conditions that made it possible for European states to adopt policies on contagious diseases and disseminate the principles of hygiene among the public.

This raising of awareness of hygiene concurred along with wider changes in the perceptions of childhood. During this period, childhood becomes the age category which most claimed the attention of the state. This state protection of children was necessitated not only by the concerns raised by dire mortality rates, but also by a desire to save "the seed" and by feelings of national inferiority that were fed by the projection of sickly children in the future.

War reverberations heightened the interest in improving children's health at the end of the nineteenth and the beginning of the twentieth century. It was not accidental then that during this period an attempt was made for the first time in medical discourse to link the high rates of physically incapable conscripts with high rates of student morbidity. The first studies on school age children revealed the high number of pupils who suffered from conditions caused by school attendance such as myopia, scoliosis, headaches, and fatigue and from conditions like tuberculosis and adenopathy. In addition, the rates of infant mortality, which remained high until the end of the nineteenth century, led to an international infant welfare movement whose goal was to educate mothers and establish consultation centers (gouttes de lait). Campaigns to make mothers aware of their maternal duties did so by trying to eradicate the traditional views on child-rearing. The importance attached to the health of their children is evident in that the first congresses on eugenics dealt with the medical supervision of children. At the end of the nineteenth and at the beginning of the twentieth century, nationalism, physical vigor and the improvement of the condition of children's health were closely linked.

The institutionalization of the first school hygiene services and the foundation of the first paedological laboratories in Western Europe were presented by state officials and doctors as a model to emulate. Large scale welfare services for children, the operation of nurseries, and most importantly the spread of school hygiene services were all the outcome of a combination of factors: the growing influence of the medical elite in the public sphere, the work of voluntary organizations, the state's adoption of policies that aimed at growing and improving the population, the acculturation of the public to hygiene and the preparation of a strong race.

In Greece three factors played a crucial role in the growing awareness of children's health problems at the beginning of the twentieth century: the reports of the school officers that brought to light the high rates of children who suffered from various diseases; the medical studies carried out on school students especially in relation to tuberculosis; and the regular articles featured in pedagogical and medical journals, which tended to highlight the danger of degeneration among youth. In the medical discourse of the early twentieth century school was pointed to as a dangerous place not only for children, but also for the future of the nation. Mental fatigue, the unhygienic condition of most school buildings and the high number of students that carried the bacillus of tuberculosis were considered the most important risks for the degeneration of youth. In their discourse on the vulnerability of children, doctors shaped a field that legitimized their intervention in the public sphere. The frequency of publications related to the health of children ought to be examined in parallel with the strengthening of doctors' presence in the public sphere, the organization of Pan-Hellenic medical congresses, the publication of scientific journals and the establishment of medical societies.

By stressing the impact the school environment had on children's health and the health of the nation and considering its role instrumental in the progress achieved in school medical inspection by neighboring Balkan countries, physicians and educators intentionally fuelled national fears to highlight state indifference. The arguments they deployed were inscribed in a traditional nationalist rhetoric that developed in the last quarter of the nineteenth century, which presented neighboring countries as lagging behind Greece culturally. Due to its historical past and its contribution to the development of the Western European culture, Greece appeared to be superior to its neighbors. Seen through this lens, the doctors utilized national antagonisms to make apparent the necessity for modernizing public health. Thus, at the turn of the century, doctors and social thinkers pressured the government to draw policies that would control and improve the physical health of children.

Our study revealed the importance war had on heightening people's collective fears that led to the formulation of measures for the medical inspection of childhood in Greece. First and foremost, the Greek defeat in the Greco-Turkish War in 1897, revealed the issue of children's health and paved the way for the first laws on school hygiene. Greece's participation in World War I, the Asia Minor Disaster and most importantly the influx of refugees were the turning point in the history of children's medical care. As was the case in other countries, the postwar period in Greece changed the way health was approached. The intensification of the social problems and the deterioration of working-class living conditions, especially in cities, after 1922, made the reorganization of public health imperative. To achieve this aim the Greek government resorted to international organizations for help. The rise in infant mortality and the lack of consultation centers in particular made the necessity for state policy on mothers and children obvious so as to repair the war's damage and improve the quality of the biological capital. Finally, the atmosphere of intense war preparation on the eve of World War II did not leave the policy of Metaxas's dictatorship on children's health unaffected.

Over the span of the fifty years, covered in this study, we followed the many political meanings attached to children's care. The central place reserved for the child in the state social policy became more evident in the interwar period. This happened for two reasons: firstly, population policy became more important and was linked with policy on family and births; and secondly, youth occupied a more prominent place in different political ideologies. The measures that the Venizelos government took at the end of the 1920s and the authoritarian 4th of August regime's policy illustrate two characteristic phases of state policy regarding children's welfare. Both governments articulated a child-centered discourse that linked the improvement of the conditions for child-rearing with increasing productivity and improving national defense. For Venizelos's liberal government, the children's care was the basis of its health policy. The establishment of modern institutions specially designated for children, as well as the collaboration of Greek agencies with international organizations created in the spirit of the Geneva Declaration were the main directions liberal policy took in the 1920s and 1930s. In the case of the Metaxas dictatorship, children's care was crucial for the legitimization of the regime. For this reason we examined it together with the regime's general policies and with its establishment of a national youth organization.

Our research points to the continuities and discontinuities of the efforts undertaken either in relation to school hygiene by state agencies or in relation to the protection of children and mothers by voluntary societies in collaboration with the state. Although many issues in the history of children's health remain unexplored—both due to the lack of sources and to the nature of the questions raised—we mainly attempted to provide the context in which these efforts took place; to detect the scope and the limits of these efforts as well as their impact on fighting disease and on the understanding of health itself.

As has already been stressed, circumstances improved at the beginning of the twentieth century enough that the Greek state could adopt the first measures for children's welfare. In an attempt to periodize state policy in this sector, three phases that are linked to wider social and political changes can be distinguished. The first measures for the formulation of school hygiene were inscribed within the efforts made by the liberal governments to modernize the state in the 1910s. We examined these efforts, which had been made by doctors and educators intervening in the public sphere in the previous decade, in correlation with the contemporary reform in education and legislation on the improvement of work conditions. 1914 to 1920 were critical for the School Hygiene Service. Sixty school doctors and health officers who staffed the twelve educational districts had to meet a wide array of duties from defining the requirements of the building and inspecting school premises, to controlling students and protecting them against contagious diseases. The protection of children could be achieved by means of mass vaccination and the spread of hygienic habits, but mainly through the inspection and recording of measurable evidence for the physical health of children.

The statistics of student morbidity revealed the extent of the spread of infectious diseases among students as well as the indifference with which parents regarded doctors' advice. According to these statistics, the spread of infectious diseases, the outbreaks of children's diseases and various epidemics were the main characteristics of student health in the early twentieth century. Despite the efforts made by successive Greek governments, the rates of students that fell prey to tuberculosis, malaria and trachoma remained high until the mid-twentieth century.

Although the high rates of morbidity and mortality pointed to the dire living conditions of the working-class, doctors in the early twentieth century stressed instead the importance of hygiene education for the working-class, highlighting the responsibility of the individual not only for their health but also for the health of the others. From this perspective, the medical discourse of the early twentieth century bears similarities to the discourse of the philanthropists as regarded the moralization of the working-class. Hygiene instruction in schools was a method for educating the working-class family in hygiene, a method that worked complementarily with other measures such as the inspection of students' individual hygiene, the distribution of popular leaflets for the fight against contagious diseases and the instruction of women in the principles of "scientific motherhood." Due to meagre funding for health care and the low level of medical knowledge, hygiene policies focused on popularizing hygienic principles, as was the case in other countries. The cooperation of doctors with poor families was of crucial importance for the success of preventative methods and therefore for the consent or even for the instruction of the patient, in other words on aspects of human relations that had to be cultivated or modified to facilitate the contact of scientists with the illiterate. If doctors had not earned the trust of the lower class, preventive measures would have had a limited effect. A series of changes in cultural health practices were a prerequisite for the penetration of doctors into the private sphere. Due to the immense size of the public, schools made the spread of these practices possible.

The bureaucracy that funneled into the School Hygiene Service proved useful on many levels. First of all, it contributed to the planning of hygiene policies fighting epidemics. Knowledge of statistics and the detection of the primary carriers of infection were of the utmost importance for controlling the spread of disease. On the other hand, recording students' physical data on individual health cards led to the classification of bodies by health, drawing for the first time a line between health and disease, as well as determining the normal pace at which the mind and body of the child should develop. In an effort to medicalize childhood in schools, medical officers derived their practices from military medicine or from the scientific organization of industrial work as the body of the child was perceived in relation to the future performance of its biological capital. The medical discourse and the measurements of the child body contributed to growing eugenic concerns and to stereotypes about the physiology of the sexes. The imposition of a physical culture of childhood extended into mental health, diet, exercise and individual hygiene. The tools used for the inspection and discipline to the commands of a bio-political power point to the total control of the body-as-machine.

Despite the expectations for the first school hygiene institutions, they did not bring the expected results due to limited state funding. School doctors understood that without welfare institutions that could treat students and given the financial inability of many families to cover the cost of treatment, the spread of contagious diseases was a given. The solution was to resort to philanthropy. The cooperation of the Ministry of Education with the Patriotic League of Greek Women, set up on the initiative of Queen Sofia during World War I to offer aid to the families of conscripts, was an attempt to fill the gap. In 1915 the League responded to the request of the School Hygiene Service's director to establish student polyclinics, an open-air school and summer camps which would treat the sick children of Athens and strengthen their constitution. For the success of these institutions high-ranking state officials, female volunteers, doctors and educators cooperated to implement modern medico-pedagogical methods, which they had become familiar with while studying in Western Europe. Questions were raised regarding the range and the effectiveness of these efforts for the health of the urban working-class in a period when a system of social insurance was yet to be introduced.

A few years later, in 1917, Venizelos's government dissolved the royalist voluntary association of the Patriotic League to replace it with a semi-state foundation for the protection of mothers and children, widening its responsibilities to include birth, infant care and the instruction of women in their maternal duties. These institutional changes illustrate the extent to which welfare was politicized during this period. Despite the Foundation's instability during the National Schism, it gradually became the main institution for social policy on mothers and children, while maintaining the characteristics of a mixed welfare economy. Its operation was based on state and private funding, as well as on the cooperation among state officials, doctors and urban, upper-class women who worked as volunteers.

Around 1920, the conditions had improved enough that the Greek state could undertake children's care more efficiently. Success in foreign affairs and the increase of the population in the aftermath of World War I, as new regions had been annexed to the national territory, posed the issue of modernizing state public health policy in accordance with progress made in Europe. The law establishing the Ministry of Health and Social Welfare, to which all health services would belong, did not pass because of the influx of refugees. The political and social upheavals brought about by the Asia Minor Disaster in 1922 made it impossible for children's state welfare to come full circle. Yet, the foundations for a future approach had been laid.

The spread of contagious diseases, the drop in births, the increase in infant mortality, and the curbs on government spending on school hygiene vividly illustrate the strained atmosphere that characterized the 1920s. However, despite the numerous difficulties faced by the state and the political upheavals of the period, policy makers continued to explore solutions inspired by developments in public health in the postwar period. Greece did not remain unaffected by the important changes that came about in public health internationally. It was mainly affected by three trends: the turn of medical interest to the social analysis of health, which led to the standardization of individual and public health; the creation of international health organizations that spread hygiene models internationally and reformed the health systems in various countries; and the increase of biological concerns involved in interwar national antagonisms. Eugenic concerns fed into the

discussion about the quality of the nation's biological capital, thus contributing to the ever growing involvement of the state in health issues related to
citizens. Either as a national or as a social issue, health became an index of
prime importance for the interwar policy.

Despite the discontinuities in the first years after the arrival of the refugees, the work accomplished in the medical inspection of children during
the last Venizelos's government (1928–1932) lightened the negative atmosphere of the period. The foundation of institutions for children's health,
which took into account the social dimensions of health, signified the interest the Liberals took in completing the modernization attempts they
had undertaken during the 1910s. The establishment of summer camps
and school meals in the 1930s was inscribed in the larger efforts to curb the
high rates of student tuberculosis in the light of the newer more sociological interpretations of the disease. The law on the protection of childhood
and the transformation of the Patriotic Foundation of Welfare into the Patriotic Foundation for the Protection of the Child, which had the sole aim
of protecting motherhood and childhood, were inscribed within the same
context. Staffed with eminent pediatricians, the Patriotic Foundation promoted programmes that laid the foundations for the instruction of women
in scientific motherhood. These pediatricians, who were members of international societies for the protection of children, devised new tools of observation, recording and technical control of families, and began new ways of
collaboration between the doctors and their patients. They adopted modern means of approaching mothers i.e., the Child's Week and health prizes
for the healthiest babies which had already been successfully introduced in
other countries. They promoted the professionalization of health care with
the gradual replacement of female volunteers by professional social workers.
The latter attempted to get into the private lives of their subjects to record
and guide their behavior. The medicalization of birth, the observation of infants and visiting nurses were some of the methods used to approach working-class families.

Despite the concerns voiced by some pediatricians about the racial degeneration of youth and the low biological quality of refugees, the discussion about eugenics in the 1920s revolved around heredity, the decrease in
infant mortality and the diffusion of scientific knowledge about birth and
child-rearing among the population. Most of them were not in favor of neg-

ative eugenic measures. Since they considered high infant mortality to be the most serious problem the Greek race faced, the discussion focused on more mild means such as securing better conditions for childbirth, better child-reading, and the inspection of children's mental and physical health. Reservations were expressed by some pediatricians about sterilization and compulsory prenuptial health certification because of the limits posed by the human rights and the ethics of the medical profession, which dictated discretion in the management of the citizens' personal data. Proposals inspired by fascist states, such as the one by Apostolos Doxiadis, minister of Hygiene and president of the Patriotic Foundation for the Protection of the Child, for the creation of a biological data bank and the taxation of the unmarried were examined by the government, but did not materialize. On the contrary, more consent was granted for instructing couples in their biological duties and for the optional use of prenuptial health certification. In the 1930s hygiene propaganda was extended to the field of sexual relations.

Like other authoritarian regimes of the period, the 4th of August regime laid great emphasis on social policy for children's health, seeking to reap multiple benefits from its application. Although one can detect much resemblance with Venizelos's policy Ioannis Metaxas tried to make his policy seem different. The welfare policy he adopted was presented as a rupture with the past and was meant to make the regime appear radical and legitimize its overthrow of democracy. The "New State" was represented in propaganda as a new start for Greece, a different system both from the liberal state, which had been indifferent to the interests of the working-class, and from communism, which took advantage of this indifference to seize power. Stressing his interest for the health of the people, Metaxas tried to gain a strong foothold among the working-class, which he needed. In addition, the creation of a robust youth was linked to the cultural superiority of Greece and its long standing history. The establishment of the national youth organization (EON) in which a large number of children and adolescents participated was the most obvious manifestation of Metaxas's interest in children and a characteristic it shared with other interwar fascist regimes.

In the four years of Metaxas's dictatorship there was a trend of the state's increasing involvement in social welfare. The centralization of services, the planning of social policy by Metaxas himself, a series of regulations meant to change the landscape of health care, the restrictions on the action of volunteers and the formation of hospital and institutional boards that comprised members loyal to Metaxas were some of the changes that point to the transition towards a personal-centered perception of power. Faith in the regime was taken for granted not only for the ones involved in the administration of the welfare institutions but also for its recipients.

Mothers and children were central to the regime's regenerative efforts as these two groups were thought to be connected to the nation's biological and historical continuity. However, the emphasis was placed on the health of children rather than the protection of mothers. The establishment of sanatoriums, children's athletic and welfare centers and the spread of school meals and summer camps absorbed majority of funds allotted to social welfare as a whole. Although the decline in infant mortality was among the goals of the regime, its policy on mothers was limited to the establishment of a few nurseries and a maternity clinic in Athens. Instead, the regime emphasized educating mothers on their duties to their children and to the race. Although many elements of social policy were derived from fascist Italy, the regime did not take measures to increase Greece's population. Neither did it adopt a family policy on providing young couples with incentives, as it did not share the same demographic concerns as fascist Italy.

The regime's emphasis on improving the position of mothers in rural areas did not translate into securing better conditions for childbirth and introducing new institutions for the welfare of mothers. The institutions in the capital adsorbed the lion's share of the state funding. The lack of policy on state allowances or maternity benefits aligned with the regime's general financial policy regarding farmers and the working-class, and was characterized by rhetorical flourishes and a lack of substantial help. In reality, projects for the protection of children proved to be more useful for the regime's goals. The ideological inculcation of children in the ranks of the National Youth Organization and the social welfare projects intended for children were meant to cement Metaxas's bonds with children. In other words, it was through youth that the dictator attempted to fulfil his dream for the country's cultural and racial regeneration.

PRIMARY SOURCES AND BIBLIOGRAPHY

Primary Sources

1. (Archives)

1) Apostolos Doxiadis's Archive, files no. 2, 3, 7, 8, 9, 10, 11, 16, 17, 18, 19, 20, 21, 22, 23, 24. *The Benaki Museum's Historical Archives.*
2) Emmanouil Benaki's Archive, file no. 9. *The Benaki Museum's Historical Archives.*
3) Eleftherios Venizelos's Archive, files no. 74, 131–135. *The Benaki Museum's Historical Archives*
4) Alexandros Koryzis's Archive, files no. 16, 21, 23, 24, 25, 26. *The Benaki Museum's Historical Archives.*
5) Emmanouil Lambadarios's Archive, unclassified. *Hellenic Literary and Historical Archive (ELIA).*
6) Archive of the Ministry of Social Welfare, unclassified, *Hellenic Literary and Historical Archive (ELIA).*
7) Elefterios Venizelos's Archive, I/S, *Ekthesis Pepragmenon tis eis tin Konstantinoupolin kai Ponton Apostolin tou Patriotikou Idrymatos Perithalpseos, Athens, May 20, 1919,* Ypourgeion Pronoias [Ministry of Welfare] 1919. *Hellenic Literary and Historical Archive (ELIA).*
8) Archive of the Technical Service of the Ministry of Education, Series: architectural plans and statistics, 1929 Nomikos's Buildings in Patisia, Ypaithrio Scholeio para ti Skholi Evelpidon [Open air school near Evelpidon school], file no. 540. *General State Archives (GAK).*
9) Mathitika Syssitia [Soup kitchens], files no. 1093–1094. *General State Archives.*
10) Khatzipanagiotou Archive, file 46 (ΠΙΚΠΑ Oreinai Paidikai Exokhai Pentelis, 1937–1938) [Summer schools on Mountain Penteli]. *Architectural Archives of Benaki Museum.*
11) Nikolas Tzelepis's Archive, file no. 445 (1938–1940) *Architectural Archive of Benaki Museum.*
12) Ioannis Metaxas's Archive, *General State Archives (GAK).*

2. Newspapers

Athinai, 1916.
Akropolis, 1911–1914, 1936.
Asty, 1903–1906.
Ethnos, 1916.
Eleftheron Vima, 1927–1932.
I Elliniki, 1928.

Embros, 1908.
Efimeris tis Etairias tis Ygieinis, 1884.
Kathimerini, 1935.
Pamprosfygiki, 1925–1928.
Patris, 1928.
Prosfygikos Kosmos, 1926–1928.

3. Journals

In Greek

Arkheia Iatrikis, 1912, 1915–1917, 1922.
Arkheia Ygieinis, 1936–1939.
O Agonas tis Gynaikas, 1923–1936.
Dimosia Ygieini, 1931.
Dimotiki Ekpaidefsis, 1899–1904.
Ethniki Agogi, 1897–1903.
Ekpaideftiki Epitheorisis, 1917–1920.
Ellniki Iatriki, 1927–1928.
Ellinis, 1921–1934.
Ergasia, (M. Papamavrou), 1923–1924.
Ergasia, 1930–1935
Erythros Stavros Neotitos, 1925–1932.
Iatriki Epitheorisis, 1918–1920.
Iatriki, 1926–1928.
Kliniki, 1925–1928.
Nea Agogi, 1922.
Neolaia, 1938–1940.
Skholiki Praxi, 1927–1928.
Skholiki Ygieini, 1936–1939.
To Paidi, 1930–1944.
To Neon Kratos, 1937–1940.
Paidologia, 1920–1921.
Iatrika Khronika, 1928–1935.
Ygeia, 1924– 1931.
Ygeionomikos Kosmos, 1931.

In French

La Médecine Scolaire, 1909–1914.
L'Hygiène Scolaire, 1906–1920.

4. Congress Proceedings and Bulletins of Scientific Societies and Public Services

Deltion tou Ypourgeiou ton Ekklisiastikon kai tis Dimosias Ekpaidefseos, 1919–1924.
Deltio tou Ekpaideftikou Omilou, 1912, 1913, 1920.
Deltion tou Patriotikou Syndesmou ton Ellinidon 1916–1917.
Ygeionomikon Deltion Iatrosynedriou 1919–1920.
Praktika tis Akadimias Athinon 1926–1935.
Praktika tis Anthropologikis Etaireias 1925–1932.
Praktika Iatrikis Etaireias Athinon 1926–1932.
Praktika tou A΄ Panhelliniou Synedriou kata tis Phymatioseos, May 6–10, 1909. Athens: 1909.

Praktika tou B' Panhelliniou Synedriou kata tis Phymatioseos, May 20–23, 1912. Athens: 1912.
Praktika Synedriou Prostasias tis Mitrotitos kai ton Paidikon Ilikion. Athens: 1930.
Congrès Balkanique de la Protection de l' Enfance, Premier Congrès, Athènes, April 5–9, 1936. Athens: 1936.
Deuxième Congrès Balkanique de la Protection de l'Enfance, Compte Rendu, Belgrade, Octobre 1–7, 1938. Genève: 1939.

5. Special Publications

Ektheseis ton kata to 1883 pros Epitheorisin ton Dimotikon Skholeion Apestalmenon Ektakton Epitheoriton. Athens: n.d.
Ekpaideftika Nomoskhedia I. Aitiologiki Ekthesis kai Agorefseis peri Dimotikis Ekpaidefseos. Athens: 1899.
Ekthesis ton Pepragmenon en to Oikonomiko Syssitio. Apo tin 1h Ianouariou eos tin 31h Dekemvriou 1905. Athens: 1906.
Katastatikon tis Etaireis Ygieinis en Athinais. Athens: Typografika Katastimata Tsaousoglou, 1916.
Patriotikos Syndesmos Ellinidon, Etkthesis ton Pepragmenon ypo tou Tmimatos tis Ygieinis, etos 1915. Athens: 1916.
Patriotikos Syndesmos Ellinidon, I Paidiki Exokhi Falirou, Theros 1921. Athens: 1922.
Efimeris ton Syzitiseon tis Voulis, B' Dipli Anatheoritiki Vouli 1911, vol. 1, 1051–52.
Ta Pepragmena kata to Skholikon Etos 1914–1915, ypo Ioanni Fassaneli, Skholiatrou A' Ekpaideftikis Perifereias. Athens: 1915.
Eniafsia Ekthesis peri tis Ygieinis Katastaseos ton Skholeion, ypo Akhillea Armodiou, Skholiatrou IB' Ekpedeftikis Perifereias. Athens: 1918.
Etisia Ekthesis tou Ygeionomikou Epitheoritou Khristou Georgakopoulou, Skholiatrou D' Ekpedeftikis Perifereias, 1923–1924. Athens: 1924.
Etisia Ekthesis tis Ypiresias Skholikis Ygieinis. Athens: 1926–1927.
Etisia Ekthesis ton Pepramgenon tis Ygeionomikis Ypiresias ton Skholeion A' Ekpaideftikis Perifereias dia to Skholikon Etos 1927–1928, ypo L.N. Khristopoulou. Athens: 1928.
Ekthesis ton Pepragmenon tou Patriotikou Idrymatos Koinonikis Pronoias kai Antilipseos, 1934–1935 kai 1935–1936. Athens: 1938.
Panellinios Syndesmos kata tis Phymatioseos (Phthiseos), Logodosia 1918. Athens: 1919.
Panellinios Syndesmos kata tis Phymatioseos. Ta ypo tou Syndesmou Pepragmena (1h Ianouariou-31h Dekemvriou 1919). Athens: 1920.
Diagramma Katapolemiseos tou Trakhomatos eis ta Skholeia. Athens: 1925.
Ta Pepragmena tis Ygeionomikis Ypiresias tou Ypourgeiou ton Esoterikon kata tin Dekaetian 1911–1921, ypo K.N. Kyriazidou. Athens: 1929.
I Etisia Ekthesis peri tis Ygieinis Katastaseos ton Skholeion. Skhedion Organoseos tis Skholiatrikis Ypiresias, 1926–1927. Athens: 1927.
Praktika ton Synedriaseon tis Voulis. Athens: 1929.
L'Organisation d'Hygiène de la Société des Nations. Genève: 1923.

Special Publications of Ministries and Organisations

Dodekalogos Paidikis Exokhis Patriotikou Idrymatos Prostasias tou Paidiou, n.d.
O Dromos pros tin Ygeian. Athens: Greka, 1930,
I Phymatiosis. Athens: Syllogos pros Diadosin Ofelimon Vivlion, 1906.
Ygieini tou Mathitou. Athens: Erythros Stavros Neotitos, 1928.
Ypourgeio Ygieinis, Pos Prepei na Ziseis gia na Therapefteis. Athens: 1930.
Kanonismos Mathitikon Syssition. Athens: 1938.
Ekpaideftika Nomoskhedia Ypovlithenta eis tin Voulin ton Ellinon ypo tou epi ton Ekklisiastikon kai tis Dimosias Ekpaidefseos Ypourgou Georgiou Theotoki tin 4h Dekemvriou 1889. Athens: 1899.

Publications of The Metaxas Regime

Oi Arithmoi Omiloun dia to Ergon tis 4is Avgoustou, 4h Avgoustou 1938–1939. Athens: 1939.
Oikogeneia. Athens: EON, 1940.
Ypothikai tou Arkhigou. Kathikonta ton Goneon pros ta Paidia ton. I Skhesis ton Goneon pros tin Neolaian. Athens: EON, 1939.
4h Avgoustou. O Apologismos mias Dietias 1936–1938. Athens: 1938.
Deftera Diaskepsis Perifereiakon Dioikiton kai Dioikitrion Ethnikis Organoseos Neolaias Ellados (19–26 Maiou, 1940). Athens: EON, 1940.

BIBLIOGRAPHY

A. In Greek or in translation until 1940

Agapitos, Spyros. "H Hygieini ton Poleon" [Hygiene in towns]. *Ergasia,* no. 1 (May 3, 1930), 9–11.

———. "H Hygieini ton Poleon" [Hygiene in towns]. *Ergasia,* no. 2 (May 10, 1930), 10–2.

———. *Ergatika Spitia* [Working class houses]. Athens, 1918.

Alivizatos, Gerasimos. "Epidioxeis, Epitefxeis kai Provlepseis en ti Hygeini" [Aims, accomplishments and predictions in hygiene]. *Kliniki,* no. 8 (April 15, 1939): 297–309.

Anonymous. "Ta Nea Ktiria ton Dimotikon Skholeion" [The new buildings of primary schools]. *Ethniki Agogi,* no. 2 (March 15, 1898): 17–9.

Anonymous. "Ta Oikimata ton Ellinikon Skholeion" [The buildings of Greek schools]. *Ethniki Agogi,* no. 23 (December 1, 1902): 265–67.

Anonymous. "Entyposeis apo ta Skholeia tou Dimou Athinaion" [Impressions from the schools in the municipality of Athens]. *Deltio tou Ekpaideftikou Omilou,* vol. 2 (November 1912): 176–201.

Anonymous. "O Skopos tis Ellinikis Paidologikis Etaireias" [The aim of the Greek paidological society]. *Paidologia,* no. 2 (May 1920): 73.

Anonymous. "Paidologikon Kentron Athinon, Examinaia Ekthesis Pepragmenon," [Paedology centre of Athens] *Skholiki Ygieini,* no.7 (May 1937): 37–9.

Anonymous. "Symvoulion Skholikis Ygieinis," [School hygiene board]. *Skholiki Ygieini,* no. 31 (September 1939): 10–13.

Anonymous. "Ta Pepragmena apo tis 4is Avgoustou kai Entefthen. Diefthynsis Skholikis Ygieinis," [Accomplishements of the school hygiene service of the 4th of August regime]. *Skholiki Ygieini,* no. 31 (September 1939): 13–14.

Anonymous. "I Nomothesia peri Skholiatrikis Ypiresias. Aitiologiki Ekthesis epi tou Skhediou Anagkastikou Nomou 'Peri Organoseos tis Skholiatrikis Ypiresias'," [Regulations on the school medical service. Preamble to the draft of Emergency Law on "The organization of the school hygiene service"]. *Skholiki Ygieini,* no. 31 (September 1939): 15–41.

Anonymous. "I Eklaikefsis tis Paidokomikis. Ai Dialexeis tou Tmimatos 'Laikis Diafotiseos' tou Patriotikou Idrymatos," [Popularisation of puericulture. Lectures of the Department of Popular Education at the Patriotic Foundation]. *To Paidi,* no. 66 (March 1940): 15.

Anonymous. "To Sanatorion Paidon tou Patriotikou Idrymatos eis tin Pentelin," [Children's sananatorium of the Patriotic Foundation in Penteli]. *To Paidi,* no. 71, (October 1940): 27.

Anonymous. "I Titaneios Prospatheia pros Anatasin tis Phylis," [The titanic effort for the regenaration of the race]. *To Paidi,* no. 64, (March 1940): 4.

Aravantinos, Ioannis. "I Symvoli tou Patriotikou Idrymatos eis tin Exygiansin tis Neas Genias" [The contribution of the Patriotic Foundation to strengthening the health of the young generation]. *To Paidi,* no. 67 (June 1940): 3–5.

Doxiadis, Apostolos. *Grammata pros Miteras* [Letters to mothers]. Athens: Greca, 1927.

———. "Paidologia kai Evgonia" [Paedology and eugenics]. *Paidologia* 2, no. 12 (April 1921): 14–22.

————. "To Dimografikon Provlima" [The demographic problem]. *Ellinika Grammata* 3, no. 2 (July 1928): 49–51.

————. "Arkhai Eygonikis" [Eugenic principles]. *To Paidi* 1, no. 2 (July-August 1930): 31–7.

————. "Evgoniki kai Paidokomia" [Eugenics and puericulture]. *Ygeia*, no. 7 (July 1931):153–4.

————. "Evgonia" [Eugenics]. *To Paidi* no. 26 (December 1934): 5–15.

————. "To Paidi os Klironomikon Kefalaion" [The child as inheritable capital]. *To Paidi*, no. 55 (June 1939): 3–5.

Drakoulidis, Nikos. *I Sexoualiki Diapaidagogisis* [Sex education]. Athens: Ekdotiki Etaireia A.N. Kontomari, 1930

————. *I pro tou Gamou Iatriki Exetasis* [The pre-marital medical examination]. Athens: 1933.

Drosinis, Georgios. "Ta Skholeia tou Dimou Athinaion" [The schools of the municipality of Athens]. *Ethniki Agogi*, no. 19 (January 1, 1903): 223–24.

————. *Skorpia Fylla tis Zois mou* [Scattered papers of my life] vol. 2, Athens: Syllogos pros Diadosin ton Ofelimon Vivlion, 1982.

Elefteriadis, Dimitrios. *Ygieonologiki Politiki* [Hygiene policy]. Athens, 1929.

————. "To Progamiaion Iatrikon Pistopoiitikon" [The pre-marital medical certificate]. *Dimosia Ygieini*, no. 6 (March 21, 1931): 164–69.

Evelpidis, Khrysos. *To Agrotiko mas Provlima* [The agriculture problem]. Athens: 1944.

Exarkhopoulos, Nikolaos. *Somatologia tou Paidos* [Somatology of the child]. Athens: 1928.

————. "Psykhologia ton Atomikon Diaforon. I Diagnosis tou Vathmou tis Noimosynis epi ti Vasei Peiramatikon Erevnon. Nea Morfi tis Klimakos Binet-Simon" [Psychology of individual differences. The diagnosis of the intelligence on the basis of experimental research. New form of the Binet-Simon scale]. *Praktika tis Akadimias Athinon* 5 (November 1931): 356–74.

————. *Psykhikai Diaforai ton Paidon kai I Diagnosis Afton* [Mental differences of the children and their diagnosis] vol. 1. Athens: 1932.

Fabri, Sileno. "To Ethnikon mas Idryma Prostasias Mitrotitos kai Paidikis Ilikias" [Our national foundation for the protection of motherhood and childhood], transl. Kharilaos Prokopidis, *To Paidi*, no. 54 (May 1939): 24–7.

Flora-Karavia, Thalia. *Vivlion tis Ygeias* [The book of health]. Athens: 1890.

————. "Liges Ores stis Paidikes Exokhes tis Voulas" [Spending some time at the summer camps of Voula]. *To Paidi* no. 71 (October 1940):16–8.

Fotakis, G.N. "Pos na Organothomen Ygeionomikos" [How we can be organized from a hygienic point of view]. *Iatriki Kinisis* no. 6–7 (1927): 153–56.

Fragou, Zoi. *I Mitera kai to Paidi* [The mother and the child]. Athens: 1925.

Gedeon, Sophia. *Paidometrikai Erevnai en Elladi* [Paedometric research in Greece]. Athens: 1931.

Iliadis, Panagiotis. "I Paidiki Eglimatikotis kai ai Prospathiai tou Neou Kratous" [Child delinquency and the efforts of the new state]. *To Neon Kratos* 4, no. 29 (January 31, 1940): 304–5.

Iliou, Mikhail. "I Eniskhysis tis Zotikotitos tis Fylis mas" [Strengthening the vitality of our race]. *Ygeia*, September 15, 1925.

Imvrioti, Rosa. "Eidika Skholeia gia ta Anomala kai Kathysterymena Paidia," [Special schools for the anomalous and mentally impaired children]. *Paidagogiki*, no. 13 (May 25, 1937): 180–93.

————. "Ekthesis peri tis Leitourgias tou Eidikou Scholeiou Athinon. Apo 1ois Maiou mekhri 20is Iouniou," [Report on the operation of the special school in Athens]. *Skholiki Ygieini*, no. 8 (June 1937): 22–38.

————. "I Ergasia tou Protypou Eidikou Skholeiou Athinon (1937–1938)" [The work of the model special school in Athens]. *Skholiki Ygieini*, no. 18–19 (September–November 1938): 18.

————. *Anomala kai Kathysterimena Paidia. Protos Khronos tou Protypou Eidikou Skholeiou Athinon* [Anomalous and mentally impaired children. The first year of the model special school in Athens]. Athens: Elliniki Ekdotiki Etaireia, 1939.

————. "Ta Anomala kai Kathysterimena Paidia" [The anomalous and mentally retarded children]. *To Paidi*, no. 66 (May 1940): 6–7.

Ioannidis, Theodoros. "Skholeio dia Trakhomatika Paidia" [School for children with trakhoma]. *To Paidi*, no. 62 (January 1940): 4–6.

Kalyvas, G. "Ecoles nouvelles en Grèce," *L'Architecture d'Aujourd'hui*, no. 2 (1933): 68–70.

Karanikas, Konstantinos. *La crise de la population en Europe et les données démographiques de la Grèce*. Athens: Flamma, 1937.

Karantinos, Patroklos. *Ta Nea Skholika Ktiria*. [The new school buldings]. Athens: Ekdosis Tekhnikou Epimelitiriou tis Ellados, 1938.

Karapanagiotis, Giorgos. *Ygieini Proliptiki tis Mathitikis Myopias* [Preventive hygiene of students' myopia]. Athens: 1898.

———. *Enkheiridion Praktikis Ygieinis pros Khrisin ton Didaskaleion Amfoteron ton Fylon* [Manual of practical hygiene for use in female and male teachers' training college]. Athens: 1894.

———. *Gnoseis Praktikis Ygieinis pros Khrisin ton Gymnasion kai Parthenagogeion* [Knowledge of practical hygiene for use in secondary schools and female seconadary schools]. Athens: 1889.

Kardamatis, Ioannis. *Pragmateia peri Eleiogenon Noson* [Study on malarial diseases]. Athens: Typografeion Paraskeva Leoni, 1908.

———. *Ta Pepragmena pros Peristolin tis Elonosias en to Kratei kata to 1922* [Proceedings for the control of malaria in the country during 1922]. Athens: Ypourgeion Syngoinonias. Tmima Ygieonomikon, 1924.

———. *Ai Athinai Elonosiopliktoi* [Malaria-stricken Athens]. Athens: 1927.

Kariofyllis, Georgios. *Dialexeis peri Profylaxeos tis Dimosias Ygeias apo ton Loimodon Noson* [Lectures on the protection of the public health from contagious diseases]. Athens: Etaireia Ygieinis Athinon, 1917.

Katsigra, Anna. *Nea Ygieini* [New hygiene]. Athens: 1915.

———. *Stoikheia Ygieinis kai Nosileias* [Elements of hygiene and treatment]. Athens: 1929.

———. *Proetoimasia tou Koritsiou sta Genetisia Zitimata* [Preperation of girls on sex matters]. Athens: Typois A.B. Paskha, 1932.

Kharitakis, Kostis *Ygieini Stoikheiodis kai Skholiki*. [Basic hygiene and school hygiene]. Athens: 1914.

———. *Stoikheia Nipiokomias se 6 Mathimata. Skholi Episkeptrion Adelfon tou Ellinikou Erythrou Stavrou*. [Elements of nursing in six lessons. School of visiting vurses of the Hellenic Red Cross]. Athens: 1924.

———. "Koinoniki Ygieini." [Social hygiene]. *O Agonas tis Gynaikas* no. 104 (November 15, 1928): 3–5.

———. *Kodix tis Deontologias kai Nomothesias ton Iatrikon Epangelmaton* [Ethical and legal code of the medical professions]. Athens: 1928.

———. "Koinoniki Ygieini" [Social hygiene]. Athens: Erevna, 1928.

———. "Koinoniki Ygieini" [Social hygiene]. *Ellinis* no. 11 (November 1927): 233–35; no. 12 (1 December 1927): 259–62; no. 13 (January 1928): 10–2.

———. *Ta Neotata Dedomema tis Koinonikis Ygieinis* [The latest findings about social hygiene]. Athens: 1929.

———. "Ta Zitimata tis Ygeiaς os Kolyma Gamou. I Evgonia, i Syzygiki Molynsis kai to Progamiaio Pistopoiitiko Ygeias" [Health issues as an impediment to marriage. Eugenics, the conjugal contagion and the prenuptial certificate]. *Dimosia Ygieini*, no. 1 (January 10, 1931): 13–6.

———. "Ta Zitimata tis Ygeias os Kolyma Gamou" [Health issues as an impediment to marriage]. *To Paidi*, no. 6 (March-April 1931): 22–32.

———. "To Provlima tis Maias idia eis tas Agrotikas Periokhas. Dynatai I Maia na Ekteli kai Ergon Adelfis Episkeptrias?" [The problem of the midwife especially in rural areas. Can she undertake the duties of the visiting nurse?]. *Arkheia Ygieinis* 3, no. 6 (June 1939): 248–51.

Khoremis, Konstaninos. "Epi tou Provlimatos tis Diatrofis tou Ellinopaidos" [Concerning diet of the Greek child]. *Kliniki* no. 15 (August 1, 1939): 519–28.

———. "I Paidiatriki en ti Iatriki Etaireia" [Pediatrics in the Medical Society]. *Elliniki Iatriki* (1930): 400–90.

Khristopoulos, P. *Mathimata Ygieinis* [Courses on hygiene]. Athens: 1924.

Khryssaki, Margarita. "Ai Peristerai tou Politismou. I Episkeptria Adelfi apo Arkhaiotaton Khronon Mekhri Simeron" [The apostles of culture. The visiting nurse from ancient times to date]. *To Paidi*, no. 66 (May 1940): 20–3.

Khryssafis, Mikhail. "Ai Paramorfoseis tou Kormou kata tin Paidikin Ilikian. Sykhnotis, Aitia, Mesa, Therapeia" [Deformation of the spine during childhood. Frequency, reasons, treatment]. Athens: 1920.

———. "I Somatiki Askisis os Meson tis Ygieinis" [The physical exercise as a means of hygiene]. *Iatrika Khronika* (May 1930): 428–32.

Kopanaris, Fokion. *I Dimosia Ygeia en Elladi* [Public health in Greece]. Athens: 1933.

Koromilas, Georgios. "Peri tis mi en Khrono kai Rythmo Physikis Ekpaideyseos os Aitiou Prodiatheseos eis Nosous kai di eis tin Phthisin" [Concerning physical education as a contributory factor to tuberculosis]. *Dimotiki Ekpaideysis*, no. 16 (February 15, 1903): 246–53.

Koutsoumaris, Aristotelis. "I Koinoniki Pronoia gia tin Prostasia tou Paidiou ston Topo mas" [The social welfare for the protection of children in our country]. *To Paidi*, no. 41 (January-February 1937): 5–17.

Kyriakidis, Kyriakos. *Ta Pepragmena tis Ygieonomikis Ypyresias tou Ypourgeiou ton Esoterikon kata tin Dekaetian 1911–1921* [The accomplishemnts of the hygiene service of the Ministry of Interior during the decade 1911–1921]. Athens: Typografeion Estia, 1929.

———. *I Thessaloniki apo Ygieinis Apopseos* [Thessaloniki from a hygienic perspective]. Athens: 1917.

Lagakos, Ilias. "To Progamon Pistopoiitikon. Nomikai kai Koinoniologikai Apopseis" [The prenuptial health certificate. Legal and sociological views]. *To Paidi*, no. 2 (July–August 1930): 3–23.

Lambadarios, Emmanouil. "Organosis kai Therapeftika Apotelesmata tis A' Ellinikis en Vouliagmeni Paidikis Exokhis" [Organisation and treatment results of the first summer camp in Vouliagmeni]. In *Praktika tou B' Ellinikou Synedriou kata tis Phymatioseos, en Volo 20–23 Maiou 1912*, 243–60. Volos: 1912.

———. *Peri tis en Elladi Skholioseos*. [Concerning scholiosis in Greece]. Berlin: Archiv fuer Schulhygiene, 1913.

———. *I Skholiosis* [Scoliosis]. Athens: 1915.

———. *Organosis ton Paidikon Exokhon Vouliagmenis kata tin 4etian 1911–1914* [The organization of the children's summer camps in Vouliagmeni during the four-year period 1911–1914]. Athens: 1915.

———. *Stoikheia Paidologias. Geniki Eisagogi eis tin Paidologian, Somatologian kai Ygieinin. Dia tin Didaskalian toy Mathimatos tis Ygieinis eis ta Didaskaleia, Gymnasia kai Loipa Skholeia* [Elements of pedology. General introduction to pedology, somatology and hygiene. For the teaching of the hygiene in teacher's training colleges, Secondary schools and the rest of schools.] vol. 1. Athens: Sideris, 1916.

———. *I Ygieini tou Skholeiou kai to Ergon ton Skholikon Iatron* [The hygiene of school and the work of the school doctor]. Athens: Ypourgeion Esoterikon, 1918.

———. *Odigiai pros Profylaxin ton eis ta Skholeia Foitonton apo ton Loimodon Noson meta ton Skhetikon Egyklion* [Instructions for the protection of students from contagious diseases accompanied with the relevant circulars]. Athens: Ypourgeion ton Ekklisiastikon kai tis Dimosias Ekpaideyseos, 1920.

———. "Ai Paidologikai Epistimai kai I Simerini afton Apopsis" [The paedological sciences and their current views]. *Paidologia*, no. 1 (April, 1920): 3–7.

———. "Ai Paidologikai Epistimai kai I Exhelixis afton eis Diafora Krati [The paedological sciences and their evolution in various countries]. *Paidologia*, no. 2 (May, 1920): 54–9.

———. "Peri tou Anthifthysikou Agonos kata tin Paidikin Ilikian" [Concerning the anti-tuberculosis fight in childhood]. *Paidologia*, no. 4 (August 1920): 116–24.

———. "I Kinisis ton Mathitikon Polyklinikon Athinon, Pireos, Smyrnis tou Patriotikou Idrymatos Perithalpseos: A' Ekthesis peri ton Ergasion tis Mathitikis Polyklinikis kata to Skholikon Etos 1919–1920" [The movement of the student polyclinics of the Patriotic Foundation of Welfare in Athens, Piraeus, Smyrna: The first report on the work of the student polyclinic during the year 1919–1920]. *Paidologia*, no. 4 (August 1920): 141–3.

———. "I Somatiki Anaptyxis tou Paidiou" [The physical development of the child]. *Paidologia*, no. 6 (October 1920): 184–88.

———. "I Somatiki Anaptyxis tou Paidiou" [The physical development of the child]. *Paidologia*, no. 5–8 (May-August, 1921): 129–39.

———. "I Somatiki Anaptyxis tou Paidiou (kai idia tou Ellinos Mathitou)" [The physical development of the child (and especially of the Greek student)]. *Paidologia*, no. 9 (September, 1921): 2–5.

———. *Kodix Skholikis Ygieinis* [Code of school hygiene]. Athens, 1922.

———. *Ipaithria Skholeia* [Open-air schools]. Athens: 1923.

———. *Mathimata Skholikis Ygieinis* [Lessons on school hygiene]. Ellinikos Erythros Stauros. Skholi Episketrion Adelfon Athens: 1923.

———. *Diagramma Katapolemiseos tou Trakhomatos eis ta Skholeia* [Plan for the fight against trachoma at schools]. Athens: 1927.

———. *O Kinimatographos kai I Paidiki Ilikia* [Cinema and childhood]. Athens-Alexandreia: Kasigoni, 1928.

———. "I Somatiki Exelixis tou Ellinos Mathitou: Anthropologiki Afxisiologia" [The physical development of the Greek student: Anthropological auxology]. *Iatrika Khronika*, no. 6 (December 1928): 354–56.

———. "Prostasia tis Ygeias tou Mathitou" [The protection of the student's health]. In *Praktika tou A´ Panelliniou Synedriou Prostasias Mitrotitos kai Paidikon Ilikion*, October 19–26, 1930. (Athens, 1930): 108–12.

———. "Peri tou Antiphthisikou Agonos kata tin Paidikin Ilikian" [Concerning the fight against tuberculosis in childhood]. *To Paidi*, no. 4 (November 1930): 48–58.

———. "To Ygieionomikon Programma" [The hygiene programme]. *Ergasia*, no. 28 (July 19, 1930): 21–3.

———. "I Ygeia tou Ellinos Mathitou" [The health of the Greek student]. *Ergasia*, no. 18 (June 1930): 16–9.

———. *Ygieinai Synitheiai* [Healthy habits]. Athens: Ekdotikos Oikos Dimitrakou, 1931.

———. "I en Elladi Efarmogi tou Antiphymatikou Emvoliou BCG en Elladi" [The application of the BCG vaccine in Greece]. In *Praktika tou Synedriou gia tin Prostasia tis Mitrotitas kai tis Paidikis Ilikias*, 358–85. Athens: 1930.

———. *To Antifymatikon Emvolion BCG kai ta Apotelesmata tis en Elladi Efarmogis tou ypo tou Ellinikou Erythrou Stavrou* [The BCG vaccine and the results of its application by the Hellenic Red Cross in Greece]. Athens: Ekdotikos Oikos Dimitrakou, 1931.

———. *Peri tou Antidiptheritikou Emvoliasmou eis ta Imetera Skholeia* [Concerning the vaccination against diftheria in our schools]. Athens: Reprinted from the journal *Kliniki*, 1932.

———. *I Skholiki Antilipsis kai idios peri ton Mathitikon Syssition en Elladi* [The students' welfare, concerning especially the school meals in Greece]. Athens: 1934.

———. *Skholiki Ygieini meta Stoikheion Paidologias* [School hygiene with elements of paedology]. Athens, 1934.

———. *I Ygieini ton Skholeion en Anglia* [School hygiene in England]. Athens: *Deltion tis Paidiatrikis Etaireias Athinon*, 1934.

———. "I Skholiki Antilipsis kai Pronoia kata tas Simerinas Antilipseis tis Epistimis," [Students' welfare and relief according to the current views of science]. *To Paidi*, no. 25 (May–June 1934): 5–15.

———. "Symvoli eis tin Psykhometrian tou Anomalou Ellinos Mathitou kai Arkhai Organoseos tou Protou Skholeiou Anomalon Paidon par' Imin" [Contribution to the psychometrics of the anomalous Greek student and organization of the first school for anomalous children in our country]. *Skholiki Ygieini*, no. 7 (May 1937): 5–16.

———. "I Prostasia tis Ygeias tou Mathitou" [The Protection of the Student's health]. *Skholiki Ygieini*, no. 4 (February 1937): 3–10.

Lambrinoulos, Georgios. "Iliotherapeia i Iliosis" [Sunbathing or sunstroke]. *Ygeia*, no. 1 (January 1928): 1–4.

Leka, Vertha. "I Anagki tis Idryseos enos Paidikou Asylou" [The need for the establishment of a children's asylum]. *To Paidi*, no. 11 (January–February 1932): 33–4.

Livadas, Grigorios A., and Ioannis K. Sfangos. *I Elonosia en Elladi 1930–1940: Erevna, Katapolemisis* [Malaria in Greece 1930–40: Research, fight against it]. Athens: Pyrsos, 1940.

Mantoudis, Manolis. "Les Bâtiments Scolaires en Grèce," *L'Hellénisme Contemporain*, no. 7 (1936): 633–39.

Makkas, Georgios. *I Thnisimotis tis Paidikis Ilikias en Elladi. Aitia kai Mesa pros Peristolin.* [Child mortality in Greece. Causes and means of restraint]. Athens: Vassilikon Typografeion Nikolaou Khioti, 1911.

———. I Prostasia tou Paidiou [The protection of the child]. Athens: 1921.

Makridis, Nikolaos. *Ai Ypiresiai Ygieinis en Elladi: Apo tis Idryseos tou Ellinikou Vasileiou mekhri ton Imeron mas* [Hygiene services in Greece. From the foundation of the Greek Kingdom till today]. Athens: Typografika Katastimata Adelfon Gerardou, 1933.

Mastrogiannis, Ioannis D. *Istoria tis Koinonikis Pronoias tis Neoteris Ellados (1821–1960)* [History of the social welafare in modern Greece (1821–1960). Athens: 1960.

Messinezis, Dimitrios. *I Protypos Ygeionomiki Organosis Ambelokipon tou Dimou Athinaion kai tis Ygeionomikis Skholis. To Programma kai ta Pepragmena mias Topikis Ygeionomikis Ypiresias. Octovrios 1935–Dekemvrios 1936* [The model health care organization of Ambelokipi in the city of Athens and of the school of hygiene. The programme and the accomplishments of a local hygiene service, October 1935–December 1936]. Athens: 1937.

Mitropoulos, Panagiotis. "Skopos kai Organosis ton Paidikon Exokhon." [Aim and organization of summer camps]. *To Paidi,* no. 59 (October 1939): 8–9.

Moutousis, Konstantinos. "I Ygieini kai i Evgonia eis tas Synkhronous Koinonias." [Hygiene and eugenics in contemporary societies]. *Kliniki,* 9, no. 47 (November 25, 1933): 863–74.

Moysidis, Moysis. *I Kallipaidia. Allote kai Simeron* ["Kallipaidia" in the past and today]. Constantinople: 1912.

———. "Evgonismos kai Gamos." [Eugenics and marriage]. *Ygeia* no. 1 (1 January 1924): 2–4.

———. *Evgoniki kai Paidokomia para tis Arkhaiois Ellisin.* [Eugenics and puericulture in ancient Greece]. Athens: 1925.

———. *I Gyni: Ygieini tou Gamou kai tis Eggamou Gynaikos* [The woman: hygiene of the marriage and of the married woman]. Athenes: Kasigonis, 1925.

———. *Genetisios Paidagogiki.* [Sexual pedagogy]. Alexandreia: Kassigonis, 1927.

———. *Ygieini tis Egkyou, tis Epitokou, tis Lechoydou kai tis Galoukhousis* [Hygiene of the pregnant women, of mothers during the puerperium and of breastfeeding mothers]. Alexandreia: Kassigonis, 1927.

———. *Ygieini ton Phylon.* [Gender hygiene]. Athens: Kasigonis, 1929.

———. "I pro tou Gamou Iatriki Exetasis" [The pre-martital medical examination], *Ergasia,* no. 1 (April 29, 1930): 19

———. "I Iatriki, Koinoniki kai Nomiki Apopsi tou Progamiaiou Iatrikou Pistopoiitikou." [The medical, social and legal dimensions of the prenuptial health certificate]. *Dimosia Ygieini* no. 5, (March 7, 1931): 134–42.

———. "Genikotites peri Afxiseos." [General issues concerning growth]. *To Paidi* no. 12, (January-February, 1932): 3–17.

———. *O Malthousianismos Allote kai Nyn* [Maltousianism in the past and in the present]. Athens: 1932.

———. *Evgoniki Aposteirosis* [Eugenic sterilisation]. Athens: Kassigonis, 1934.

Nikolaidis, Th. *Ygieini ton Paidon (apo tis Genniseos mechri tis ek tou Skholeiou Apofoitiseos)* [Hygiene of children (from birth till graduation from school)]. Mytilini: 1916.

Offner, Max. *I Pnevmatiki ton Mathiton Koposis kata tas Erevnas kai ta Porismata tis Peiramatikis Psykhologias met' Efarmogon eis tin Didaskalian.* Transl. D. M. Georgakaki [Students' mental fatigue according to the research and the findings of experimental psychology]. Athens: Estia, 1915.

Oikonomopoulos, N. B. *Koinoniki Ygieini, Koinoniki Pronoia, Kratiki Merimna* [Social hygiene, social welfare, state care]. Athens: Petrakos, 1922.

———. *I Phthisiogenesis.* [The genesis of the tuberculosis]. Athens: 1916.

————. *I Elefthera Nosileia ton Phymatikon. Koinonikoygieini Apopsis.* [The free hospitalization of tuberculars. The socio-hygienic aspect]. Athens: Pergamalis, 1927.

————. *I Ygeionologiki Politiki eis tin Khoran mas.* [The hygienic policy in our country]. Athens: 1933.

————. "I Endeiknyomeni Kratiki Merimna dia ton kata tis Phymatioseos Agona en Elladi." [Proper state policies for the fight against tuberculosis in Greece]. Athens: 1929.

Pamboukis, P. *O Agon kata tis Phthiseos. Prophylaxeis-Therapeia.* [The fight against tuberculosis. Prophylaxis-treatment]. Athens: 1927.

————. "Pos Prepei na Diexakhthei o kata tis Phthiseos Agon. To Programma tis Ellinikis Antipthysikis Etaireias." [How the fight against tuberculosis should take place. The programme of the Greek Anti-Tuberculosis Society]. *Ygeia* no. 20 (October 15, 1925): 399–402.

Panagiotakos, Panagiotis, G. "Statistikai Erevnai epi tis Phymatioseos kai Thnitotitos en to Dimo Athinaion kata to Etos 1930" [Statistical research on tuberculosis and mortality in the municipality of Athens during 1930]. *Iatrika Khronika* no. 6 (1931): 385–93.

Panagiotakos, Konstantinos. "Systimatiki Egairos Diagnosis tis Pnevmonikis Phymatioseos kata tin Skholikin kai Metaskholikin Periodon os Vasis tis Skholikis kai Epangelmatikis Ygieinis" [Systematic on-time diagnosis of pulmonary tuberculosis as a basis of school and professional hygiene]. *Iatrika Khronika* no. 6 (Decembre 1928): 338–44.

————. "Koinoniki Iatriki I Koinoniki Ygieini." [Social medicine or social hygiene]. *Iatrika Khronika* no. 2 (August 1928): 92–5.

Panagiotatou, Aggeliki. *Ta Mathimata tou Savvatou i Mathimata Ygieinis.* [Saturday courses or hygiene courses]. Alexandreia: 1913.

Papagiannis, Konstantinos. "Peri tis Ygieinis ton Skholeion en Elladi." [Concerning school hygiene in Greece]. In *Praktika Panelliniou Iatrikou Synedriou en Athinais 6–11 May 1901*, 155–67. Athens: 1903.

Papadakis, Antonios. *Prophylaktika Metra kata ton Loimikon Nosimaton.* [Preventive measures against infectious diseases]. Athens: 1900.

Papadimitriou, Anna. "I Prostasia tou Paidiou eis to Exoteriko kai eis ton Topon mas." [Child's protection abroad and in our country]. *To Paidi* no. 1 (May–June 1930): 4–9.

Papadopoulou, Mikhail. "I Koinonia ton Ethnon en ti Prostasia Mitrotitos kai Paidiou" [The role of the League of Nations in the protection of mothers and children]. *To Paidi* no. 30 (March–April 1935): 5–22.

Papakostas, Georgios. "Organosis Antiphymatikou Agonos," [Organisation of the anti-tuberculosis struggle]. *Arkheia Ygieinis*, no. 9 (December 1937): 333–84.

Papamavrou, Mikhalis. "O Dr. Lietz kai to Ergo tou" [Dr. Lietz and his work]. *Deltio Ekpaidetikou Omilou* no. 8 (1920): 100–15.

Papanagiotou, Alkiviadis. "I Thnitotis ton Paidon en Athinais" [Child mortality in Athens]. *Imerologion Efimeridos ton Kyrion tou 1891* no. 5 (1890): 36–40.

Patridis, S. *Stoikheia Ygieinis. Pros Khrisin ton Mathiton ton Gymnasion* [Elements of hygiene. For the use of students in secondary schools]. Athens: Sideris, 1931.

Patrikios, Vassilios. *Nosimata kai Mikrovia* [Diseases and viruses]. Athens: Syllogos pros Diadosin Ofelimon Vivlion, 1901.

————. *Ta Asklipeiia i Phthisiatreia* [Asklipeiia or TB infirmaries]. Athens: 1902.

————. *I Phthisis en Elladi.* [Tuberculosis in Greece]. Athens: 1903.

Peridis, P.B. *Enkheiridion Stoikheiodous Ygieinis.* [Textbook of elementary hygiene]. Athens: 1890.

Pyrlas, I.P. *Synekdimos Ygieini. Pros Khrisin Ekastou.* [Hygiene for everybody]. Athens: 1864.

Roussopoulou, Agni. "To A' Valkanikon Synedrion Prostasias tou Paidiou" [The first Balkan congress on child protection]. *To Paidi* no. 53 (April 1930): 8–11.

————. "Ti Apefasisen to Synedrion tou Veligradiou gia tin Prostasia tou Paidiou stin Ypaithro Khora" [What the Belgrade Congress decided about the child protection in the countryside], *To Paidi* no. 58 (September 1939):14–6.

Sakellariou, Georgios. *Ygieini tou Mathitou* [Student's hygiene]. Athens: Ellninikos Erythros Stavros, 1926.

———. *I Metrisis tis Efyias met' Efarmogon eis tin Ekpaidefsin, ton Straton, tin Epangelmatikin Katefthynsin kai tin Poinikin Dikaiosinin* [The measurement of intelligence applied in education, the army, the professional orientation and the criminal justice]. Athens: 1928.

———. *Psykhogia tou Paidos* [Child psychology]. Athens: 1930.

———. *I Metrisis tis Efiias Atomikos kai Omadikos*. [The measurement of intelligence individually and in groups]. Athens: 1952.

Saranti, Alexandra. "I Metarythmisi tou Astikou Kodika. Ta Kolymata tou Gamou" [The reform of the civil code. The impediments to marriage]. *O Agonas tis Gynaikas*, no.141 (March 15, 1931): 3–6

Saratsis, Dimitris. *Mathimata Laikis Ygieinis*. [Courses on popular hygiene]. Athens: 1936.

Saroglou, Konstantinos. "I Prostasia tou Paidiou en Elladi." [Child protection in Greece]. *To Paidi* no. 4 (November-December 1930): 59–79.

———. *Pos tha Profylaxete ta Paidia sas apo ti Phthysi*. [Protecting your children from tuberculosis]. Athens: Makris, 1932.

———. "Psykhiki kai Somatiki Ygieini tou Paidiou sto Skholeio." [Mental and physical child hygiene in school]. *To Paidi* no. 16 (November-December, 1932): 11–28.

———. "Pshykhikoi Paragontes kai Paidiki Ygieini." [Mental factors and child hygiene]. *To Paidi* no.11 (January–February, 1932): 18–25.

———. "Anagki Diethnous Synergasias dia tin Prostasian tis Mitrotitos kai tou Paidiou." [Need of international cooperation for the protection of mothers and children]. *To Paidi* no. 37–38, (May-August 1936): 58–70.

Savvas, Konstantinos. *Odigiai peri Apolymanseos*. [Instructions on disinfection]. Athens: 1902.

———. "Nyxeis Tines pros Veltiosin tis Skholikis Ygieinis en Elladi." [Some thoughts on the improvement of school hygiene in Greece]. *Dimotiki Ekpaidefsis*, no. 22 (April 10, 1904): 337–57.

Savvas, Konstantinos and Kardamatis Ioannis. *I Elonosia en Elladi kai ta Pepragmena tou Syllogou* [Malaria in Greece and the accomplishments of the anti-malaria association]. Athens: Syllogos pros Peristolin ton Ellodon Noson, 1907.

———. "Ypomnima peri Idryseos Ypourgeiou Ygeias kai Koinonikis Pronoias Ypovlithen eis ton Kyrion Proedron tis Kyverniseos kata Mina Dekemvrion 1920," [Memorandum on the establishment of the Ministry of Health and social welfare addressed to the president of the gvernement on December 1920]. *Arkheia Iatrikis* no. 3 (March 1922): 65–72.

———. *O pros Peristolin ton Elodon Noson Syllogos, 1905–1928*. [The anti-malaria association, 1905–1928]. Athens: 1928.

Stefanou, Dimitrios. "Pro pantos na Eklaikefthei I Ygieini. Anagki na Eisakhthei eis ola ta Skholeia os Kyrion Mathima" [The popularisation of hygiene comes first. The need to introduce hygiene as a main course in all types of schools]. *Ygeia* no. 8 (April 15, 1925): 161–64 and no. 9 (May 1, 1925): 186–90.

———. "Istoria Syssition" [History of school meals]. *Dimosia Ygieini* (1931): 268–71.

———. "Ta Mathitika Syssitia" [The school meals]. *Skholiki Ygieini*, no. 4 (February 1937): 13–9.

———. "Skopoi kai Simasia ton Mathitikon Syssition" [Aims and significance of the school meals]. *Skholiki Ygieini*, no. 31 (December 1939): 34–42.

Sotiriadis, Dimitrios. *I Dimosia Ygeia en Elladi kai I Eklaikefsis tis Ygieinis*. [Public health in Greece and the popularization of hygiene]. Athens: Etaireia Ygieinis Athinon, 1917.

———. "To Ergon tis Etaireias Ygieinis" [The work of the hygiene society]. *Iatrika Khronika* no. 1 (January 1930): 66–7.

Triantafyllidis, Nikolaos. *Enkheiridion Skholikis Ygieinis met' Eikonon* [Textbook of school hygiene with illustrations]. Constantinople: 1911.

Trimis, Georgios. *Ai Dieikdikiseis ton Ergazomenon* [The claims of the workers]. Athens: 1948.

Tsourouktsoglou, Stavros. "Geniki Ygieini. Apo ta Synkhrona Provlimata tis Koinonikis Ygieinis. I Evgonia" [General hygiene. Contemporary problems of social hygiene. Eugenics]. *Ygeia* no. 11 (June 1, 1925): 221–24; and no. 12 (June 15, 1925): 246–48.

———. "Peri Evgonias" [Concerning eugenics]. In *Praktika Ellinikis Anthropologikis Etaireias*. Athens: 1925.

Vafas, Georgios. *Ai Athinai apo Iatrikin Apopsin: I Polis* [Athens from the doctors' point of view: the city] vol. 1, Athens: 1878.

Valaoras, Vassilios. *To Dimografikon Provlima tis Ellados kai I Epidrasis ton Prosfygon* [The demographic problem of Greece and the impact of refugees]. Athens: 1939.

———. "To Provlima tis Thnisimotitos en Elladi" [The problem of mortality in Greece]. In *Praktika tis Akadimias Athinon*, 15 (1940): 205–18.

Vamvas, Ioannis. *Peri tis Katastaseos en I Diatelei I Dimosia Ygieini en Athinais* [Concerning the condition of public hygiene in Athens]. Athens: 1882.

Varouxaki, Aikaterini. *Ygia Somata, Ygieis Psychai* [Healthy bodies, healthy minds]. Athens: 1911.

Variot, Gaston Felix-Joseph. *O Iatros ton Paidon. Pros Khrisin ton Miteron kai Paidagogon* [The handbook of medicine for children. For the use of mothers and educators]. Athens: 1893.

Veglidis, Ioannis. "O Agon kata tis Phthiseos" [The fight against tuberculosis]. *Ygeia* 1, no. 11 (June 1, 1924): 180–4.

———. "O Agon kata tis Phthiseos" [The fight against tuberculosis]. *Ygeia* 1, no. 12 (June 15, 1924): 204–7.

———. "O Agon kata tis Phthiseos" [The fight against tuberculosis]. *Ygeia* 1, no. 13 (July 1, 1924): 220–3.

———. "O Agon kata tis Phthiseos" [The fight against tuberculosis]. *Ygeia* 1, no. 14 (July 15, 1924): 239–41.

Veras, Solon. *I Hygieini tou Paidiou. Omiliai dia tas Miteras* [The child's hygiene. Lectures for mothers]. Athens: Syllogos pros Diadosin Ofelimon Vivlion, 1927.

———. *Ai Laikai Prolipseis oson Afora tin Ygieinin tou Paidiou* [Popular superstitions concerning the hygiene of the child]. Athens: 1932.

———. *I Anagki dia to Paidi na Zei eis to Ypaithron* [The child's need to live in the countryside]. Athens: 1932.

———. "To Paidi, o Iatros tou kai I Oikogeneia" [The child, its doctor and the family]. *To Paidi* 5, no. 24 (March–April 1934): 5–9.

Vlavianos, Georgios. "I Hiliotherpaeia kai I Megisti Diaititiki kai Therapeftiki tis Axia" [Sunbathing and its optimal dietary and treating value]. *Nea Anatoli*, no. 1. Athens: Kallergis, 1917.

Vlamos, Georgios. *I Ygieini tou Skholeiou* [The school hygiene]. Athens: P.D. Sakellariou, 1904.

Vrontakis, Emmanouil. "Irkhisen I Leitourgia ton Paidikon Exokhon tou Patriotikou Idrymatos eis Olin tin Ellada" [Summer camps of the Patriotic Foundation open all around Greece]. *To Paidi* no. 67 (June 1940): 24–7.

B. In Greek or in translation after 1940

Ackerknecht, Eewin H. *Istoria tis Iatrikis* [A short history of medicine]. Athens: Marthia, 1998.

Aggelis, Vaggelis. *"Giati Khairetai o Kosmos kai Khamogela Patera..." Mathimata Ethnikis Agogis kai Neolaiistiki Propaganda sta Khronia tis Metaxikis Diktatorias* [Courses on national education and youth propaganda during the Metaxas's dictatorship]. Athens: Vivliorama, 2006.

Alexiou, Thanasis. *Perithoriopoiisi kai Ensomatosi. I Koinoniki Politiki os Mikhanismos Elenkhou kai Koinonikis Pitharkhisis* [Marginalization and integration. Social policy as a mechanism of control and social discipline]. Athens: 1999.

Antoniou, David. *Ta Programmata tis Mesis Ekpaidefsis (1833–1929)* [Curricula in secondary education (1833–1939)]. Athens: IAEN, 1987.

———. *Diadromes kai Staseis sti Neoelliniki Ekpaidefsi 19os-20os Aionas* [Milestones in the modern Greek education, 19th and 20th centuries]. Athens: Metaikhmio, 2008.

———. *Ta Programmata tis Mesis Ekpaidefsis (1833–1929)* [Secondary school curricula]. Athens: IAEN, 1987.

Avdela, Efi, Kharis Exertzoglou and Khristos Lyrintzis, eds. *Morfes Dimosias Koinonikotitas stin Ellada tou Mesopolemou* [Forms of public sociality in interwar Greece]. Athens: Panepistimiakes Ekdoseis Kritis, 2015.

Avdela, Efi, Dimitris Arvanitakis and Eliza-Anna Delveroudi, eds. *Fyletikes Theories stin Ellada:*

Proslipseis kai Khriseis stis Epistimes, tin Politiki, ti Logotekhnia kai tin Istoria tis Tekhnis kata ton 19o kai 20o Aiona [Racial theories in Greece: Perceptions and uses in sciences, politics, literature and the history of art during the 19th and 20th centuries]. Heraklion: Panepistimiakes Ekdoseis Kritis, 2017.

Bournazos, Stratis. "I Ekpaidefsi sto Elliniko Kratos." [Education in the Greek state]. In *Istoria tis Elladas tou 20ou Aiona: Oi Aparkhes 1900–1922* [History of Greece in the 20th century. The beginnings 1900–1922], edited by Khristos Khatziiosif, vol. A2, 189–281. Athens: Vivliorama, 1999.

Bouzakis, Sifis. *Georgios A. Papandreou, 1888–1968*. vol.2. Athens: Gutenberg, 1997.

Bregianni, Katerina. "I Politiki ton Psevdesthiseon: Kataskeves kai Mythoi tis Metaxikis Diktatorias" [The politics of illusions: Constructs and myths of the Metaxas' dictatorship], *Istorika* 16 no. 30 (June 1999): 171–98.

Dafnis, Kostis. *Apostolos Doxiadis, o Agonistis kai o Anthropos.* [Apostolos Doxiadis, the fighter and the man]. Athens: 1974.

Dimaras, Alexis. *I Metarrythmisi pou den Egine* [The reform that did not happen]. Vol.1, 2 Athens: Ermis 1974–1986.

Dimaras, Alexis and Vasso Vasilou-Papageorgiou, eds. *Apo to Kontyli ston Ypologisti* [From the slate to the computer]. Athens: Metaikhmio-ELIA, 2007.

Exertzoglou, Kharis. *Ethniki Taftotita stin Constantinoupoli ton 19o Aiona: O Ellinikos Filologikos Syllogos Constantinoupoleos 1861–1912* [National identity in Constantinople during the 19th century. The Hellenic Philological Society]. Athens: Nefeli, 1996.

Fournaraki, Eleni. *Ekpaidefsi kai Agogi ton Koritsion: Ellinikoi Provlimatismoi (1830–1910): Ena Anthologio* [Female education and instruction: Greek concerns (1830–1910): An anthology]. Athens: IAEN, 1987.

———. "Somatiki Agogi ton dyo Phylon stin Ellada tou 19ou Aiona" [Physical education for both females and males in Greece in the 19th century]. In *Praktika tou Diethnous Symposiou Oi Khronoi tis Istorias: Gia mia Istoria tis Paidikis Ilikias kai tis Neotitas*, 293–317. Athens: IAEN, 1988.

———."O Olympismos ton Kyrion: Oi Diethneis Olympiakes Diorganoseis (1896, 1906) kai i *Efimeris ton Kyrion*" [Olympism of the ladies: the international Olympic events (1896, 1906) and the journal *Efimeris ton Kyrion*]. In *Athina, Poli ton Olympiakon Agonon 1896–1906*, edited by Khristina Koulouri, 337–80. Athens: Diethnis Olympiaki Epitropi, 2004.

Giakoumatos, Andreas. "I Skholiki Arkhitektoniki kai I Empeiria tou Monternou stin Ellada tou Mesopolemou." [The school architecture and the experience of the modern in interwar Greece]. *Themata Khorou kai Tekhnon*, no. 18 (1987): 50–61.

———. *Stoikheia gia ti Neoteri Elliniki Arkhitektoniki. Patroklos Karantins* [Elements of Greek architecture. Patroklos Karantinos]. Athens: Morfotiko Idryma Ethnikis Trapezas, 2003.

Giannitsiotis, Giannis. *I Koinoniki Istoria tou Peiraia. H Syngrotisi tis Astikis Taxis 1860–1910* [The social history of Pireaus. The shaping of the middle class 1860–1909]. Athens: Nefeli, 2006.

Gizeli, Vika. *Koinonikoi Metaskhimatismoi kai Proelefsi tis Koinonikis Katoikias stin Ellada, 1920–1930* [Social tranformations and the origins of the social housing in Greece, 1920–1930]. Athens: 1984.

Glinos, Dimitirs. *Apanta,* [Collected works], vol. 1: 1890–1910. Athens: Themelio, 1983.

Kalafati, Eleni. *Ta Skholika Ktiria tis Protovathimas Ekpaidefsis, 1821–1929* [The school bulidings for the primary education, 1821–1929]. Athens: IAEN, 1988

———. "Istoriko ton Skholikon Ktirion tis Dimotikis Ekpaidefseos (1821–1940)," [History of the school bulidings of the primary education (1821–1940)]. *O Politis* no. 67–68 (1984): 34–40.

Karas, Giannis, ed. *Istoria kai Filosofia ton Epistimon ston Elliniko Khoro. (170s-190s Aionas)* [History and philosophy of sciences in Greece (17th-19th century)]. Athens: Metaikhmio, 2003.

Kazolea-Tavoulari, Panagiota. "Psykhologia kai Evgoniki stin Ellada." [Psychology and eugenics in Greece]. *Tetradia Psykhiatrikis* no. 78 (April-May-June 2002): 52–65.

———. *I Istoria tis Psykhologias stin Ellada, 1880–1987* [The history of psychology in Greece, 1880–1987]. Athens: Ellinika Grammata, 2002.

Kharisi, Antonia. *I Rosa Imvrioti sto Protypo Eidiko Skholeio (1937–1940)* [Rosa Imbrioti at the model special school (1937–1940)]. Athens: Epikentro, 2013.

Kharitakis, Kostis. *To Vivlio tis Miteras. Ygieini kai Diaititiki tis Miteras kai tou Paidiou* [The mother's handbook. Hygiene and nutrition of the mother and the child]. Athens: 1945.

Kharitos, Kharalambos. *To Parthenagogeio tou Volou* [The secondary school for girls in Volos]. Athens: IAEN, 1989.

Khatziiosif, Khristos. "Koinovoulio kai Diktatoria" [Parliament and dictatorship]. In *Istoria tis Elladas tou 200u Aiona*, edited by Khristos Khatziiosif, vol. B2, 114–22. Athens: Vivliorama, 2004.

Kokkinos, Giorgos. "Ygeia, Alki, Kalokagathia: Orthodoxi Ekklisia kai Somatiki Agogi. Oi Antistaseis kai I Vathmiaia Prosarmogi." [Health, robustness and good disposition: the Orthodox Church and physical education. Resistances and progressive adaptation]. In *Praktika Diethnous Symposiou Oi Khronoi tis Istorias. Gia mia Istoria tis Paidikis Ilikias kai tis Neotitas*, 317–39. Athens: IAEN, 1988.

―――. *I Evgoniki Dystopia* [The eugenic dystopia]. Athens: Thines, 2017.

Kontogiorgi, Elsa. "I Apokatastasi. 1922–1930" [The resettlement. 1922–1930]. In *Istoria tou Neou Ellinismou 1770–2000*. Edited by Vasilis Panagiotopoulos, vol. 7, 101–18. Athens: Ellinika Grammata, 2004.

Korasidou, Maria. *Otan I Arrostia Apeilei: Epitirisi kai Elenkhos tis Ygeias tou Plithysmou stin Ellada tou 190u aiona* [When the disease threatens: Inspection and control of the populations' health in Greece at the 19th century]. Athens: Typothito, 2002.

Kotsi, Agapi. *Nosologia ton Paidikon Ilikion kai tis Neotitas (200s Aionas)* [Childhood and youth diseases (20th century)]. Athens: IAEN/EIE, 2008.

Koulouri, Khristina. *Athlitismos kai Opseis tis Koinonikotitas: Gymnastika kai Athlitika Somateia 1870–1922* [Sport and aspects of sociability. Associations of gymnastics and sports 1870–1922]. Athens: IAEN/EIE, 1997.

Kritsotaki, Despo and Vassia Lekka, "Noimata kai Embeiries ton Nevrologikon kai Psykhikon Diatarakhon kai Praktikon. Paidia kai Neoi sta Exoterika Iatreia tou Eginitiou Nosokomeiou (1904–1940) [Meanings and experiences of neurological and pschychiatric illnesses and practices. Children and adolescents in the outpatient clinic of Eginiteio hospital (1904–1940)]. *Synapsis* 8, no. 25 (2012): 48–53.

Kountouras, Miltos. *Kliste ta Skholeia: Ekpaideftika Apanta* [Close the schools: Collected works]. Athens: Gnosi, 1985.

Lambraki-Paganou, A. *I Sofia Gedeon kai I Aikaterini Striftou-Kriara* [Sofia Gedeon and Aikaterini Striftou-Kriara]. Athens: Mikros Romios, 1998.

Leontidou, Lila. *Poleis tis Siopis: Ergatikos Epoikismos tis Athinas kai tou Peiraia 1909–1940* [Cities of silence: The "colonization" of Athens and Piraeus by workers, 1909–1940]. Athens: ETVA Politistiko Tekhnologiko Idryma, 1989.

Liakos, Antonis. *Ergasia kai Politiki stin Ellada tou Mesopolemou: To Diethnes Grafeio Ergasias kai i Anadysi ton Koinonikon Thesmon* [Labour and politics in Greece in the interwar: The international labour office and the emergence of social Instutitons]. Athens: Idryma Erevnas kai Paideias tis Emporikis Trapezas tis Elladas, 1993.

Makhaira, Eleni. *I Neolaia tis 4is Avgoustou. Fotografes* [Youth and the 4th of August regime]. Athens: IAEN 1987.

Mavrogordatos, Giorgos and Khristos Khatziiosif, eds. *Venizelismos kai Astikos Eksynkhronismos* [Venizelism and urban modernization]. Heraklion: Panepistimiakes Ekdoseis Kritis, 1988.

Mavrogordatos, Giorgos. "Metaxy dyo Polemon" [Between two wars]. In *Istoria tou Neou Ellinismou 1770–2000* [History of the new Hellenism, 1770–2000], edited by Vassilis Panagiotopoulos, vol. 7, 9–32. Athens: Ellinika Grammata, 2003.

Metaxas, Ioannis. *To Prosopiko tou Imerologio* [Metaxas's personal diary]. Athens: Govostis, 1960.

―――. *Logoi kai Skepseis* [Discourses and thoughts]. Athens: 1938.

Papastefanaki, Lyda. "Dimosia Ygeia, Phymatiosi kai Epangelmatiki Pathologia stis Ellinikes Poleis stis Arkhes tou 200u Aiona. I Antifatiki Diadikasia tou Astikou Eksynkhronismou" [Public health, tuberculosis and professional pathology in the Greek cities at the beginning of the 20th century. The problematic urban modernization]. In *Praktika Synedriou Eleftherios Venizelos kai Elliniki Poli: Poleodomikes Politikes kai Koinonikopolitikes Anakatataxeis*, 155–70. Athens: Ethniko Idryma Erevnvon kai Meleton Eleftherios Venizelos, 2005.

————. *Ergasia, Tekhnologia kai Fylo stin Elliniki Viomikhania* [Labour, technology and gender in the Greek industry], Heraklion: Panepistimiakes Ekdoseis Kritis, 2009.

Papastefanaki, Lyda, Manolis Tzanakis and Sevasti Trubeta, eds. *Dierevnontas tis Koinonikes Skheseis me Orous Ygeias kai Astheneias. I Koinoniki Istoria tis Iatrikis os Erevnitikio Pedio* [Researching the social relations in terms of health and disease. The social history of medicine as a research field]. Heraklion: Panepistimio Kritis, 2013.

Paxton, Robert. *I Anatomia tou Fasismou* [The anatomy of fascism], transl. Katerina Khalmoukou. Athens: Kedros, 2006,

Riginos, Mikhalis. *Paragogikes Domes kai Ergatika Imeromisthia stin Ellada, 1909–1936* [Structures of production and the workers' wages in Greece, 1909–1936]. Athens: Idryma Erevnas kai Paideias tis Emporikis Trapezis tis Ellados, 1987.

Sarantis, Konstantinos. "The Ideology and Character of the Metaxas Regime" in *Aspects of Greece 1936–1940: The Metaxas Dictatorship*, edited by Robin Higham and Thanos Veremis, 152–63. Athens: ELIAMEP-Vryonis Center 1993.

————. "I Ideologia kai o Politikos Kharaktiras tou Kathestotos Metaxa" [Ideology and the character of Metaxas' regime]. In *O Metaxas kai I Epokhi tou*, edited by Thanos Veremis, 45–71. Athens: Evrasia, 2009.

Skopetea, Elli. "Oi Ellines kai oi Ekhthroi tous. I Katastasi tou Ethnous stis Arkhes tou Eikostou Aiona" [The Greeks and their enemies. The nation at the beginning of the 20th century]. In *Istoria tis Elladas tou 200u Aiona: Oi Aparkhes 1900–1922*, edited by Khristos Khatziiosif. vol. A2, 9–35. Athens: Vivliorama, 1999.

Soutzoglou-Kottaridou Pelagia. *Paidi kai Ygeia sta Prota Khronia tis Anexartitis Elladas, 1830–1862. Mia Istoriko-koinoniki Prosegisi mesa apo ton Periodiko Typo tis Epokhis* [Child and health during the early years of the Greek Independent State, 1830–1862. A historico-social approach through contemporary journals]. Athens: Idryma Erevnon gia to Paidi, 1991.

Stasinos, Dimitris. *I Eidiki Ekpaidefsi stin Ellada* [Special education in Greece]. Athens: Gutenberg, 1991.

Svolopoulos, Konstantinos, ed. *Konstantios B. Gontikas, 1870–1937. Thesmikes Allages kata ton Mesopolemo* [Konstantinos Gontikas, 1870–1937. Institutional refoms during the interwar]. Athens: Etaireia Meletis Ellinikis Istorias, 2003.

Theodorou, Vassiliki. "Oi Giatroi apenanti sto Koinoniko Zitima: O Antifymatikos Agonas stis Arkhes tou 200u Aiona (1901–1926)" [Doctors and the social issue: The anti-tuberculosis battle at the beginning of the 20th century (1901–1926)]. *Mnimon* no. 24 (2002): 145–78.

————. "Prostasia tis Mitrotitas kai tis Paidikis Ilikias ston Mesopolemo: Ethnikes Proteraiotites, Koinoniki Politiki kai Diekdikiseis gyro apo ti Syngrotisi tis Ennoias tou Physikou Kathikontos ton Gynaikon" [Protection of mothers and children in the interwar: National priorities, social policy and claims concerning the meaning of the natural duty of women]. In *Praktika tou Diethnous Symposiou, Logos Gynaikon*, edited by Vassiliki Kontogianni, 639–56. Athens: ELIA, 2008.

———— "Prospatheies Metarrythmisis tis Dimosias Ygeias stin Ellada tou Mesopolemou: Emblokes kai Oria" [Reform attempts in public health in interwar Greece: objections and limits]. In *I Ellada sto Mesopolemo*, edited by E. Avdela, D. Kousouris and M. Kharalambidis, 233–59. Athens: Alexandreia, 2017.

Theodorou, Vassiliki and Despina Karakatsani. 'Ygieinis Parangelmata'. *Iatriki Epivlepsi kai Koinoniki Pronoia gia to Paidi tis Protes Dekaeties tou Eikostou Aiona* [Hygiene orders. Medical inspection and social welfare for children in the early twentieth century]. Athens: Dionikos, 2010.

Trikha, Lydia. "Synthikes Ygeias kai Ygieinis kata ti Dekaetia tou 1880." [Health and hygiene conditions during the 1880s]. In *O Kharilaos Trikoupis kai I Epokhi tou: Politikes Epidioxeis kai Koinonikes Synthikes* [Charilaos Trikoupis and his times: political pursuits and social conditions], edited by Kaiti Aroni-Tsikhli and Lydia Trikha, 379–400. Athens: Papazisis, 2000.

Tsoukalas, Giorgos, Mexis P. and I. Tsoukalas. "I Paidiatriki mesa apo ti Drasi tis Iatrikis Etairias Athinon 1835–1930" [Pediatrics through the activity of the medical society of Athens, 1835–1930], *Deltio A' Paidiatrikis Klinikis Panepistimiou Athinon* 50, no. 2 (2003): 170–79.

Tzedopoulos, Giorgos, ed. *Pera apo tin Katastrofi: Mikrasiates Prosfyges stin Ellada tou Mesopole-mou* [Beyond the catastrophy: Refugees from Asia Minor in interwar Greece]. Athens: Vouli ton Ellinon, 2003.

Vasileiou, Georgios, E. *Ta Ekpaidefsima Noitika Kathisterimena Paidia kai Efivoi* [Mentally retarded children and adolescents that can be educated]. Athens: Ellinika Grammata, 1998).

Vatikiotis, Panagiotis. *Mia Politiki Viografia tou Ioanni Metaxa. Filolaiki Apolytarkhia stin Ellada. 1936–1941* [A political biography of Ioannis Metaxas. A popular authoritarian system in Greece, 1936–1941]. Athens: Evrasia, 2005.

Vigarello, Georges. *To Katharo kai to Vromiko. I Somatiki Ygieini apo ton Mesaiona os Simera* [The clean and the dirty from the middle-ages to date]. Transl. by Sp. Marketos. Athens: Alexandreia, 2000.

Vladimiros, Lazaros. *Ioannis Kardamatis: O Protergatis tou Anthelonosiakou Agona* [Ioannis Kardamatis: the pioneer in the anti-malaria fight]. Athens: 2006.

Zivas, Dionysios, A. and Maro Kardamitsi-Adami. "Syntomo Istoriko ton Skholikon Ktirion stin Ellada," *Arkhitektonika Themata* 11(1979):174–83.

C. In English and French until 1960

Armand-Dellile, P., "L'oeuvre Grancher, préservation de l'enfance contre la tuberculose," *Bulletin du Comité National de Défense contre la Tuberculose*, no. 1(1920): 217–21.

Badeau, John and Georgianna Stevens, eds. *Bread from Stones: Fifty Years of Technical Assistance.* New Jersey: Prentice-Hall Inc., 1956.

Barton, James. *Story of Near East Relief, 1925–1930. An Interpretation.* New York: The Macmillan Company, 1930.

Barbatis, Phocion. *L'inspection médicale des Écoles.* Paris: Vigots Frères, 1917.

Binet, Alfred, and Henri Victor. *La fatigue intellectuelle.* Paris: Schleicher, 1898.

Doxiades, Apostolos. *La situation des réfugiés en Grèce.* Genève: 1924

Fosdick, Raymond. *The Story of the Rockefeller Foundation.* New York: Harper and Brothers, Publishers, 1952.

Godin, Paul. *Manuel d'anthropologie.* Paris: 1921.

Goodman, Neville, M. *International Health Organizations and their Work.* Edinburgh and London: 1952.

Hogarth, Archibald Henry. *Medical Inspection of Schools.* London: County Council, 1909.

Jebb, Englantyne. *Cambridge: A Brief Study in Social Question.* Cambridge: 1906.

Lacassagne, Alexandre. *Précis d'hygiène privée et sociale.* Paris: Masson Éditeur, 1879.

Lambadarios, Emmanouil. "La vaccination préventive des nouveaux-nés contre la tuberculose par le BCG en Grèce," *Revue de Phtisiologie Médico-Sociale*, vol. 9, 1928.

———. *Les écoles de plein air.* Athens: 1923.

———. "L'evolution du cinema educatif en Grèce," *Revue Internationale du Cinema Educatif*, no. 6 (1929): 634–37.

———. *L'organisation de l'hygiène scolaire en Grèce.* Athens: Pyrsos, 1933.

———. "Quelques faits relatifs à la vaccination contre la tuberculose par le BCG en Grèce," *Annales de l'Institut Pasteur*, vol. XLV (1930).

League of Nations. *Greek Refugee Settlement.* Genève: 1926.

Mosso, Angelo. *La fatigue intellectuelle et physique.* Paris: 1908.

Panayotatou, Aggeliki. "Sur la prophylaxie antituberculeuse dès le premier age," Conférence donnée à l'Institut Rousseau de Genève, Suisse, Juin 1927. Paris: Vigot Frères Editeurs, 1927.

Premier Congrès International des Ecoles de Plein Air en la Faculté de Médecine de Paris, 24–28 Juin 1922. Paris: A. Maloine, 1925.

Rey-Hermé, Philippe Alexandre. *Les colonies de vacances en France: origines et premiers développements (1881–1906).* Saint-Étienne: Imprimerie de Dumas, 1954.

Riant, Aimé. *Hygiène scolaire, influence de l'école sur la santé des enfants.* Paris: Hachette 1874.

Sacorrafos, Menelaos. "L'hérédité de la tuberculose," *Presse Médicale*, no. 76, 1929.

Stefanou, Dimitris. *Les écoles de plein air.* Athens: 1948.

Variot, G. *Projet d'un institut du puericulture aux enfants assistés.* Paris: Imprimerie A. Davy, 1908

Zinnis, A. *Etude sur les principales causes léthifères chez les enfants au-dessous de cinq ans et plus spécialement chez ceux de 0-1 an à Athènes.* Athens: 1880.

D. In English, French and German after 1960

Adams, Mark, ed. *The Wellborn Science: Eugenics in Germany, France, Brazil, and Russia.* Oxford: Oxford University Press, 1990.

Aisenberg, Andrew R. *Contagion: Disease Government and the 'Social Question' in Nineteenth Century France.* London: Stanford University Press, 1999.

Apple, Rima D. *Mothers and Medicine. A Social History of Infant Feeding, 1890–1950.* Madison: University of Wisconsin Press, 1987

———. "Constructing Mothers: Scientific Motherhood in the Nineteenth and Twentieth Centuries." *Social History of Medicine,* no. 8 (1995): 161–78.

Ariès, Philippe. *L'enfant et la vie familiale sous l'Ancien Regime.* Paris: Editions du Seuil, 1973.

Armstrong, David. *Political Anatomy of the Body: Medical Knowledge in Britain in the Twentieth Century.* Cambridge: Cambridge University Press, 1983.

———. "The Invention of Infant Mortality," *Sociology of Health and Illness* 8, no. 3, (1986): 211–32.

Avdela, Efi, and Aggelika Psarra. "Engendering "Greekness": Women's Emancipation and Irredentist Politics in Nineteenth-Century Greece." *Mediterranean Historical Review* 20, no. 1 (June 2005): 67–79.

Balinska, Martha A. "The National Institute of Hygiene and Public Health in Poland, 1918–1939," *Social History of Medicine* 9, no. 3, (1996): 427–45.

———. *For the Good of Humanity: Ludwik Rajchman, Medical Statesman.* Budapest: Central European University Press, 1998.

———. "The Rockfeller Foundation and the National Institute of Hygiene, Poland, 1918–1945," *Stud. Hist. Biol.&Biomed. Sci.* 31, no. 3, (2000): 419–32.

Ball, St. ed. *Foucault and Education: Disciplines and Knowledge.* London: Routledge Press, 1990.

Bardet, Jean Pierre, Patrice Bourdelais, Pierre Guillaume, François Lebrun and Claude Quétel, eds. *Peurs et terreurs face à la contagion.* Paris: Fayard 1988.

Barraque, B. "L'école de plein air de Suresnes, symbole d'un projet de réforme sociale par l'espace?" in *La banlieue Oasis. Henri Sellier et les cités-jardins, 1900–1940,* edited by Katharine Burlen, 221–31. Saint Denis: Presses Universitaires de Vincennes, 1987.

Bock, Gisela, and Patricia Thane, eds. *Maternity and Gender Policies. Women and the Rise of the European Welfare State 1880s-1950s.* London and New York: Routledge, 1994.

———. "Antinatalism, Maternity and Paternity in National Socialist Racism." In *Maternity and Gender Policies. Women and the Rise of the European Welfare State 1880s-1950s,* edited by Gisela Bock and Pat Thane, 233–255. London and New York: Routledge, 1994.

Borowy, Iris. "Continuing Death and Disease: Classification of Death and Disease in the Interwar Years, 1919–1939," *Continuity and Change* 18, no. 3 (2003): 457–481.

———. "The Health Organisation of the League of Nations." In *Alcohol and Temperance in Modern History: An International Encyclopaedia,* edited by Jack Blocker. Santa Barbara and Oxford: ABC-Clio, 2003.

Borowy, Iris, and Gruner, Wolf D. eds. *Facing Illness in Troubled Times. 1918–1939.* Franfurt am Main and New York: Peter Lang, 2005.

Borowy, Iris and Anne Hardy, eds. *Of Medicine and Men. Biographies and Ideas in European Social Medicine between the Two Wars.* Frankfurt am Main: Peter Lang, 2008.

Bourdelais, Patrice, ed. *Les hygiènistes: Enjeux, modèles et pratiques.* Paris: Belin 2001.

———. *Les epidémies terrassées.* Paris: Éditions de la Martinière, 2004.

Bourdelais, Patrice, and Jean-Yves Raulot. *Une peur bleue. Histoire du choléra en France 1832–1854.* Paris: Payot, 1987.

Bourdelais, Patrice and Olivier Faure, eds. *Les nouvelles pratiques de santé. Acteurs, objets, logiques sociales (XVIIIe-XXe siècles).* Paris: Belin, 2004.

Bryder, Lynda. *Below the Magic Mountain: A Social History of Tuberculosis in Twentieth Century Britain*. Oxford: Clarendon Press, 1988.

———. "The First World War: Healthy or Hungry?" *History of Workshop Journal*, vol. 24 (1987): 141–157.

———. "'Wonderlands of Buttercup. Clover and Daisis': Tuberculosis and the Open-air school Movement in Britain, 1907–39." In *In the Name of the Child, Health and Welfare, 1880–1940*, edited by Roger Cooter, 72–95. London- New York: Routledge, 1992.

Carol, Anne. "Médecine et eugénisme en France ou le rêve d'une prophylaxie parfaite, XIXe - première moitié du XXe siècle," *Revue d'Histoire Moderne et Contemporaine*, vol. 43–44, (October–December 1996): 618–631.

———. *Histoire de l'eugénisme en France*. Les Médecins et la Procréation XIXe-XXe Siècle Paris: Edition du Seuil, 1995.

Cassata, Francesco. *Building the New Man. Eugenics, Racial Sciences and Genetics in Twentieth-Century Italy*. Budapest: Central European University Press, 2011.

Chassaigne, Philippe. "La politique sociale à Londres 1850–1914. Charité privée et public welfare," in *Le Social dans la Ville en France et en Europe 1750–1914*, edited by Jacques-Guy Petit et Yannick Marec. Paris: Les Editions de l'Atelier, 1996.

Châtelet, Anne Marie, Dominique, Lerch and Jean Noel, eds. *L'École de plein air. Une expérience pédagogique et architecturale dans l'Europe du XXe siècle*. Paris: Editions Recherches, 2003.

Châtelet, Anne-Marie. "A Breath of Fresh Air. Open Air Schools in Europe." In *Designing Modern Childhoods. History Space and the Material Culture of Children*, edited by Marta Gutman and Ning de Coning-Smith, 108–11. Brunswick, New York and London: Rutgers University Press, 2008.

Clark, Anne. "Compliance with Infant Smallpox Vaccination Legislation in Nineteenth-Century Rural England Hollinbourne 1876–88," *Social History of Medicine* 17, no. 2 (2004): 175–198.

Cooter, Roger, ed. *In the Name of the Child: Health and Welfare 1880–1940*. London and New York: Routledge 1992.

Cooter, Roger and John Pickstone, eds. *Companion to Medicine in the Twentieth Century*. Rootledge: London and New York, 2003.

Corsini, Carlo. "Enfance et famille au XIXe siècle." In *Histoire de l'Enfance en Occident du XVIIe Siècle à Nos Jours*, edited by Egle, Becchi and Dominique Julia, 273–301. Paris: Éditions du Seuil, 1998.

Cova, Anne and Costa Pinto A. "Women under Salazar's Dictatorship," *Portuguese Journal of Social Science* 2, no.1 (2002): 129–46.

Cruickshank, M. "The Open-air School Movement in English Education," *Paedagogica Historica* 17, no. 1 (1977): 62–74.

Cunningham, Andrew and Andrews Bridie, eds., *Western Medicine as Contested Knowledge*. Manchester and New York: Routledge 1997.

Cunningham, Hugh. *The Children of the Poor: Representations of Childhood since the Seventeenth Century*. Oxford: Blackwell, 1991.

———. *Children and Childhood in Western Society since 1500*. London: Pearson Longman, 2005.

———. "Saving the Children c. 1830–1920," In *The Global History of Childhood Reader*, edited by Heidi Morrison, 341–59. London and New York: Routledge, 2012.

Cupers, Kenny. "Governing through Nature: Camps and Youth Movements in Interwar Germany and the United States," *Cultural Geographies* 15, no. 2 (2008):173–205.

Daniel, Hameline, "Adolphe Ferrière (1879–1960)." *Prospects: the Quarterly Review of Comparative Education*. Paris, UNESCO: International Bureau of Education, vol. 23, no. 1–2 (1993): 373–401.

Dekker, Jeroen. "The Fragile Relation between Normality and Marginality: Marginalization and Institutionalization in the History of Education. In "Beyond the Pale, Behind Bars: Marginalization and Institutionalization from the 18th to the 20th Century," special issue, *Paedagogica Historica* 26, no. 2 (1990): 15–8.

De Luca, V.B. *Les familles nombreuses. Une question demographique, un enjeu politique, France (1880–1940)*. Rennes: Presses Universitaires de Rennes, 2008.

Desse, D. "Un bicentenaire oublié: la médicine scolaire en France ou deux siècles de luttes incertaine." PhD diss., Université de Caen, 1993.

Dessertine, Dominique and Olivier, Faure. *La maladie. Entre libéralisme et solidarités (1850–1940)*. Paris: Mutualité Française, Racines Mutualistes, 1994.

Donzelot, Jacques. *L'Invention du social*. Paris: Seuil, 1994.

Duval, Nathalie. "L'École des Roches, phare français au sein de la nébuleuse de l'Education nouvelle (1899–1944)," *Paedagogica Historica* 42, no. 12 (February 2006): 63–75.

Dwork, Deborah. *War is Good for Babies and Other Young Children: A History of the Infant and Child Welfare Movement in England, 1898–1918*. London and New York: Tavistock, 1987.

Dzelepy, Panos. *Villages d'enfants*. Paris: Albert Morange, 1966.

Faure, Olivier. *Histoire sociale de la médecine (XVIII-XXe siècles)*. Paris: Anthropos-Economica, 1994.

———. "Demande sociale de santé et volonté de guérir en France au XIXe siècle. Réflexions, problems, suggestions," *Cahiers du Centre de recherches historiques* (en ligne) Paris: EHESS, no. 12, 1994.

———. "Médicalisation et professions de santé XVI –XXe siècles." *Revue d'Histoire Moderne et Contemporaine* no. 43–44 (October–December 1996): 571–77.

Ferrière, Adolphe, *L'école active*. (Preface by Daniel Hameline). First edition 1922. Paris: Faber, 2004.

Fildes, Valerie, Lara Marks and Hilary Marland eds. *Women and Children First: International Maternal and Infant Welfare, 1870–1945*. London and New York: Routledge, 1992.

Foucault, Michel. *Surveiller et punir: Naissance de la prison*. Paris: Gallimard, 1975.

Fournaraki Eleni and Zinon Papakonstantinou, eds. *Sport, Bodily Culture and Classical Antiquity in Modern Greece*. New York: Routledge, 2014.

Fox, Daniel M. *Health Policies, Health Politics: The British and American Experience, 1911–1965*. Princeton: Princeton University Press, 1986.

Fox, Jean E. "The English Day TB Schools 1910–39," *History of Education* 21, no. 4 (1992): 405–20.

Freeden, Michael. "Eugenics and Ideology," *The Historical Journal* 26, no. 4 (1983): 959–62.

———. "Eugenics and Progressive Thought: A Study in Ideological Affinity." *The Historical Journal* 22, no. 3 (1979): 645–71.

Frost, Nick, and Milke Stein. *Child Welfare: From Politics to Practice*. London: Routledge, 2003.

Frost, Nick, ed. *Major Themes in Health and Welfare: Child Welfare*. London: Routledge, 2005.

Gale, C.R. and C.N. Martyn. "Dummies and the Health of Hertfordshire Infants, 1911–1930." *Social History of Medicine* 8, no. 2 (November 1995): 231–55.

Guillaume, Pierre. *Le rôle social du médecin depuis deux siècles (1800– 1945)*. Paris: Association pour l'Etude de l'Histoire de la Sécurité Sociale, 1996.

———. "L'hygiène à l'école et par l'école," in *Les nouvelles pratiques de santé. Acteurs, objets, logiques sociales (XVIII-XXe siècles)*, edited by Patrice Bourdelais and Olivier Faure, 213–226. Paris: Belin, 2004.

Guy, Donna. "The Pan American Child Congresses." *Journal of Family History* 23, no. 3 (1998): 272–91.

Gijswijt-Hofstra, Marijke and Hilary Marland, eds. *Cultures of Child Health in Britain in the Nineteenth and Twentieth century*. Amsterdam and New York: Rodopi, 2003.

Gleason, Mona. "Disciplining the Student Body: Schooling and the Construction of Canadian Children's Bodies, 1930–1960." *History of Education Quarterly* 41, no. 2 (Summer 2001): 189–205.

———. "Race, Class and Health: School Medical Inspection and 'Healthy Children" in British Columbia, 1890 to 1930," *Canadian Bulletin of Medical History/Bulletin Canadien d'Histoire de la Médecine* vol. 19 (2002): 95–112.

Goodman, Neville, M. *International Health Organisations and their Work*. Philadelphia: The Blakiston Co., 1971.

Grier, Julie. "Eugenics and Birth Control: Contraceptive Provision in North Wales, 1918–1939." *Social History of Medicine* 11, no. 3 (December 1998): 443–48.

Grmek, Mirko, ed. *Histoire de la pensée médicale en Occident*. Vol. 3: *Du romantisme à la science moderne*. Paris: Le Seuil, 2000.

Goubert, Jean-Pierre. *La conquête de l'eau. L'avènement de la santé à l'âge industriel*. Paris: Laffont, 1986.

Greenless, Janet and Linda Bryder, eds. *Western Maternity and Medicine, 1880–1990*. London and New York: Routledge, 2016.

Guerrand, Roger Henri. *Hygiène*. Paris: Éditions de la Villette, 2001.

Guy, Donna. "The Pan-American Child Congresses 1916 to 1942: Pan-Americanism, Child Reform and the Welfare State in Latin America." *Journal of Family History* 3, 23 (1998): 272–91.

Hameline, Daniel ed. *L'éducation nouvelle et les enjeux de son histoire: Actes du colloque international des Archives Institut Jean-Jacques Rousseau*. Berne: Peter Lang, 1995.

Hamlin, Christopher. *Public Health and Social Justice in the Age of Chadwick: Britain 1800–1854*, Cambridge, Cambridge University Press, 1998.

Hardy, Anne. "Rickets and the Rest: Child-care, Diet and the Infectious Children's Diseases 1850—1914." *Social History of Medicine* 5, no. 3 (December 1992): 389–412.

———. *Epidemics Streets: Infectious Diseases and the Rise of Preventive Medicine. 1856–1900*, Oxford: Clarendon Press, 1993.

Harris, Bernard. *The Health of the Schoolchild: A History of the School Medical Service in England and Wales*. Buckingham: Open University Press, 1995.

———. "Health, Height, and History: An Overview of Recent Developments in Anthropometric History." *Social History of Medicine* 7, no. 2 (August 1994): 297–320.

Hays, J.N. *The Burdens of Disease: Epidemics and Human Responses in Western History*. New Brunswick, N. J.: Rutgers University Press, 1998.

Hendrick, Harry. *Child Welfare: England 1872–1989*. London: Routledge, 1994.

———. *Child Welfare. Historical Dimensions, Contemporary Debate*, Bristol: The Policy Press 2003.

Hirst, J.D. "The Growth of Treatment through the School Medical Service, 1908–1918." *Medical History* no. 33 (1989): 318–42.

———. "Public Health and the Public Elementary Schools, 1870–1907." *History of Education* 20, no. 2 (1991): 107–18.

Horn, Pamela. *Children's Work and Welfare 17801890*. Cambridge: Cambridge University Press, 1995.

Horn, Margo. *Before It's Too Late: The Child Guidance Movement in the United States, 1922–1945*. Philadelphia, Penn.: Temple University Press, 1989.

Houssaye, Jean. "Le centre de vacances et de loisirs prisonnier de la forme scolaire. *Revue française de pédagogie*, no 125 (October–November 1998): 95–107.

Hughes, David. "Just a Breath of Fresh Air in an Industrial Landscape? The Preston Open Air School in 1926: A School Medical Service Insight," *Social History of Medicine*, 17 no. 1 (December 2004): 443–61.

Hutchinson, John F. *Champions of Charity: War and the Rise of the Red Cross*, Boulder & Oxford: Westview Press, 1996.

———. "The Junior Red Cross Goes to Healthland." *American Journal of Public Health*, no. 87 (1997): 1816–23.

———. "Promoting Child Health in the 1920s: International Politics and the Limits of Humanitarianism." In *The Politics of the Healthy Life. An International Perspective*, edited by Esteban Rodriguez Ocana, 131–50. Sheffield: European Association for the History of Medicine and Health Publications, 2002.

Jones, Greta. "Eugenics and Social Policy between the Wars." *Historical Journal*, no. 25 (1982): 717–28.

———. "Infant and Maternal Health Services in Ceylon, 1900–1948: Imperialism or Welfare?" *Social History of Medicine* 15, no. 2 (August 2002): 263–89.

Jones, Kathleen. *Taming the Troublesome Child: American Families. Child Guidance and the Limits of Psychiatric Authority*. Cambridge, MA: Harvard University Press, 1999.

Kelly, Peter. "Youth at Risk: Processes of Individualisation and Responsabilisation in the Risk Society," *Discourse: Studies in the Cultural Politics of Education* 22, no. 1 (2001): 23–5.

Kevles, Daniel. *In the Name of Eugenics: Genetics and the Uses of Human Heredity*. New York: Alfred A. Knopf, 1995.

Klein, Alexandre and Séverine Parayre, eds. *Histoire de la santé (XVIII-XXe siècles). Nouvelles recherches francophones*. Quebec: Presses de l'Université Laval, 2015

Knibielher, Yvonne and Catherine Fouquet. *Histoire des mères*. Paris: Éditions Montalba, 1977.

Knibielher, Yvonne. "La lutte antituberculeuse, instrument de la médicalisation des classes populaires, 1870–1930." *Annales de Bretagne et des Pays de l'Ouest* 86, no. 3 (1979): 321–34.

Koerrenz, Ralf. *Hermann Lietz: Einführung mit Zentralen Texten*, Paderborn: Verlag Ferdinand Schöningh, 2011.

Kontogiorgi, Elsa. *Population Exchange in Greek Macedonia.The Rural Settlement of Refugees 1923–1930*. Oxford: Oxford Historical Monographs, Clarenton Press, 2006.

Labisch, Alfons. *Homo Hygienicus. Gesundheit und Medizin in der Neuzeit*. Frankfurt, New York: Campus Verlag, 1992.

―――. "Doctors, Workers and the Scientific Cosmology of the Industrial World. The Social Construction of Health and the Homo Hygienicus." *Journal of Contemporary History*, no. 20 (1985): 599–615.

Ladd- Taylor, Molly. "'Fixing Mothers': Child Welfare and Compulsory Sterilisation in the American Midwest, 1925–1945." In *Child Welfare and Social Action from the Nineteenth Century to the Present*, edited by Lawrence Jon and Starkey Pat, 219–33. Liverpool: Liverpool University Press, 2001.

Lawrence, J., and P. Starkey, eds. *Child Welfare and Social Action in the Nineteenth and Twentieth Centuries. International Perspectives*. Liverpool: Liverpool University Press, 2001.

Lee, Downs L. *Children in the Promised Land, Working-Class Movements and the Colonies de Vacance in France, 1880–1960*. Durham and London: Duke University Press, 2002.

Leichter, Howard M. *A Comparative Approach to Policy Analysis. Health Care Policy in Four Nations*. Cambridge: Cambridge University Press, 1979.

Leonard, Jacques. *La France médicale. Médecins et malades au XIXe siècle*. Paris: Collection Archives Gallimard, 1978.

―――. *La médécine entre les pouvoirs et les savoirs*. Paris: Aubier, 1981.

―――. "Les origines et les consequences de l'eugenique en France." *Cahiers du Centre de Recherches Historiques*. Paris: EHESS 1985, 203–313.

―――. *Les archives du corps. La santé au XIXème siècle*. Paris: Aubier, 1986.

Lewis, Jane. *The Politics of Motherhood: Child and Maternal Welfare in England, 1900–1939*. London: Croom Helm, 1980.

Littig, P. *Reformpaedagogische Erfahrungen der Landerziehungsheime von Hermann Lietz und ihre Bedeutung fuer Aktuelle Schulentwicklungsprozesse*. Bern: Peter Lang, 2004.

Loewy, Ilana and Patrick, Zylberman. "Medicine as a Social Instrument. Rockefeller Foundation, 1913–1945." *Studies in History and Philosophy of Biological and Biomedical Sciences* 31, no. 3 (September 2000): 365–79.

Loudon, I. *Death in Childbirth: An International Study of Maternal Care and Maternal Mortality 1800–1950*. Oxford: Clarendon Press, 1992.

Lowe, Roy A. "The Medical Profession and School Design in England." *Paedagogica Historica* 13, no. 2 (1973): 425–44.

―――. "Eugenicists, Doctors and the Quests for National Efficiency: an Educational Crusade, 1900–1939." *History of Education* 8, no. 4 (1979): 293–306.

Loyer, Fr. "Architecture de la Grèce contemporaine (1834–1966)." PhD diss., Université Paris IV Sorbonne, 1966.

Lubeck, Sally and Patricia Garrett. "The Social Construction of the "At-risk" Child," *British Journal of Sociology of Education* 11, no. 3 (1990): 327–40.

Luc, Jean-Noël. "Open-Air Schools: Unearthing a History." In *Open-Air Schools: An Educational and Architectural Venture in Twentieth-Century Europe*, edited by Anne-Marie Châtelet, Dominique Lerch and Jean-Noël Luc, 14–20. Paris: Éditions Recherches, 2003.

Macnicol, John. "Eugenics and the Campaign for Voluntary Sterilization in Britain Between the Wars." *Social History of Medicine* 2, no. 2 (August 1989): 147–69.

Marland, Hilary, "The Medicalization of Motherhood: Doctors and Infant Welfare in the Netherlands, 1901–1930." In *Women and Children First. International Maternal and Infant Welfare, 1870–1945.* Edited by Valerie, Fildes, Lara Marks and Hilary Marland, 74–96. London and New York: Routledge, 1992.

———. "A Pioneer in Infant Welfare: the Huddersfield Scheme 1903–1920." *Social History of Medicine* 6, no. 1 (April 1993): 25–50.

———. *Health and Girlhood in Britain, 1874–1920.* New York: Palgrave Macmillan, 2003.

Marshall, Dominique. "The Construction of Children as an Object of International Relations: The Declaration of Children's Rights and the Child Welfare Committee of the League of Nations, 1900–1924." *The International Journal of Children's Rights,* no. 7 (1999): 103–47.

Minesso, Michela, ed. *Stato e Infanzia nell' Italia Contemporanea: Origini, Sviluppo e Fine dell' Onmi, 1925–1975.* Bologna: il Mulino, 2007.

———. *Madri, Figli, Welfare. Istituzioni e Politiche dall'Italia Liberale ai Giorni Nosrtri.* Bologna: il Mulino, 2011.

Morrison, Heidi, ed., *The Global History of Childhood Reader.* London and New York: Routledge, 2012.

Mouret, Arlette. "L'Imagerie de la lutte contre la tuberculose: le timbre antituberculeux, instrument d'education Sanitaire." *Cahiers du Centre de Recherches Historiques* 12 (1994): 1–12.

Murard, Lion and Patrick Zylberman, *L'hygiene dans la Republique, 1870–1918.* Paris: Fayard, 1996.

Nardinelli, Clark. *Child Labour and the Industrial Revolution.* Bloomington and Indianapolis: Indiana University Press, 1990.

Nash, Mary. "Pronatalism and Motherhood in Franco's Spain," in *Maternity and Gender Policies. Women and the Rise of the European Welfare State 1880s-1950s,* edited by Gisela Bock and Pat Thane, 160–77. London and New York: Routledge, 1994.

Naumovic, Slobodan and Miroslav Jovanovic, eds. *Childhood in South East Europe. Historical Perspectives on Growing Up in the 19th and 20th Century.* Graz and Belgrade: 2001.

Nourrisson, Didier, ed. *Éducation à la santé, XIXe-XXe siècle.* Rennes: Éditions de l'École Nationale de la Santé Publique, 2002.

Nourisson, Didier, ed. *À Votre Santé! Éducation et santé sous la IVe république.* Saint-Étienne: Publications de l'Université de Saint-Étienne, 2002.

Ocanã, Esteban Rodriguez, ed. *The Politics of the Healthy Life: An International Perspective,* Sheffield: European Association for the History of Medicine and Health Publications, 2002.

Oelkers, Juergen. "Break and Continuity: Observations of the Modernization Effects and Traditionalization in International Reform Pedagogy," *Paedagogica Historica* 31, no. 3 (1995): 675–713.

Parayre, Séverine "L'hygiène à l'école aux XVIIIe et XIXe siècles: vers la création d'une éducation à la santé." *Recherches & Éducations,* no. 1 (2e semestre 2008): 177–193.

———. *L'hygiène à l'école. Une alliance de la santé et de l'éducation (XVIIIe-XIX siècles).* Saint Etienne: Presses Universitaires de Saint Etienne, 2012.

———. "L'hygiène scolaire en congrès international: Du biopouvoir légitimé et partagé à ses inégales applications pédagogiques (1852–1913)." *Canadian Bulletin of Medical History/Bulletin Canadien d' Histoire de la Médecine* 34, no. 1 (Spring/Printemps 2017): 88–121.

Parker, David. "A Convenient Dispensary': Elementary Education and the Influence of the School Medical Service, 1907–1939." *History of Education* 27, no. 1 (1998): 59–83.

Pelling, Margaret. "Child Health as a Social Value in Early Modern English." *Social History of Medicine,* vol. 1, no. 2, (August 1988): 135–64.

Pentzopoulos, Dimitris. *The Balkan Exchange of Minorities and its Impact upon Greece.* The Hague: Mouton and Co, 1962.

Perrenoud, Alfred. "La mortalité des enfants après 5 ans aux XVIII et XIXième siècle." In *Lorsque l'enfant grandit. Entre dépendance et autonomie,* edited by Jean-Pierre, Bardet, Jean-Noël, Isabelle Robin-Romero and Catherine Rollet, 107–32. Paris: Presse de l'Université Paris- Sorbonne, 2003.

Peyrenne, J., *Le mobilier scolaire du XIX siècle a nos jours.* Villeneuve d'Ascq: Presses Universitaires de Septentrion, 2001.

Peyronnet, Jean Claude. "Les enfants abandonnés et leurs nourrices à Limoges au XVIII siècles." *Revue d'Histoire Moderne et Contemporaine,* no. 22 (1976): 418–30.

Pinard, Adolphe. "De l'eugenique," *Bulletin Médical* no. 26 (1912): 1123–27.

Popova, Kristina. "From "Save the Children" to "Save the Tribe." Child Care in Yugoslavia and Bulgaria 1919–1939," Sofia: Cas Working Paper Series, Centre for Advanced Studies Sofia, 2007, https://tinyurl.com/ycmdnc9o

———. "Combatting Infant Mortality in Bulgaria. Welfare Activities, National Propaganda and the Establishment of Pediatrics 1900–1940." In *Health, Hygiene and Eugenics in Southeastern Europe to 1945,* edited by Christian Promitzer, Sevasti Trubeta and Marius Turda, 143–63. Budapest: Central European University Press, 2011.

Porter, Dorothy. "The History of Public Health: Current Themes and Approaches." *The Hygeia Internationalis,* 2 (2002): 9–21.

———. *The History of Public Health and the Modern State.* Amsterdam: Editions Rodopi B.V., 1994.

———. *Health, Civilisation and the State: A History of Public Health from Ancient to Modern Times.* London: Routledge 1999.

———. *The Cambridge Illustrated History of Medicine,* Cambridge: Cambridge University Press, 2001.

Porter, Roy. "History of the Body Reconsidered," in *New Perspectives on Historical Writing,* edited by Peter Burke, 233–61. Cambridge: Polity Press, 1992.

Porter, Roy, ed. *The Cambridge Illustrated History of Medicine,* Cambridge: Cambrode University Press, 2001.

Promitzer, Christian, Sevasti Trubeta and Marius Turda, eds. *Health, Hygiene and Eugenics in Southeastern Europe to 1945.* Budapest: Central European University Press, 2011.

Quine, Maria Sophia. *Population Politics in Twentieth-Century Europe.* London: Routledge, 1996.

———. *Italy's Social Revolution. Charity and Welfare from Liberalism to Fascism.* New York: Palgrave, 2002.

Richardson, Theresa. *The Century of the Child: The Mental Hygiene Movement and Children's Policy in the United States and Canada.* Albany, New York: State University of New York Press, 1989.

Roemer, Milton I. *National Health Systems of the World.* Oxford: Oxford University Press, vol. I, 1991, vol. II, 1993.

———. "Internationalism in Medicine and Public Health," In *Companion Encyclopedia of the History of Medicine,* vol. 2, edited by W.F. Bynum and Roy Porter, 1417–35. London and New York: Routledge, 1997.

Rollet, Catherine. "The Fight against Infant Mortality in the Past: An International Comparison," in *Infant and Child Mortality in the Past,* edited by A. Bideau, B. Desjardins and H. Perez Brignoli, 38–60. Oxford: Clarendon Press: 1997.

Rollet-Echalier, Catherine. *La politique à l'égard de la petite enfance sous la IIIe République 1870–1940.* Paris: PUF/INED, 1990.

Salomon-Bayet, Claire. *Pasteur et la révolution pastorienne.* Paris: Payot, 1986.

Saraceno, Chiara. "Redefining Maternity and Paternity: Gender, Pronatalism and Social Policies in Fascist Italy." In *Maternity and Gender politicies. Women and the Rise of the European Welfare State 1880s-1950s* edited by Gisela Bock and Pat Thane, 196–212. London and New York: Routledge: 2008.

Sarasin, Philip and Tanner, Jakob eds. *Physiologie und Industrielle Gesellschaft. Studien zur Verwissenschaftlichung des Koerpers im 19. und 20.* Jahrhundert, Frankfurt am Main: Suhrkamp Verlag, 1998.

Schnabel, Elmer. *Soziale Hygiene zwischen Sozialer Reform und Sozialer Biologie. Fritz Rott (1878–1959) und die Saeuglingsfuersorge in Deutschland.* Husum: Matthiesen Verlag, 1995.

Schneider, William. "The Eugenic Movement in France 1890-1940," In *The Wellborn Science. Eugenics in Germany, France, Brazil and Russia,* edited by Mark B. Adams, 69–109. New York–Oxford: Oxford University Press: 1990.

Schultheiss, K. *Bodies and Souls: Politics and the Professionalization of Nursing in France, 1880–1922.* Cambridge-Massachusetts: Harvard University Press, 2001.

Serge, Nicolas and Bernard Andrieu, eds., *La mesure de l'intelligence (1904–2004)*. Paris: L'Harmattan, 2005.

Stern, Alexandra Minna. "Responsible Mothers and Normal Children: Eugenics, Nationalism and Welfare in Post-revolutionary Mexico, 1920–1940." *Journal of Historical Sociology* 12, no. 4 (1999): 369–97.

Stern, Alexandra Minna and Howard, Malkel, eds. *Formative Years: Children Health in the United States. 1880–2000*. Ann Arbor: The University of Michigan Press, 2002.

Stewart, John. "The Campaign for School Meals in Edwardian Scotland." In *Child Welfare and Social Action*, edited by Jon Lawrence and Pat Starkey, 174–94. Liverpool: Liverpool University Press, 2001.

———. "Child Guidance in Inter-War Scotland: International Context and Domestic Concerns." *Bulletin of the History of Medicine* 80, no. 3 (2006): 513–39.

Stoeckel, Sigrid. *Saeuglingsfuersorge zwischen sozialer Hygiene und Eugenik. Das Beispiel Berlins im Kaiserreich und in der Weimarer Republik*. Berlin: De Gruyter,1996.

Swaan, Abram de. *In Care of the State: Health Care, Education and Welfare in Europe and the USA*. Cambridge: Polity Press, 1988.

Tennant, Margaret. "Children's Health Camps in New Zealand: The Making of a Movement, 1918–1940," *Social History of Medicine* 9, no. 1 (April 1996): 69–87.

Theodorou, Vassiliki and Despina Karakatsani. "Health Policies in Interwar Greece: the Intervention by the League of Nations Health Organisation." *Dynamis*, no. 28 (2008): 53–75.

———. "École de plein air et education nouvelle au début du XXe siècle en Grèce: Influences et limites d'une tentative." *Carrefours de l'Education*, no. 23 (January–June 2007): 187–204.

———. "Eugenics and Puericulture in Greece in Interwar Years: Medical Concerns about the Amelioration of the Biological Capital." In *Health, Hygiene and Eugenics in Southeastern Europe to 1945*, edited by Christian Promitzer, Sevasti Trubeta and Marius Turda, 299–323. Budapest: Central European University Press, 2011.

Thompson, F.M.L. ed. *The Cambridge Social History of Britain*, vol. 3. *Social Agencies and Institutions*. Cambridge: Cambridge University Press, 1990.

Thuillrer, Guy. *Pour une histoire du quotidien au XIXe siècle en Nivernais*. Paris: EHSS, 1977.

Thyssen, Geert. "Visualising Discipline of the Body in a German Open-Air School (1923–1939): Retrospection and Introduction," *History of Education* 36, no. 2 (March 2007): 247–64.

———. "The 'Trotter' Open-air School, Milan (1922–1977): a City of Youth or Risky Business?" *Paedagogica Historica* 45, no. 1–2 (February–April 2009):157–70.

Trubeta, Sevasti. *Physical Anthropology, Race and Eugenics in Greece (1880–1970s)*. Chicago: Brill, Balkan Studies Library, 2011.

Turda, Marius. "Public Health and Social Politics in Southeast Europe in the 1920s." In *Dimosia Ygeia kai Koinoniki Politiki: o Eleftherios Venizelos kai I Epokhi tou*, edited by Giannis Kyriopoulos, 517–22. Athens: Papazisis, 2008.

———. "'To End the Degeneration of a Nation': Debates on Eugenic Sterilisation in Interwar Romania." *Medical History*, no. 53 (2009): 77–104.

———. *Modernism and Eugenics*. New York: Palgrave Macmillan, 2010.

———."Controlling the National Body: Ideas of Racial Purification in Romania, 1918–1944." In *Health, Hygiene and Eugenics in Southeastern Europe to 1945*, edited by Christian Promitzer, Sevasti Trubeta and Marius Turda, 325–50. Budapest: Central European University Press, 2011.

———. "Ancients and Moderns: the Rise of Social History of Medicine in Greece and the Balkans." *Deltos: Journal of the History of Hellenic Medicine*, special issue: "Private and Public Medical Traditions in Greece and the Balkans 1453–1920," Winter 2012: 13–7.

———, ed. *Crafting Humans: From Genesis to Eugenics and Beyond*. Gottingen: V&R Unipress, 2013

———. *Eugenics and Nation in Early Twentieth Century Hungary*. Basingstoke: Palgrave Macmillan, 2014.

———, ed. *East Central European Eugenics 1900–1945. Sources and Commentaries*. London and New York: Bloomsbury, 2017.

Turda, Marius and Paul J. Weindling, eds. *Blood and Homeland: Eugenics and Racial Nationalism in Central and Southeast Europe (1900–1940)*. Budapest: Central European University Press, 2006.

Turda, Marius and Aaron Gilette, eds. *Latin Eugenics in Comparative Perspective*. London, New Delhi, New York, Sydney: Bloomsbury, 2014.

Turner, D. "The Open-air School Movement in Sheffield." *History of Education*, 1 (1972): 58–78.

Vigarello, Georges. Le propre et le sale. L'hygiène du corps depuis le Moyen Age. Paris: Editions du Seuil. 1985.

———. *Histoire des pratiques de santé: Le sain et le malsain depuis le Moyen Age*. Paris: Editions du Seuil, 1993.

Viner, Russell. "Abraham Jacobi and the Origins of Scientific Pediatrics in America." In *Formative Years: Children Health in the United States, 1880–2000*, edited by Alexandra Minna Stern and Howard Markel, 23–46. Ann Arbor: University of Michigan Press, 2002.

Watts, Sheldon. *Epidemics and History: Disease, Power and Imperialism*. London: Yale University Press, 1997.

Webster, Charles, ed. *Caring for Health: History and Diversity*. Buckingham: Open University Press, 1993.

———. "Healthy or Hungry Thirties." *History Workshop Journal* 13, no.1 (1982): 110–29.

———. "The Health of the Schoolchild during the Depression." In *The Fitness of the Nation. Physical and Health Education in the Nineteenth and Twentieth Centuries*, edited by Nicolas Parry and David McNair. 70–85. Leicester: History of Education Society, 1983.

Weindling, Paul. *Health, Race and German Politics between National Unification and Nazism, 1870–1945*. Cambridge: Cambridge University Press, 1993.

———. "From Isolation to Therapy: Children's Hospitalisation and Diphtheria in Fin de Siècle Paris, London and Berlin." In *In the Name of the Child: Health and Welfare 1880–194*, edited by Roger Cooter, 124–45. London and New York: Routledge 1992.

———. "Social Medicine at the League of Nations Health Organisation and the International Labour Organisation Compared." In *International Health Organisations and Movements 1918–1939*, edited by Paul Weindling, 134–53. Cambridge: Cambridge University Press, 1995.

———. "The Role of International Organisations in Setting Nutritional Standards in the 1920s and 30s." In *The Science and Culture of Nutrition*, edited by Harmke Kamminga and Andrew Cunningham, 319–22. Amsterdam: The Wellcome Institute Series in the History of Medicine, 1995.

———. "Philanthropy and World Health: the Rockefeller Foundation and the League of Nations Health Organisation." *Minerva* vol. 35, (1997): 269–81.

———. "Health and Medicine in Interwar Europe." In *Companion to Medicine in the Twentieth Century*, edited by Roger Cooter and John Pickstone, 39–50. London-New York: Taylor & Francis, 2003.

Welshman, John. "Physical Education and the School Medical Service in England and Wales, 1907–1939." *Social History of Medicine* 9, no. 1 (1996): 31–48.

———. "Child Health, National Fitness and Physical Education in Britain, 1900–1940." *Clio Medica* 71 (2003): 61–84.

———. "Public Health and Political Stabilization: The Rockefeller Foundation in Central and Southeast Europe Between the Two World Wars," *Minerva* 31, no. 3 (1993): 253–67.

Westwood, L. "Care in the Community of the Mentally Disordered: The Case of the Guardianship Society, 1900–1939." *Social History of Medicine* 20, no. 1 (April 2007): 57–72.

Wolf, Theta, H. *Alfred Binet*. Chicago: The University of Chicago Press, 1973.

Woods, Robert. "La santé publique en milieu urbain XIXe-XXe siècle: hygiène et mesure d'assainissement." *Annales de Démographie Historique*, no. 3 (1989): 182–95.

Worboys, Michael. *Spreading Germs: Disease Theories and Medical Practice in Britain 1865–1900*. Cambridge: Cambridge University Press, 2000.

Zelizer, Viviana. *Pricing the Priceless Child: The Changing Social Value of Children*. New York: Princeton University Press, 1985.

NAME INDEX

SUBJECT INDEX